Nature Has A Remedy

A book of remedies for Body,
Mind and Spirit gathered
from all corners of the
world.

Published By

Dr. Bernard Jensen
Rt. 1 Box 52
Escondido, California 92025

ISBN 0-913300-19-5

Second Printing – November 1979
Third Printing – August 1981
Fourth Printing – March 1984

DEDICATION

This book is dedicated to doctors and people throughout the world who are interested in healing as an art. The remedies contained herein are for those who would like to see that their body follows the holistic path; they are for the doctor who puts the whole of life together for his patients, using every appropriate remedy for the building and repair of the human body. Everything must be united in wholeness — a healthy body and mind lay the foundation for the serenity and peace we need as we develop a deeper appreciation of our Golden Days in God's Garden.

To Elsie and Louise

FOREWORD

Nature has a remedy — yet that a remedy can be found in nature is beyond the scope of most men's imagination, training, or education. It's more than they can conceive. But we have learned much about how to use nature. It is the great Provider — and Healer. Still, there is much we don't know. And many of the remedies we now use may become out of date as conditions change and as we learn more in the years to come. Electricity, for example, may come in and supplant many of the remedies we use at the present time. Our understanding of many other aspects of nature will develop and mature. But in the meantime there is a great deal we can do to promote our own health.

I want to emphasize that these remedies are not given with the idea that they provide a complete cure, but they are the little assists that a doctor may use who is interested in the use of the natural Healing Art.

Before we can live right we must first learn the proper methods. But where do you get the information to guide you in learning how to live? Today, as a rule, doctors are too busy taking care of the extreme cases; however, it has always been my belief that every doctor should spend one-half of his time educating and lecturing his patients so they will avoid some of the problems that buildup in their environment, in their thinking processes, at the table, at their job, in their marriage, while handling finances, or whatever man's path carries him into.

The consciousness of man today is not a healthy one. He comes to the office with bad habits; he known practically nothing about the care of his body. As long as things are white, sterilized, clean, and made by a well-known company, most people think the product should be good for them. This is a mistaken idea. We must consider our bodies as loyal servants depending upon our decisions, and know that everything that goes into the mouth has an effect upon them. Also, the body is affected by what you hear and see, by your feelings — and it can all add up to our

good or to our distraction. All of these things should be understood.

The remedies that are brought out here surely will only touch a small percentage of that which the average doctor or patient needs to know. Many of these remedies will not fit certain patients because of their temperament or feelings, because of inherent causes or inherent weaknesses and possibly because of their climate or attitude or occupation.

These remedies are approved by God and Nature. They are not fast working. They are not meant for cure, but when a patient has been given guidance and instruction, he can sometimes do a great deal for himself. Many times his hopes will be raised; his path becomes easier because he is doing some work besides what the doctor requires; possibly it is what nature demands. It is a matter of co-operation of the doctor, the patient, and nature that helps us to win.

The success of my work has been in the use of many of these remedies throughout my fifty years of practice. I have worked with over 250,000 students and patients. I did my best work when I considered the whole patient and not the disease. I looked to everything possible in the natural Healing Art to help me to raise the level of the health in my patients. And it was at those times that I have seen the patient leave the disease and come into good health. My work centers around helping a person to have new tissue, not just to control symptoms.

This book sums up my half-century of practice, traveling, learning, and seeing what other people do — bringing it together in written and picture form.

It is to raise the health level that we take these remedies and if you have to do fifty things better than you were doing before in order to get well, you have the privilege of doing that in this age. There is not reason for anyone not to have all the success he wants in any direction he may wish to go if it is a matter of education because education is open to everyone these days. There was a day when only the landlord, only the master, only the king had education, and the rest of the people were slaves. In this day we have broken that bondage and we can all be a king and no one has to be a slave to anyone. It is my hope that these remedies will not be used promiscuously as a cure for any disease but will be used as part of an effort to take the path to higher values, better health — physically, mentally, and spiritually — and greater happiness.

Above all things, these remedies are not given to use without considering the basic principles of life and following, for instance, a good diet before we try a remedy. A person drinking beer in one hand and taking a kidney remedy in the other is not following good sense. These remedies are not for people who want to live a deteriorating life and therefore will take a remedy to help them hang onto their life-style. This book is meant for the sincere student and for the person who is sick of being sick, wants to elevate himself, wants a finer way of going through life — and is willing to live some of nature's principles and possibly use some of these simple remedies in time of need.

None of these remedies is to take the place of a doctor's treatment. We need doctors. A doctor can be your best friend and in times of problems and troubles I think we should have somebody who works along with us, who sets up our program so we can do as much as we can for ourselves. Every doctor will be glad to give you something to do at home so you can help take care of yourself. But in cases of meningitis or acute fevers that are running at a very high temperature, don't try to take over the cure to heal yourself. These remedies are not meant for that purpose.

Let me emphasize that. Suppose you look to the index, for prostate gland trouble, turn to the specified page, and see that you should use pumpkin seeds for prostate gland trouble. Do you take pumpkin seed and consider yourself healed? No! Don't think for a moment that if you have a stoppage of urine and take a few pumpkin seeds that you're going to cure it or get rid of it. Each of these remedies should be used as part of a total health plan. This is what I suggest that you have a good doctor to work with.

These remedies are for those who are interested in learning about the natural Healing Art and should be used along with all the help possible. A good diagnosis, a good analysis, and a good doctor should be consulted in all of our problems.

You will find in working with nature's creative power that it exceeds man's inclination to destroy.

So be patient with nature, be patient with your fellow man, but, most of all, be patient with yourself.

Bernard Jensen
Hidden Valley
Escondido, California
November 1978

"Too many people still believe in cures and in spite of my protest that I cannot cure anything, they come and assume the attitude, 'Well, here I am and now it is up to you to cure me.' They are foolish enough to believe that a cure should be made without any effort or any trouble on their part. Living haphazardly, guessing how to live when dependable knowledge can be had is a foolish and inexcusable hazard. I repeat, I cannot cure, but I can teach all who crave knowledge how to live to cure themselves and how to live and stay well."

John H. Tilden, M.D.

Table of Contents

The nature of nature

N ATURE has been here a long time. The earth is nature; the sky is nature; the water is nature. All our resources and all of our building and repairing, whether it be in the body or out–all comes from nature. And nature always has a remedy.

The Armenians say it well: "There is not a disease that Nature doesn't have a remedy right next to it." I believe that. I also believe that we are using only eight to nine percent of the natural things we have found. The other 91 percent we haven't used or tapped yet in the realm of natural remedies.

The Seven Doctors of Nature

<u>Sunshine–Number One Doctor</u>. We know that without the proper amount of sunshine, an animal cannot have the proper fur on his back. Humans need sunshine too, of course. Authorities found a child who had been in an attic for five years. His teeth were soft and loose in the gums. It was because of a lack of sunshine. Sunshine fixes calcium in the body. You can have all the best foods, but without sunshine you will not be healthy. Sunshine is the number one doctor.

We are all children of the sun, even if our skins may be very light. We find we must have a definite amount of sunshine. Sunshine is a part of our existence. We live in the sun. We are not children of the apartment houses or underground shelters that we live in. We're not basement children. We are not meant to live in houses with closed doors and shaded windows that block out all the light of the sun. The sun is for our own good. It is for everyone's good. Those who live in the sun a lot have a pigment to keep off the sun's harmful effects.

The sun is a definite number one doctor.

<u>Water– Number Two Doctor</u>. Doctor number two would, in my opinion, be water. We can live only a few days without water. Our bodies are 85 percent fluid– a water mixture.

Even our teeth have water in them. We need this fluid. Without it we will dry up and become dehydrated. Tissues cannot be fed well without water. It is water that takes toxic material from dead tissue and brings building elements to living tissue.

Nature doesn't require distilled water to promote health. I have sought every country boasting of an old man or woman, yet never have I found one that uses distilled water. They used unadulterated water. It was pure, usually from mountain streams. In analyzing these waters I believe you will find them to be alive. And I'm positive you'll find more calcium in it than manhandled water has. It could be hard or soft water, depending on the area.

But there is a use for distilled water. An arthritic patient needs to dissolve and slough off the heavy calcium salts deposited in his joints and muscle structure. The wise doctor knows he can use distilled water to help this patient.

Water is not just a fluid within our bodies. We are beginning to realize that the vibratory forces in foods are influential.

Water carries a vibration. The salts contained in water carry a vibration, a magnetic influence. But in distilled water you won't have that influence; the salts and other helpful elements have been removed. I'm convinced the magnetic influence in water high in either sulphur, calcium , or sodium can help balance a person's body chemistry.

I would say that in extreme cases of arthritis, arteriosclerosis, or cholesterol deposits, use distilled water. Or you may use pure spring mountain water, if you wish.

Vibratory water contains inorganic dead material. But live material is also essential, because we are constantly throwing off chemicals. Your perspiration tastes salty because it's high in sodium. Salts are thrown off in the urine and by the bowel. When your chemical supply is depleted, the vibratory rate, the magnetic rate is gone. These rates are what we live on. Thus, live foods are also necessary.

Oxygen/Air– Number Three Doctor. Doctor number three is oxygen. We find that we can live only a few moments without it. We've got to have oxygen. Oxygen breaks up the waste material in the body. It gets rid of garbage and helps to keep heat in our body. We need heat to burn up our food, to "cook" it so it can be absorbed and delivered to the tissues properly. Without oxygen, we cannot build any structure in the body. Oxygen can be increased by using a chlorophyll supplement.

Carbon dioxide is constantly being thrown off into the air and purified by plant life, so that the air is kept in proper balance. Greens growing around us are also doctors. We must live where there are greens. People with troubles have gotten beautiful results by breathing the air around pine trees.

Mother Earth– Number Four Doctor. Mother Earth is our doctor number four, the beginning of everything our bodies need. We should return to Mother Earth in looking for the correction or the building and the development of a good body (or of a garden).

There is a saying that if it has the approval of God, it can be used. To identify with God makes it right. If we can identify ourselves with nature and work with the natural processes of nature, remaining with natural conditions, we shall find that we have the approval of God.

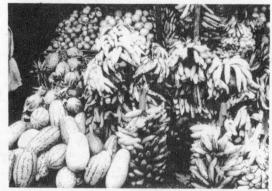

Vegetables in a market demonstrates the abundance of Mother Earth willing to give and to share all that she has.

Food– Number Five Doctor. I consider food as our doctor number five, especially foods that come directly from nature. What did God make for us in the beginning? He gave us peas with pods to use so that we get the whole thing. You don't have to eat the pea pods, but you can make a juice out of them. Put the juice in your broth, and you will get all the chlorophyll you were meant to have in the beginning. We are not meant to throw away the seeds of a watermelon. When we do, we throw away some of nature's preventive remedies. Watermelon seeds have chlorophyll, vitamin K, and iron. They are very good for kidney troubles, hypertension, and high blood pressure.

We are meant to eat the peelings of many of our foods. If they are unpleasant, we can put them into teas, make drinks out of them. We can make them into soups. There's a way to do these things; there's a way we can stay close to nature.

Life is a circle. We go from birth to adolescence, middle age, old age, mother back to the child. We go from summer to fall to winter to spring and back to summer. Our food routine should be different in the winter than it is in the summer season. We should have dissolving foods in the beginning of summer. Sodium foods like whey are cooling foods. Cucumbers are high in sodium. (They say to be cool as a cucumber). Cucumber juice with pineapple juice is cooling for the bloodstream, especially on a hot day.

Barley heats the blood. Such heating foods are winter foods.

We must consider the acid–alkaline balance. The 80 percent alkaline and 20 percent acid diet is based on the assumption that a person is being active, creating many health acids in the body in order to balance at 50/50. The pH or acid/alkaline condition is a very difficult balance to determine. I don't think any doctor knows it well. I feel we may measure the urine as supposing to be acid and find it to be alkaline. It has been held too long. There's a possibility the blood has an alkaline condition. It is also possible that no two people are exactly alike. There are some people who can hold the alkaline condition in their body better than others. There is a possibility dietary differences make for different conditons. But you must create a supposed norm as a guideline. Not everyone should be a dray horse and not everyone should be a race horse.

There is a uniqueness in nature. You can't expect a flat program to fit every human being. You can't expect that everyone has the identical acid/alkaline balance. Even skin and hair differ.

Whole foods are necessary in all seasons of the year. We must build a reserve. We build a house in six months. It can burn down in about ten minutes. *Building takes longer than burning.*

When all the chemicals are in reserve, the body can go to work in building a good sound structure.

One of the most important considerations in rebuilding the body is to allow ample time. Don't expect an overnight miracle. Plan on a minimum of one year–each of the four seasons, to get the benefits of all seasonal foods. The wise doctor uses foods as medicine and works with the patient in attaining body balance.

Nothing in nature's realm is more healthful than proteins. However, some proteins are heavier than others. Some are much heavier than some mineral salts and vitamins.

Fruits contain more vitamins than vegetables. Some vegetables, such as turnips and carrots, may be very high in vitamins. But we find the vegetable kingdom is much higher in mineral content than fruits. Fruits stir up body acids. Vegetables carry off acids. In the instance of kidney trouble, fruit juice can be aggravating. Fruits work on every organ, stirring up the acids present in those organs. How are the acids removed? The kidneys carry them off. The kidneys must be strong to handle the overload.

Color and Vibration– Number Six Doctor. I consider the number six doctor to be color and vibration. There are definite laws of nature that lead us to health. Man just hasn't become acquainted with them as yet.

One of these days man is going to seriously study color and vibration as related to the seasons and the certain foods a person needs.

There's a vibratory state of the body. The vibratory state is made up of the body's chemical structure. When the chemical structure is perfectly balanced and functioning properly, the vibratory rate is working with full life, accomplishing and progressing. In a fast, the body is balanced as best it can be, but if the person returns to the old way of living, he is worse off for the effort. Maybe he is rid of some of the toxins but he is back to creating new ones again.

Many people are constantly fasting, or on all- cleansing diets, so to speak. The program I recommend is divided into three stages: cleansing, transition, and building. The body constantly goes through these cycles, moving

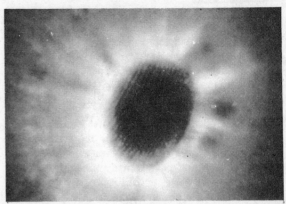

I was told by one of my great teachers that the New Age will come in with color, vibration and photography. And it certainly is coming about. Here we have the emanations from a thumbprint as it is photographed. This is Kirlian photography. More wll be heard in the future about this.

into the various changes normal to the human body but we often ignore this process.

Color is important also. For instance, we should keep the color of the urine on the light side. It cannot be dark and odorous. When it is, we know that the body metabolism isn't right that we're not eliminating toxic chemicals properly. Water helps us in our attempt to have light-colored urine.

Emotions– Number Seven Doctor. Our emotions can kill us or cure us. I consider emotions to be doctor number seven.

People can try to kill us, warp us, disturb us, yet if our emotional nature is secure we have a natural doctor. It gives us the ability to relax even when conditions are not right for us. We can know what it is to be quiet even during distressing times. During relaxation and quietness repair is done in the body.

The mind has to have a harmonious activity, a harmonious environment, a harmonious atmosphere for our life to continue in freedom, peacefulness, and joy. We find that many people interfere with that joy. We see financial problems, marital problems, children problems, school problems, many disturbances.

Emotional balance and a good mental philosophy keep the mind repairing and rebuilding as fast as you break it down. But a proper food program including appropriate mind foods, is essential. Without such a program the mind force may go down, resulting in a breakdown or a mental depletion.

On Beliefs and On Faith
It is an impossiblity to learn everything there is to know in this lifetime, so we go through life believing, having faith. We are living on beliefs and faith always.

3

When I say you can trust in nature, I go back to many original beliefs. I go back to Zoroaster, who started a good number of our religious ideas. He worshipped the sun and he believed in the sun. You can believe in the sun. It is always there. It gives life. The sun keeps things in good order. This I believe.

God and Nature Never Let Man Down

There are many reasons for returning to nature. God and nature never let a man down. I've seen that proven many times. We have to believe in things according to their past performances. I believe that my apple trees will come out again in the spring because they did it before. I believe I can get well again because I have seen cuts healed before. I believe I can continue to have good joints because they have served me well for many years and I continue to take care of them.

Change Is Permanent

I believe that the body is in a state of flux. You can't hold anything. The only thing that is permanent in life is change. I believe this because I see it working right before my own eyes. I work my beliefs into what I am doing. I cannot believe in devitalizing foods. I cannot believe in white flours, because I have seen what white flours can do. I've seen the experiments on dogs with flour. I've seen experiments where they can live longer on water than on white flour. In other words, there are a whole lot of people believing in the wrong things. They are misled. They are believing in what man has told them. But, man has often been mistaken.

You Have to Believe in Nature

You don't have to believe in God, but I'll say you have to believe in nature.

I realize a lot of people don't want to believe in God. But man by nature is a being that must worship something, and if he doesn't worship God, he will invent his own god or gods. Man knows something is actually behind it all, repairing all growth, all life. He knows that something gave a first shove to get things started even before man was around. We have to believe that, if we go way back.

Personally, though I have doubted many times that God was around, I can never say I've been an atheist. But I've had experiences that have led me to believe in prayer and God. Now I want to live the Godly principles of truth, joy, and happiness in having a loving Father. I know He wants his children healthy and harmonious. I live in His teachings, but I don't put it on a religious basis.

The universe itself teaches us these beliefs. Dr. Wernher von Braun said:

Anything as well ordered and perfectly created as is our earth and universe must have a maker, a master designer. Anything so orderly, so perfect, so precisely balanced, so majestic as this creation, can only be the product of a Divine Idea. There must be a maker. There can be no other way.

Astronaut Eugene A. Cernan looked at this earth a little differently than we do. He said:

When you get out there- a quarter of a million miles away from home you look at earth with a little different perspective. The earth looks big and beautiful and blue and white, and you can see from the Antarctic to the North Pole and the continental shores. The earth looks so perfect. There are no strings to hold it up, no fulcrum upon which it rests. You think of the infinity of space and the infinity of time. I didn't see God but I am convinced of God by the order in space. I know it didn't happen by accident.

Spiritual Aliveness

A person must be spiritually alive. I'm not speaking of religion; but we do need the spiritual things for our health.

To be spiritually alive is to be truthful. To get the truth we aren't looking for who is right, but what is right. Man goes with truth because it feels good inside, because he knows he is doing the right thing, even if he has to go alone. He knows that by doing the right thing he has relief of tension in his body; he has relief of animosity; relief of anxiety.

Man knows to do the right thing before God and to leave the rest to God. He realizes that living as only a human being he is limited and his life is in a limited sphere, and he can live only past the next week. Some people can't think past tomorrow afternoon.

The spiritual things have to be developed. Some people have more spiritual awareness than others. If you have this spiritual awareness, you have to be touched a few times by spiritual phenomena and it moves you.

Some people are so coarse, so calcified in their thinking that they wouldn't give in to any spiritual experience or phenomena whatsoever. Their awareness has to come through some great extremity--like the man who was buried in a mine for thirty-one days recognizing for the first time in his life his need for

4

God. As Robert Ingersoll, the famous nineteenth century lawyer and agnostic, said in his last moments, "Life, or nobody can help you, let us pray." Eddie Rickenbacker, out on a raft for twenty-one days on the Pacific, did not believe in God. Yet he finally reached his extremity as he was starving to death.

When man needs water, when he needs people, when he needs to have his life spared, then he looks up. He looks up in some direction for a moment that will save him. And that moment comes along. The sight of a ship to a castaway is greater than all the money in the world, greater than any woman he has ever met. The ship becomes the greatest thing in the world. Some people say that God intervened; some people say God appeared; some people say that man's extremities are God's opportunities.

So we need to believe in these things and be grateful for the lovely things that come to us all day long. This is part of good health. We live to be grateful for each day, this is healthy. A healthy spiritual attitude is just as important as having a good working body.

My Favorite Poem

I asked God for strength that I may achieve;
I was made weak that I might learn humbly to
  obey.
I asked for health that I might do greater
  things;
I was given infirmity that I might do better
  things:
I asked for riches that I might be happy;
I was given poverty that I might be wise.
I asked for power that I might have the praise
  of men;
I was given weakness that I might feel the
  need of God;
I asked for all things that I might enjoy life;
I was given life that I might enjoy all things.
I got nothing that I asked for but everything
  that I had hoped for.
Almost despite myself my unspoken prayers
  were answered.
I am, among all men, most richly blessed.
          (Author Unknown)

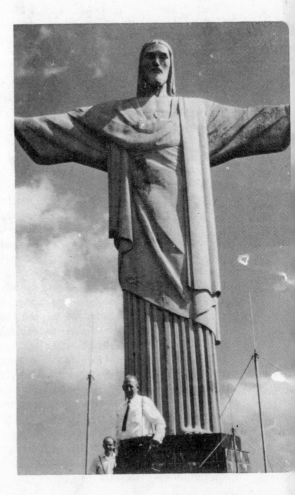

A sculptured model of the Christ spreading protective arms out over the city of Rio de Janeiro in South America.

TWO

The world around us

MANY experiements have been performed to show that certain environments are better than others for our good health. For instance, studies with rats and other animals show that different altitudes and climates have definite effects on lung structure, heart movement, and the water balance of the body.

Certain types of people do better in one environment than in another. With high blood pressure you should not go to a high altitude, and sometimes a too dry climate is not good.

Each person is different, and will be uniquely affected by his particular environment: climate, altitude, temperature, humidity, and so forth.

The Air We Breathe. The air is composed of one part oxygen and four parts nitrogen. There is one percent of a gas called argon, and a small percentage of neon, krypton, and xenon. Our air contains close to 21 percent oxygen; if the oxygen is increased very slightly, we do not thrive well. Nitrogen exists in our air to the amount of a little more than 78 percent. Of course, the air can also contain dust, insect wings, gases, water vapors, smoke, coal tar, fumes, ammonia, nitrous acid, sulphuric acid, nitric acid, bacteria, earth gases, bacterial gases, disease fumes, perfumes, odors, and other impurities.

We need to learn to breathe properly. Oxygen, when inhaled into the lungs, is attracted by the hemoglobin of the red corpuscles of the blood and is carried by the blood into every organ, tissue, fiber, and cell of the body for purposes of oxidation. Blood also carries carbon dioxide from the tissues to the lungs, where the carbon dioxide is extracted and sent out into the air through the nose. When the breathing function is not efficiently developed, the carbon dioxide in the tissues and blood is not carried away. This results in bloating, an overacid blood,

and carbonosis– causing gas generation, gastritis, and carbon dioxide poisoning symptoms. This is why it is necessary to breathe vigorously in high altitudes, together with the exercising of the muscular tissue in vital organs.

A man at rest uses about 580 to 1,000 litres of air. A heavy man of 250-300 lbs. doing physical work uses more than 1,000 litres in 24 hours. An office worker who uses only about 400 litres of air each day will soon suffer from bad blood, gas acidity, bloating, brain fag, and sleeplessness.

Respiration can vary from three breaths a minute to 30 breaths a minute. The respiration can vary in the same man at different times according to his state of health, the development of his chest and brain, the presence of gases in his system, the amount of food in his stomach, the degree of his physical and mental depression, the condition of his lungs, his state of mind, and the size of his chest, his disposition, his intensity of emotion, his age, his state of activity, and many other conditions. The more powerful the lungs, the more reposed the individual will feel at any given time and the fewer breaths each minute. But the weaker the man and the more emotional, mental, nervous, and sensitive he is, the greater the number of breaths each minute.

We know that the air in an unventilated room is unfit for breathing. But did you know that those who have a lot of sugar, starch, and fat in their bodies produce more carbon dioxide in the blood and tissues and therefore need more oxygen? The more carbohydrate foods we eat, the more carbonic acid gas we make. This gas does not allow the proper amount of oxygenation to take place in our bodies. Eventually oxygen hunger develops and disease results. When we begin to need more oxygen in the body, we should leave sugars, starches, and fats alone and seek a higher altitude with dry air.

6

Without air, light, heat, moisture, and plants, animals would not exist very long. We should realize that the plant and vegetable kingdom is a manufacturing concern which gives us a new supply of oxygen- and therefore life. Men, birds and animals utilize oxygen and exhale carbonic acid. Plants need carbon dioxide and nitrogen and give off oxygen for us to breathe. Here we can see the wisdom of the great World Builder. The more abundant the garden around us, the more trees, plants and flowers, the more oxygen and ozone in the air. Wind and light help to purify the air and are therefore great blessings to us. Carbon dioxide decreases as we ascend into higher altitudes but increases enormously in crowded cities because of the many lungs and factories and lack of vegetable life.

Carbonic acid is more abundant close to water surfaces, but at higher elevation it decreases. There are some people who benefit by carbonic air and moisture while others improve in localities where carbon dioxide is minute in quantity, where the air is dry.

Air that contains 35 percent carbonic acid gas paralyzes the lung centers and kills at once. A strong healthy man cannot live more than five minutes in such air. Carbon dioxide in excess in the blood, stomach tissues, secretions, and waste matter is one common cause of varied blood pressure, acid formation, and gas generation. Odors can stimulate the lungs, brain, chest, and vital faculties, and often carry the dust containing deadly bacteria. The more dust in the atmosphere, the more germs in the air. In a big dusty city, mouth breathers are never safe!

In analyzing the air, Ehrenberg found some 460 different organic substances in it. It's no wonder we are sick, taking in all the metal dust, smoke, chalk, clay, wood fibres, disease vapors, sand, scales, capsules, legs and wings of insects, vapors, odors, and so forth. It is a wonder that we live at all, especially in our cities with the modern automobile and the lack of vegetation.

There is more carbon dioxide in the city than in the country. City people therefore usually have more carbon dioxide in their systems. This leads to acidity, gas in the stomach, bloating, gastritis, rheumatism, stiffness, stomach trouble, headache, colds, catarrh, asthma, carbonosis, acidosis, and other ailments.

Living away from these conditions would lessen the number of disturbances in our

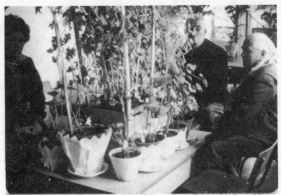

This is a room where people with various bronchial problems sit for 15 min. to half an hour breathing the very essence and aromas from various herb plants and flowers. This Healing Breath is used in a sanitarium in Southeast Russia where they have thousands of letters on file testifying to the relief of various breathing problems.

bodies and would help us to relate more to nature. A recent Associated Press piece from Tokyo told of one Chen Chu, who has developed that kind of closeness to nature:

"Chen Chu, an ordinary 48 year-old peasant, has been issuing weather forecasts with 95 percent accuracy on the basis of cloud movements, animal behavior and other natural phenomena, the China's Hsinhua news agency said."

Electricity and Climate. Electricity is said to be one of the forces of nature. In reality it is God at work in nature. It is God's power house. The air is charged with electricity. There is more in the air in summer than in the winter. Plant growth is, of course, much greater in the summer. And, under the influence of heat, light, and sunshine, the vegetable kingdom generates electricity. (Electricity can be manifested in the forms of light and heat and motive power.) When there is an increase of electricity, growth

Here we see the black soot coming from a bus, polluting our air and then man has to breathe this. No wonder we have to seek fresh air, that we have to have the essence of plants and flowers to breathe, to clean our lung structure. No wonder we have to seek our herbs that will clean out the lung structure, or water treatments for better circulation so that toxicity can be removed from the lungs. Man has to clean up his environment before he expects to be well.

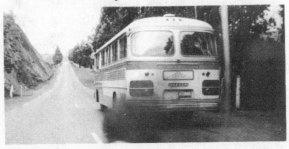

increases in many animals and vegetation.

The less light the less plant growth. The less light, the less oxygen and the more carbon dioxide there is in the body. The less light, the less electricity in the air. Thunderstorms are few in the winter, but in the summer they are numerous. Light in the oxygen makes the blood more alkaline by the removal of carbon dioxide. Light improves electrical generation in the muscles and electrical tensions in the atmosphere. Light causes a positive chemical effect upon nutritive function and plant life.

When we study climatology we are interested in the air chemistry: air pressure, winds, humidity, light and its influence, the ultraviolet effects of different altitudes, temperature and its effect upon the skin and the organic structure of the body. Those who are interested in health recognize that what we eat and drink is a necessary part of health building, but they should also realize that climatic phenomena can add to our health or take away from it.

For instance, the friction of clouds, winds, hail, evaporation, snow, and changes in gases alter the electrical tension of the atmosphere, which has a tremendous effect on the nerves, brain, and blood of certain types of people. Many cannot sleep, they cannot recuperate properly when electrical tension is high. High-tensioned people should not seek the high-tension electrical regions and high-tension electricity, with its great electrical variation, is not always favorable to nerves, mind, and the senses, especially for nervous people and for those who are inclined to develop fears easily.

During electrical storms ozone is formed. We notice this most when we go into the mountains after an electrical storm. The cerebellum, or chest brain, is stimulated in these ozone belts. Ozone is important to consumptive and to certain highly nervous people. Nervous distress is nearly always favored by a breezy climate, but oxygen must be in abundance in such a climate, and the muscular system must not be weak. Many types of paralysis, hysteria, paralytic ailments, dropsy, anemia, impotence, mental depression, tired feelings, and a weakened cerebellum can be improved in this belt. Ozone can be like a powerful tonic but too much of it can weaken the body. Ozone in excess does harm to the blood and to the pulmonary circulation.

Mountains are wonderful for a vacation. They are usually full of pine odors and have less carbon dioxide. People with a low breath capacity or consumption should go to a higher altitude where carbonic acid is less abundant. Invigorated, toned up to the point of friskiness, we feel new after a visit to the mountains. Night sweats usually disappear in the mountains. When the skin is always damp the vital organs are not protected. The system loses its heat. Health resorts owe their curative power to such agents as air, exposure to the sun, vigorous exercises, massage, ozone, climate, air pressure baths, light rays, altitude, rest, vegetable luxuriants, peace and a change of habits. Before you go on a vacation, consider the dust that is in the air, the manufacturing that is going on, the humidity, altitude, heat, cold, drafts, winds, and air pressure.

Electricity also has a very positive effect on the soil. A recent news article explained:

"Lightning helps fertilize the soil by producing up to ten million tons of nitrogen annually, according to Dr. Martin A. Uman, professor of electrical engineering at the University of Florida in Gainesville. When a thunderbolt streaks through the air, it creates a nitrogen compound, or natural fertilizer, that falls to the earth in raindrops, he explained. Dr. Uman is author of the book, *Understanding Lightning.*"

Air Pressure. The air pressure is not the same at different times of the day. It rises toward sunset; it usually falls as heat increases. Warm air expands and ascends, and cold air takes its place. This produces the air circulation or air motion called wind. Sea breezes are cold air flowing from the sea to the heat soaked land. This is why wind blows from the sea toward the land at night. Night wind is landward wind. Day wind is seaward wind. There is a constant interchange of sea air and land air, day and night.

Storms are nothing but air in motion. When the wind blows at the rate of three miles an hour or less we call it a stand-still, a calm. When air moves eight miles an hour the wind is hardly noticeable. When the air travels 13 miles an hour, we call it a pleasing breeze. Sixteen to 19 miles an hour is a gentle breeze. Air circulation at 22 to 24 miles an hour is a moderate breeze; 27 to 29 miles an hour is a fresh breeze; 34 miles an hour is a medium wind. A gale is from 38 to 42 miles an hour. In a fresh wind the air moves at 37 to 49 miles an hour. A strong wind travels 56 miles an hour. When the air moves at 64 to 68 miles an hour, we have a storm; and if it moves at 75 miles an hour, we call it a strong storm. In a hurricane the air travels approximately 88 to 130 miles an hour.

Rain is man's best friend in the sense that it purifies the air, but it can be his enemy, too, because a storm increases germ life. Microbes increase enormously when it begins to dry after a rain. In dry weather great clouds of dust are found in the air. The best time to breathe freely is in the winter, the spring, or immediately after a rain.

Rain decreases inorganic substances in the air, but it increases microorganisms almost unbelievably. Dust, dirt, and impurities, however, are more dangerous than germ life. Pathogenic bacteria never stay long in the air because of light, rain, and wind. Such bacteria are thrown to the ground by the rain. A salt moisture is found in the air to a certain extent, evaporated from the ocean, and it floats about as little salt globules and particles. Salty air has a soothing effect upon sleeplessness, nervousness, hysteria, temper, and restlessness.

The weight of air is considerable when we realize that there is an air pressure of from 11 to 15 tons bearing down on us daily, yet no one is conscious of it. Moist air is much heavier than dry air.

Gases expand upon heating, and rise. Atmospheric pressure therefore diminishes as we ascend into the air. The higher we go, the less pressure. The air is thinner, rarified; the air molecules are farther apart. And it is cooler because as gases expand, temperature drops. When we go into higher elevations we should ascend slowly, gradually.

Altitude. At sea level people are known to have about five million red blood corpuscles per cubic millimeter, but those living in high altitudes of five to six thousand feet have seven or even eight million per cubic millimeter. In the Andes Mountains in South America many people at some 10 to 12 thousand feet have blood counts of 7,500,000, which is unheard of with those living by the ocean. There may be much truth in the old Bible saying, "Go to the hills for thy strength."

Divers and others who work in dense air suffer from pain in the limbs, grow weak, and become anemic. Oxygen under high air pressure becomes toxic, and the red blood count decreases alarmingly. Mountain sicknesses, on the other hand, are peculiar to people who suddenly go to high elevations.

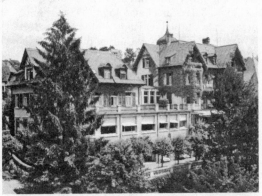

Bircher-Benner Sanitarium in Zurich, Switzerland where I have learned a great deal. It was through the counseling and the work of Dr. Ralph Benner that we have the foundation for much of our work today.

At first our nervous system is irritated by high altitude: temper increases, we become more violent, fussy, morose, and hunger and thirst increase. If the altitude is excessive to us, our digestive functions suffer. If, however, our vital functions can respond to the change of altitude, we soon feel as wonderful as if we were born anew. We become active; our functions are sharpened; the brain is clearer. We think right, concentrate better, create better, feel more important, accomplish greater deeds.

At a higher altitude and in a drier climate, we breathe differently. We have a greater expansion of the chest, oxygenation takes place more rapidly, metabolism is quickened, and the thyroid gland works at a more rapid pace.

If we go too high, however, new symptoms and ailments appear. Our red blood cells are the oxygen carriers in the body. Our lungs are actually an oxygen pantry where the red corpuscles go for their oxygen supply. The more red corpuscles we have, the more oxygen we can utilize. In a higher altitude we can become more irritable, impatient, impulsive, more thirsty and hungry, more urgent and imperative, more active in spirit, more willing to work, more inventive, and less tired. But in *too high* an altitude we can become dizzy; we can have a roaring in our ears; our senses can be impaired; our hearing and vision become dull, our minds stupid; we get sleepy and sluggish; and we can suffer from oxygen hunger.

Hens stop laying in high altitudes no matter how we feed them. Dogs do not breathe 13,000 to 16,000 feet above sea level. Trying to raise cats at an altitude of 14,000 feet will prove to you that there is a good lesson to learn in climatology. You cannot breed cats at that altitude. Muscular effort is nearly impossible. Unusually high elevations produce a high nervous pulse and increase the number of respirations per minute to the point of fevered breathing. Nervousness is increased at a high altitude and decreased at a low altitude. Unusually high altitude produces a rapid pulse and a feverish respiration, which makes the heart tumultuous and the breath as rapid as an intimidated bird. It makes all people nervous. Work that is easy at low altitudes for most people is difficult at a very high elevation. An excessive elevation may develop heart disease, lung trouble, and especially hypertrophy of the heart, owing to the fact that the blood is not sufficiently charged with oxygen. This throws an extra strain upon the valves of the heart. Send a flesh-clogged or soggy, waterlogged lady or man to a high altitude, and they will both suffer from suffocation.

Humidity. Humidity is the invisible water vapor in the air, not snow, fog, rain, or dew. Relative humidity is the vapor present in the air as compared to the vapors the air *can* hold. Cold air holds less humidity. The higher we go, the less humidity. The more the air expands, the less water vapor it can hold. If air cools after reaching its saturation point, precipitation results.

Dry air permits the sunbeams and light to pass through it. Moist air absorbs light, heat, and sunshine. When moist air moves briskly and is cold, we lose heat so rapidly that the next day we are "under the weather" with a cold, and our nasal membranes are congested. A dry climate has many changes of temperature caused by the sun's heat in the daytime and the great heat radiation at night.

There is more heat where there is more vegetation, which is especially true around the equator. Vegetable exuberance moderates both heat and cold.

Moisture intensifies both heat and cold, while dry air decreases heat. Dry air makes tissues more alkaline than any diet will. When the skin evaporation is poor, the kidneys are overworked. When the skin is sluggish, the kidneys work double shift. A moist, warm congenial climate relieves the kidneys, but a cold climate does not. An active skin relieves the kidneys. When we have a high or slightly high humidity, the skin function is always more active, as more water vapor is removed by the skin from the body. Evaporation of

bodily heat decreases as the water vapors of the air increase. Thus, we feel uncomfortable in warm, stuffy air. A high temperature and muggy air always lower respiration and functional activities; they also increase the carbon dioxide in blood and tissue. In cold weather more carbon dioxide is exhaled and breathing has a wider, deeper range.

The advice of Dr. Clarence A. Mills, (author of *Climate Makes the Man*) to some of his patients in cases of sinusitis and high blood pressure is to seek a warmer climate. In another case, he told one of his patients with high blood pressure to leave Wyoming, where he was trying to get well, and seek the relaxing warmth of southern Florida. He says that most physicians in the tropics now appreciate the importance of lowered vitality in hot climates and send their patients out to more invigorating regions as soon as tuberculosis is detected. The wise doctor will take care that his move does not plunge his patient into the respiratory hazards of winter cold and storms. Here again, the dry nonstormy Southwest is an ideal region.

Dr. Mills has shown that the blood pressure of an American usually falls during a few years' stay in Peking, and that of a Chinese rises when he comes to the northern United States even without any change in dietary or living habits. He tells how two of his Peking faculty colleagues, both native Britishers, experienced a 30 percent fall in blood pressure within a year after returning to China from furloughs spent in England or the United States. In Peking it was difficult to find enough cases of hypertension (high blood pressure) for teaching purposes. But in Cincinnati, almost a third of the hospital beds were occupied by this type of health problem.

So it is easy to see that temperature, altitude, humidity, winds, and electrical differences in the atmosphere can create a profound effect upon us, especially where disease is present.

The Seasons

Wintertime. In the wintertime we should consider taking large amounts of vitamins A and C: 30,000 mg. of vitamin A daily, and from 1,500 to 2,000 mg. of vitamin C daily.

During the wintertime many people living in foggy or smoggy areas spend too much time indoors and do not get enough winter sunshine. Heavy clothing is worn and longer hours are worked than normal. Consequently, about the month of March, lack of resistance allows colds and bronchial troubles to develop. To build natural resistance, eat plenty of oranges, grapefruit, sulphur vegetables to produce heat, and tops of vegetables. Then you are adequately supplied with winter sunshine. Sensitivity to weather changes indicates a need for potassium and calcium foods.

It is well to give children a little cod liver oil. This contains the sunshine vitamin material and will help us remain healthy if we do not get enough sunshine and are not outside enough. The best cod liver oil is obtained from Norway, and I would suggest that you take one teaspoon daily, or two capsules daily.

If you suffer from chilblains a good remedy is to apply lime water several times a day until there is relief.

Summertime. Most people get well in the summertime. Every disease is helped during the summer because this is when nature works best with all human tissues. In the summer we either naturally get well or are able to utilize a natural environment that helps us get well.

We should seek two summers in a row. There's no reason to build ourselves up 50 percent and then drop down 25 percent again in the wintertime. A lot of people who are sickly ought to go south like the birds do. If we're using natural remedies, natural foods, and so forth, let us use all the natural environment we can to add to our getting well.

Summer sunshine fixes the calcium needed by the body during the coming winter. It

Cultivating the land is the most heathful of all occupations.

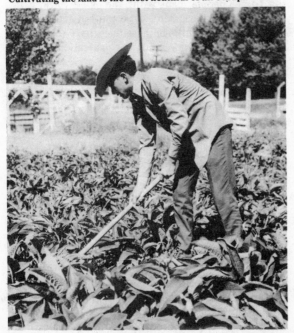

should be a recreative time in which we build up the body to carry on our life's activities.

Calcium is the healer, the knitter in the body. All sores require calcium to effect healing; therefore, get those "greens" going.

In the summer, greens are available. This is the time to eat greens because next winter you are going to need it.

We must be careful about exposure to the sun during the summer. The rays of the sun are very powerful in the summertime. If you work in the hot sunshine, protect your head with some type of covering. Wear a blue band inside your hat. We have in our bodies mineral elements which melt at a temperature of 106 degrees; therefore, we must protect ourselves from extreme heat. To maintain a good temperature your bloodstream must be more fluid, contain a greater amount of water in the summer.

Sodium is an important summer cooling element. Powdered whey is the most important food for the summer. It is highest in sodium. Sodium is eliminated through perspiration, which has a salty taste. We need to replace the salt thus eliminated, especially if one perspires freely. We can use okra and celery, which are high in sodium. Celery juice combined with pineapple juice is splendid. Juice of comfrey leaves may be added, using one-third of each with a little whey powder. Combining comfrey and strawberries is also very good.

Strawberries are high in sodium. Eating strawberries ripe does not cause hives. If you have berries that are not fully ripened, put them in a sieve under hot water. This will remove the fuzz on their skin. Rinse immediately with cold water. This should prevent any occurrence of hives. Try to get ripe berries. In fact get all fruit as ripe as possible. Our choice of foods in the summer should be those which are most easily digested and low in carbohydrates. Maintain a low starch and sugar intake during the summer months. The natural sugars of fully ripened fruits are most easily handled in digestion. Drink plenty of juices. If you are on a high intake of juices and you are losing too much weight, add a tablespoon of nut butter or sunflower seed meal (from seeds freshly ground if you use a liquefier).

Serious skin malignancies may be the result of an accumulation of inorganic elements in the body; these are drawn to the surface by excessive sun exposure. Ten minutes a day in your birthday or bathing

11

suit is sufficient when the sun's rays are the most intense during the midday hours.

Air baths are just as important as sunbaths. In privacy, practice this cosmic, vital air bathing as much as possible. This may be enjoyed indoors with benefit if you have adequate ventilation.

Today most of us have thyroid disturbances. This results from an overbalance of those things which affect the mental side of life. To balance this, get out in the air. Get a lot of fresh air upon the skin. Wear as little clothing as suitable for the occasion. This will help the nerves more than anything else. Mental and nerve depletion may be overcome by air and sunbathing.

Iced drinks are one of the worst things we can use in the summertime (or anytime). They cause the villi (the tiny fibers lining the walls of the intestines) to contract, thus impairing one's digestion. Ice cream can be good if it is made from nutritious ingredients, preferably in your own kitchen. But don't mix it with other foods and eat it slowly, allowing each spoonful to melt in the mouth. The coldness of ice cream contracts the stomach wall so that we don't secrete the hydrochloric acid needed for digestion.

For cooling the blood in the summertime, use cucumbers, lettuce, celery, parsley, tomatoes, and a low-calorie diet.

Environment and Body Heat

We need to be aware of our body heat and careful that it is at the right level. People whose internal heat is low have very sluggish skin. This is why purification of the system falls so heavily upon the liver, lungs, and kidneys. These organs become overworked and result in liver, kidney, and lung diseases. Some seven to eight percent of the bodily heat is lost through the evaporation process performed by the lungs. Muscles are the great oxidizers and heat producers in the body. When the cerebellum is weak, we suffer from cold feet, cold hands, chilly sensations, colds, catarrh, and perhaps pneumonia.

It is good that the heat generation in man is dissipated easily. More than 70 percent of bodily heat radiates through the skin. If we did not radiate this heat continually, we would come to a boiling point and be cooked in less than 40 hours. Excess body heat is lost through radiation, evaporation, perspiration, and convection. At certain altitudes we find that this takes place better than at others.

Which Climate? A cold bracing climate and high altitude (that is, from 2,000 to 6,000 feet) tone our functions, increase appetites, build new red blood corpuscles, promote oxidation in the tissues and blood. However, in high altitudes our hearts must be sound.

Weak people, old people, lazy people, and paralyzed people thrive in a warm climate; but healthy people, people of high production, muscular people, and great workers are comfortable in a cool climate. Cold increases energy, but heat decreases it. Some people are subject to infectious diseases in hot climates. Breathing is decreased in hot weather, and the removal of carbon dioxide is more difficult. People in hot climates are less energetic and more sociable. People in cold climates are greater fighters and less sociable. Cold winters lead to muscular action. Hot weather favors indolence. Moderate exercise of muscles and nerves and a breezy climate favor the muscular and nervous systems.

Normal cold increases the elasticity of arteries and the heart, but heat decreases these. People in a cold climate have a slower pulse and higher blood pressure. People in the tropics have a higher pulse and a lower blood pressure. Small people have a quicker pulse than larger people. The skin pores are always active in hot climates, but they are sluggish in cold climates. Perspiration carries off heat and moisture through the skin in a hot climate.

Some people can withstand more heat than others. Dark-skinned people can endure it better than white because they have more nitrogen in the skin and less generation of muscular electricity.

Life is less productive in cold regions. Temperatures affect the sex functions. Warmth develops sexuality unless heat is excessive. Heat increases the generative function. There is more sexual excess in hot climates than in cold climates. The menstrual function begins earlier in a hot climate. Child-bearing is attended with greater difficulty in a hot climate because of a tendency to hemorrhages. Warmth develops the sexual system and increases sexual power.

Heating foods, on the same principle, develops sexuality. Wind is bad for the sexual system and for people who suffer from sexual weaknesses. Excessive heat destroys tissue, as does excessive cold. Great heat makes the blood toxic and melts the myelin cells in the spinal cord and brain. When the myelin cells melt, the man is in danger. This can result in sunstroke. Sunstroke kills; excessive cold kills also. If the cold is excessive, all vital processes suffer, and unfavorable results follow. Cold, as you know, constricts the surface blood vessels beneath the skin, lowers skin activity, and affects the capillary function of the circulation, resulting in inadequate skin nourishment. Then the skin is robbed of its fatty principle, sebum, it cracks, and chilblains form. Wounds fail to heal because of lowered vitality and faulty circulation. Such an excessive cold climate is too severe for our wellbeing. Regenerative functions suffer in a very cold and windy climate. Male reproductive capabilities are seldom at their best. Female processes act under lower pressure, giving rise to menstrual difficulties and female ailments.

Extremes Are Dangerous. Going to extremes in climate is always dangerous. It is not wise for anyone to change climate and stay there for good. A man who goes from a hot climate to a cold climate and lives there the rest of his life may be healthy, but his offspring will suffer and die early. This holds good also for one who goes from a cold to a hot climate. A climate can be a tonic to one man, depressive to another, and even death to a third.

There are many books written on climate, but I think one of the best is the one written by Clarence A. Mills, M.D., *Climate Makes the Man*. He answers a great many of our questions about what climate does to us. Dr. Mills is one of the leading men in the field of experimental medicine and has studied climate for many years. He demonstrates that climate plays a dominating and startling role in all that we do. He shows that it affects our growth, speed of development, resistance to infection, fertility of mind and body, happiness, and length of life. He also shows that it lulls the people of the tropics into passive complacency and drives those of the temperate zone into restless activity. According to Dr. Mills, sexual development is actually retarded by extremes of heat and cold. He has worked with many rats and mice and other animals and has concluded that caffeine, alcohol, and nicotine have differing effects under different climatic conditions: he shows that hardening of the arteries, tuberculosis, sinusitis, and many other ills are related to man-made weather, air conditioning, etc. He points out that different diseases are related to various types of weather.

For instance, he has seen how breeders of small animals around Cincinnati frequently find that their animals are almost completely sterile by the end of a hot summer, while the same rabbits, mice or guinea pigs can, in cool winter, continue to reproduce profusely. One beautiful male rabbit, known to be highly fertile, was overheated in their laboratory hot-room but recovered to apparent good health; afterwards, however, repeated mating showed him to be permanently sterile. In Panama's warmth the prolific guinea pig becomes a poor breeder, improving only slightly during the short dry season when low humidity renders the warmth less depressive. Large numbers of guinea pigs are required for certain hospital and laboratory procedures in Panama, but those imported from the North endure the heat poorly and are of little value.

During the severe heat of the 1934 summer in the Middle West, fertility was sharply reduced. Kansas City showed a 30 percent reduction in conception rate during the month when day temperatures consistenly rose about 100 degrees. The usual summer decline is only 15 percent. All through the Middle West, birth certificate statistics showed the same sharp decline for conception during that period of the blazing heat.

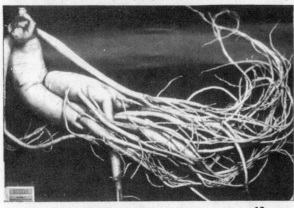

The herb Ginseng has been used for thousands of years by the people in the Far East and is purported to promote longevity. As can be seen here, the roots take on appearance of human body.

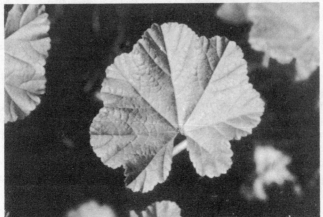

Malva grows wild and is a weed, yet it is one of the highest foods in Vitamin A—50,000 units of Vitamin A to one pound of Malva. A great catarrhal resistent food. It was this particular form of weed that we informed the King of Hunza to use more of because we found that many of the children had discharging eyes. To see these conditions leave in a short time by using this high Vitamin A product was a surprise to all. Malva is considered a weed, yet possible if we knew more about our weeds, we could get more good from weeds than some of the foods that we eat today.

Persimmons are wonderful when they are dried. They are wonderful fresh also, however, they can be taken into the body and slurped down the throat without chewing them. This fiber many times can cause many intestinal disturbances and we must make sure we break up the fiber material in chewing the persimmon. Try drying them. They are wonderful and almost like a candy for the child.

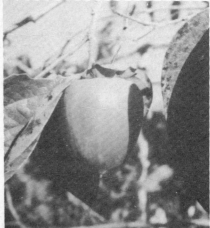

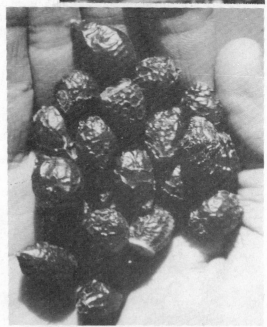

Dried Cherries are very high in iron so you can get an iron tonic for yourself during the winter. This keeps up the blood count, avoids anemia and this is the time of the year when we want the greatest amount of iron.

MIDDLE: Rose Hips: High in Vitamin C, can be made into a lovely drink, can be dropped into soup, can be used in many different ways. Helps to fight infections and comes at a time of year, the end of summer, where we can put them away and use them for resisting our diseases that are so prevalent in wintertime.

How can we live a long life? THREE

A PROMINENT San Jose pioneer was celebrating his eightieth birthday and also his fiftieth wedding anniversary. The reporters gathered around him to express congratulations. Then they asked, "What do you attribute this long span of successful living to?" He reflected for a moment and replied, "When I got married my wife and I had an agreement that any time we saw an argument coming on, I would grab my hat and walk four times around the block. You'd be surprised what fifty years of outdoor exercise will do for your health."

That's not the only method of having a long life. Dr. Frank Gallup polled 29,000 Americans who were 94 years old and older and concluded that the way to have a long life is to: 1. be a woman, 2. be born in Norway; 3. be of long-lived ancestors; 4. not worry; 5. not smoke; 6. eat wisely and lightly; 7. have enthusiasm; and 8. have a strong religious belief. Sounds good — but what if you aren't Norwegian?

Youth. The secret of a long life *can* be learned. But all is not always just as it seems. The paradox is that in regions of the world where sanitary conditions are often primitive, many persons reach a span of life beyond 100 years. How can they do that? A major reason is that their life-style makes them healthy, and a healthy body is immune to infections; harmful microbes are scavengers existing only in putrefying matter.

If a child is introduced to a natural diet after weaning, his or her intestinal flora closely resembles that of the milk diet. Fresh, uncooked, organically grown food provides the ideal nourishment. Cooking reduces food's ability to give us resistance.

Raw foods harden the gums; chewing stimulates digestion. Raw foods are often the only ones supplying the vital enzymes that protect us.

We poison ourselves. Anyone who lives on an unnatural diet of artificially grown and processed foods, who overeats meat and carbohydrates to the exclusion of fresh fruits and vegetables, who fills his mind with negative thoughts and overworks at the expense of adequate rest, who floods his body with acids (the home of pathogenic bacteria) — any man who does those things is bringing trouble to paradise. His bowels become a sewer from which poisons seep into the blood and are carried to all parts of the body. No wonder so many people try to regain health by taking strong purgatives! But they are no cure. Prevention is the wisest medicine. And prevention means to find a natural way to live, the way we *by our natures* should live. When we do, nature will reward us with a healthy, active body — a long living body. One means of finding the natural health life-style is to study peoples around the world. Is a particular people healthy? Why — or why not?

The first 40 years of life give us the text; the next 30 supply the commentary.

— Schopenhauer

FOUR

Learning from other countries

I HAVE made many travels in my fifty years of practice and I have gleaned something from each country that I believe will help you in your "health search," to put your health on a higher level.

Colombia, Heleconia — The average of life here is thirty years. The reason is they do not have enough protein. But when they have added soy milk powder to their diet great changes have taken place. *I believe soy milk powder is a great protein and a great food.* Learn how to use it in your daily menu.

Persia (Iran)- -Here they have a variety of soils, good and bad, and they also have the extremes in age. I believe the chemistry of our body depends on the chemical balance of the soil. Elderly people here live where the soil is black. Try to *eat foods from black soil, free of fertilizer or spray.*

Germany- In a sanitarium here they were using sauerkraut and tomato juice as a slight laxative. This was taken daily by people who were constipated, as part of an elimination diet program. In Woerschofen, we saw the great Kneipp baths (water treatment). The same circulation you have in your legs, you have in your head. *To improve the circulation in your head, take care of the legs and feet.* Use the Kneipp leg bath at home as follows: go out into the yard and run cold water from a hose up the back of the right leg, from the toes to the groin and down again. Repeat the same motions on the left leg. Then walk on grass or in the sand. Do this once a day.

Denmark- Here they have a wonderful broth that increases the calcium content of the body and helps growing children in proper bone development. It is made from barley and green kale.

Turkey- In Turkey, they use sesame seed mixed with a concentrated grape juice as a candy. Use sesame seed butter in one-half glass of grape juice as a tonic. *Use sesame seed daily for building a strong body.* They have men of great strength in Turkey. A man seventy-five years of age was head of Turkey's wrestling team.

Finland- The greatest lesson here was the value of *using rye to build muscle.* Wheat builds fat. The greatest runner of all time was from Finland.

New Zealand- In New Zealand they all *have a weekend holiday for rest and recuperation* and *for happy hours.* Lydiard, the great Olympic champion from New Zealand, takes people jogging through the country. Jogging began there. *Jogging is a great sport to keep one in fit condition.* Every school in New Zealand has a swimming pool. *Swimming is one of the finest of all exercises.*

Bulgaria- Bulgaria has traditionally had more people over one hundred years of age, per capita, than any other country in the world. They claim the reason is that they use a fair amount of a clabbered milk that contains the Bulgaricus acidophilous bacteria. *Everybody with any bowel trouble should take a course in acidophilous culture for at least one month, three times yearly.*

India- Sri Ahrobindo Ashram is the greatest Universal Center I ever visited; there a balance of the physical, mental, and spiritual are taught. The integration of all three was deemed most important. Sai Baba was one of the greatest individuals my group ever met. His teachings and philosophy lift everyone. He said, "Money may bring comfort, but it cannot bring you contentment; however, *your spiritual attitude can bring you contentment.*"

Russia- We met many of the oldest people in the world here. The last man we met was 153 years of age, a Mr. Gasanov. The secret of these men living to great age is the altitude, climate, a simple life and plenty of protein. The protein they use most is clabbered milk. It is a wonderful food- a complete protein and a whole food that is easy to digest. *Put a little concentrated apple juice in clabbered milk and use daily in your diet. How to make clabbered milk:* Heat two quarts raw milk to lukewarm. Stir in one cup yogurt or buttermilk. Set in oven with only pilot light on. Leave overnight. Remove from oven, leave in same pan, and place in refrigerator to thicken. If you use a starter from a health store, follow the directions included with the starter.

Spain- In Barcelona, we were entertained by the mayor, who served a delightful almond milk drink. This gave us the idea of *making milk out of seeds and nuts.* I have developed what I call "my drink." It is a complete vitality-giving protein drink. It is non-catarrhal forming and a delightful body-builder for vegetarians. My drink: Take one tablespoon of any good brand of sesame seed meal or butter, one glass of liquid (may be raw milk, fruit juice, vegetable juice, soy milk, broth, or water), ¼ avocado, and one teaspoon honey (or add honey to taste), and blend 30 seconds.

Armenia- The people here are most gracious, receive you royally, and make you feel at home. This is a necessary characteristic for good human relationships. A good idea I saw here was to fold rice in grape leaves and steam. One elderly lady, 127 years of age, told us that rose hip tea kept her well.
Egypt- *The greatest energy-giving food is the date.* I found dates and milk to be an ideal combination for people suffering with stomach trouble.

Tahiti- Relaxation and absorbing the sun was the highlight in Tahiti. They were healthier without clothes. I believe that wearing clothes is the beginning of every disease. *Those who wear clothes must get acquainted with skin brushing to keep the skin clean and healthy.* You make new skin every twenty-four hours, and the skin is only as clean as the blood is. No soap can wash the skin as clean as the new skin is, so use a skin brush to remove the top layer of old skin. This helps to eliminate uric acid crystals, catarrh, and various other acids in the body. The skin should eliminate two pounds of waste acids daily. Keep the skin active. Use a dry vegetable bristle brush with a long handle. (Do not use a nylon brush). Use the brush dry, in the morning before dressing, and before bathing. Use over the whole body for about three minutes.

Hawaii- All fruits grown in Hawaii are high in iodine because they grow close to the ocean. The people who had the best teeth chewed the natural sugar cane. *Their greatest combination is fruit and fish.*

Mexico- The word *mañana* would help to make famous men more famous by helping them live longer. To crowd too much into one day will kill anybody. *Do what you can today, but don't do tomorrow's work too.* Don't try to get a quart out of a pint bottle.
Peru- This is the country where I learned that *altitude helps to create a better blood count.* Peru developed squash, *one of the greatest of all foods.* Winter squash is one of the greatest foods for intestinal disturbances.

South Seas- *Coconut milk is a perfect protein* and should be used more in the diet. *Dried papaya seeds make a wonderful tea* which helps in digestion.

Hunzaland- One of the greatest secrets of Hunzaland (an area west of Tibet) is the apricot pit. After breaking open the apricot seeds, the Hunzas string the pits and eat them whenever they wish. They are very rich in protein and taste almost like an almond. To make an apricot drink, squeeze the dried apricots in water with your hands until they are completely dissolved. This is a splendid fruit drink. Apricots and apricot pits give one a good carbohydrate and protein combination. The Hunzaland people stuff apricots with apricot pits and eat them during the winter. They make an apricot and apricot pit soup which is very tasty, and provides them with a lot of the energy they need for the heavy work they do. The oldest man we met in Hunza was 120 years of age and still working.

Switzerland- The greatest food here is yogurt. This is good protein food that builds friendly bacteria in the bowel. Yogurt with fruit makes a good combination. One of the finest things they did in Switzerland during World War II was to establish a place in the country where each person could grow his own foods. *Everyone should grow some foods for himself. The*

Swiss grow their herbs in window boxes. These are used for flavoring salads, soups, and various other foods used in their daily meals. You could grow your own parsley, chives, rosemary, anise, etc. Everyone should grow comfrey and dry it for a winter tea. Whatever herbs are not used fresh can be dried for winter use.

Equador--This country taught me that *gravity affects our health.* Here I found a man over 130 years of age, and there were many other very old people here in Equador. You have to have good health to resist the pull of gravity. The poorer the health, the more effect gravity has on one, interfering with proper circulation in the body.

Norway- Beauty is brought out in Norway so much because of its past culture. There is beauty surrounding everything- the fjords, the mountains, the green pastures, the people- and the feeling is wonderful, which helps beauty to act as a healing factor.

Philippines- Soak *coconut pieces in honey* in a jar for one week. It makes a wonderful sweet for the children.

Sweden- The great thing here is gymnastics. *Outdoor exercise and massage are both necessary to keep man balanced.* Everyone here is very health conscious. In many places, groups go for a weekend of swimming or to the mountains to ski. They have wonderful athletic bodies, lithe and in good condition due to their participation in athletics. They use codliver oil for all their athletic patients.

France- The most wonderful thing to come out of France was their Roquefort brand cheese. This is a cheese which crumbles and was originally made from sheep milk and goat milk. *It is a great calcium builder* in the body. Always use cheese that breaks and is aged.

Japan- A wonderful soup, high in iodine, can be made with many varieties of sea weed. In Japan, they make many things from sea weed soups, candy, salads. There are over 500 varieties of sea weed that can be used.

Italy- *Sun-dried olives from Italy are the highest potassium producing foods.* Olives are cured in sea salt in Turkey and in Italy. The heart needs the potassium. A potassium broth can be made from ten sun-dried olives steeped in two cups of hot water for ten minutes. Strain and drink the liquid. Another excellent heart remedy is honey and water. Mix one teaspoon honey into a glass of water two or three times daily. A great potassium broth is made from potato peelings. We use it for extreme acids in the body and for rheumatism and arthritis. It is made this way: cut peelings of six potatoes, ¾ inches thick, simmer 20 minutes in covered pan. Strain off liquid and drink every two or three hours. Do not make too strong in a convalescing diet. Celery may be added for flavor. Add powdered okra if the stomach is irritated.

China- In the last years, there has been considerable talk about Ginseng, Gotu-Kola, and Fo-Ti-Tieng. These three herbs have been used in China for many centuries and are purported to promote longevity. For instance, a man by the name of Li Ching Yun lived in Szechuan Province. He lived to the age of 252 and it is reported he gave some 28 lectures at the University of Sinkiang when he was over 200 years old. It is claimed that the three herbs of Ginseng, Gotu-Kola, and Fo-Ti-Tieng were used in his daily diet. Whether this had anything to do with his old age or not cannot be verified; however, before he died he was asked what he attributed his long life to. I think he left a sermon for us in just two words when he said, "I attribute my long life to *inward calm.*"

What We've Learned from Experience

There is much else that we know about strengthening our health and lengthening our life through natural means. Experience teaches us much. Following is a brief catalog. *Mother's milk* is traditionally used to rejuvenate elderly persons, especially the men in Europe. When they become old and feeble and cannot move around to activate the body and keep life flowing through tissues, they pay for mother's milk to rejuvenate their bodies. John D. Rockefeller did such in his latter years, and credited the practice as part of what saved his life at that time.

Pollen and Special Herbs

Much is to be said about pollen helping glands in the body. All the experiments on animals show it prolongs life and helps to keep the glands in good order.

Ginseng, Gotu-Kola, Fo-Ti-Tieng, and Damiana have been considered long life herbs, as is the commonly known Sage.

Self-Culture and a Corrective Diet

We find that in healthy youth the inhalation is deep and rapid, while exhalation is slow. Air should enter the lungs rather quickly and with force and leave the lungs rather slowly to invite life and vigor.

Self-culture and a corrective diet are the keys to life, health, vigor, beauty, influence, and accomplishment. We find that the snatching of breath with ease and force makes men of vigor and women of beauty. You find their voices distinct, their faces bright, and their step elastic- oxygen steams them up.

My professor used to say, "Quick, deep inhalations vitalize when the air leaves the lungs silently." The most noticeable habit of the nobleman is his deep, quick, full inhalation and slow, silent exhalation. Other points of distinction are his full, large chest, lofty bearing, courteous manners, erect position, expanding nostrils, and so forth. Look at the ample nostrils of the spirited orator as he pours out his pathos. Notice the heaving bosom of the loving maiden, her springy steps, beauty of complexion, glowing eyes, and lively manners.

In fever, lung disease, flu, and low states of vitality respiration is short, shallow, and faint.

Compare the face, manners, walk, cheeks, eyes, and chest movements of vigorous men and beautiful women with those of the pessimist, cynic, and the disheartened. Self-culture *does* make a difference in health.

Invigorating Life Tonic

In the pericarp of barley we find a principle that is very invigorating to the functions of life. The same is true of the pericarp of oats.

When that pericarp essence can be extracted and mixed with the fresh raw juices from celery, parsley, thyme, beets, and spinach, it became a remarkable restorative to man in time of lassitude and fatigue.

Soaking barley- or better still barley bran- in cold water to prevent fermentation until the oily substances come to the top, enables the housewife to extract, to a certain degree, this pericarp essence in barley. A cupful of the juices mentioned and one-third cup of the barley skimming, but not the scum, gives you this pericarp essence called *avenin*. Parsley and celery contain *apeol*, beets contain *betaine*. Such food essences are a tonic and sanative for the weak and aged.

Small Meals Favor Old Age

Small meals favor old age because of a weaker digestion, sluggish bowel action, low nerve force, and reduced secretion of the digestive juices.

Use clabbered milk as you get older rather than the whole milk. Older people should never, under any circumstances, eat until they are hungry. Eat slowly and masticate foods well. Seek fresh air and breathe it deeply. Elderly people should sit and tempt their appetite at meals for some five to ten minutes before they eat in order to secrete gastric juices in abundance for good digestion.

As we get older, we must have the food salts to carry out the functions of life. These are found mainly in goat brown cheese, in berries, and in greens. We should eat some of these foods each day.

In old age, digestion and elimination (especially elimination) need constant attention.

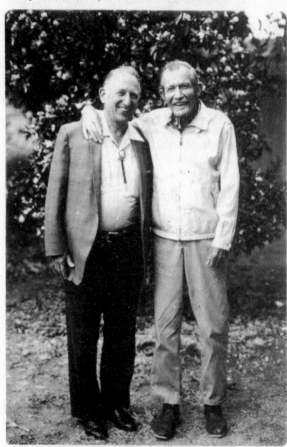

DAVID POWERS, 82 year old vegetarian, has established four records in his jogging, two of which have never been broken, in walking across the United States. We helped him get started in jogging and getting out of a serious sickness that plagued him for years. You develop records through good health.

Uric acidity, which causes neuritis, rheumatism, and arthritis, is best treated by dry, intense, local heat applied again and again.

Avoid Pronounced Changes

Vacations can favor us if we go to the right altitude and right cimate and have the proper comforts. Pronounced changes do not favor old age. As soon as our feet or knees or head, or any part of our body become cold or damp, we should do something to regain the normal heat equilibrium. Even if we have to change footwear, bedclothes, underwear, or gloves, we cannot afford to chill any part of our body, or become damp as we advance in years. We should dress so that we are comfortably warm and dry at all times. We should not stay long in sultry heat, severe cold or strong winds.

Spend Time Outdoors

Outdoor life among trees, shrubbery, and flowers, life in the fresh air and sunshine favor health in both young and old. As we get older we should spend at least six hours outdoors each day. If it is possible, go on horseback rides. They have found that this is vibratory and promotes circulation, elimination, respiration, oxidation, tissue metabolism, and nerve generation. Sleep in abundance. If you are restless, use abdominal applications, take a Swedish massage, and eat a combination salad with evening meal.

Take pleasurable walks each day after each meal to promote the vital functions. Do not sit in a rocking chair after meals. Don't work hard after meals and don't use the brain energetically after meals. Find a genial

In the little town of Villacabamba in South America where there is immunity to heart troubles, the people live to a ripe old age. José on left is 132 years of age. The woman next to him is 85 years old and jogs eight blocks every morning before breakfast.

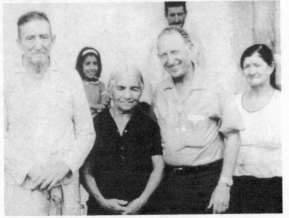

climate which is neither humid, arid, nor windy, and which is not too sunny. Avoid glaring sunlight: it can be trying on the optic nerves. The Swedish massage from a trained masseur has a wonderful effect on the tissues and function of all people, whether young or old.

It is especially important to know and live in the climate that is good for you. There you can feel pleasant and relaxed.

Light Brain Work

Excessive study, reading, talking, discussing, lecturing, teaching, or singing is not favorable to old people. These things liberate fatigue products and produce acidity and bloating. Light brain work helps to keep the brain from becoming rusty, but stop for a period when it becomes too tiring.

Staying Healthy after Forty

Men and women over forty should realize that they now have the opportunity to start enjoying the special richness of a full life that only time can bring.

There are many interesting hobbies and rewarding occupations. One of the best is gardening. (If the joints become the least bit stiff and hard, use lots of sodium and eat potassium broths.) Never retire from work— find something interesting to do. Then never lose that interest. Tissues will become flabby if you do, and circulation will decrease. Use iodine in the diet— one to three Nova Scotia Dulse tablets daily. The Dulse tablets not only help flabby tissues but also will help weight conditions. Cut down on starch and add a little more protein. Go to a temperate climate, usually at an altitude of 2,000 to 3,000 feet.

For men, if prostate gland trouble develops, if you have difficulty urinating, or if you have to get up several times in the night, consider hot and cold sitz baths. They are very good for these conditions.

Use a slant board for any prolapses of abdominal organs, if no high blood pressure exists. Consider getting a vibrating bed for internal circulation. Add vitamin E- taking one to three capsules daily or as recommneded by your doctor.

Walking, breathing pure air, is one of the best exercises for people over forty. Spend much time in the open air; partake of natural foods; avoid work in the city. Papaya and mint tea will help the secretions of the stomach to digest proteins. Avoid extreme changes in temperatures; don't become "chilled to the bone." Use distilled water when the joints become hard.

A good tonic is to use lecithin and lots of vegetable broths in the diet. Fresh goat's milk adds to the youth of the body. Drink black cherry juice along with bitter pungent salads. Eat dark cherries and strawberries. When you need fats in the diet, raw sweet cream and avocado should be used as a source of fat. Try a celery juice cocktail with wheat germ in it. Have warm drinks. Eat gruels made from barley and wheat. Plan light meals for morning and at night. Take one egg yolk in black cherry or Concord grape juice daily.

Strive for a simple life with freedom from economic pressure.

Health Vacations

Sometimes we need to take a vacation to improve or to restore our health. Seek a health vacation that rests the mind and the body. It must be a total change from the type of work you are getting away from. Seek a complete change in climate. Eat the right foods. Sometimes elimination foods are desirable.

During the vacation you should be surrounded by people who are easy to get along with; the vacation environment should be enjoyable. Spend your health vacation with people who are happy and companionable.

This vacation should be one that allows for recuperation to prepare the mind and body for the job that's waiting for them when you return.

How to Avoid Unnecessary Surgery

To help consumers combat a wave of unnecessary surgery, Herbert Denenberg, Pennsylvania Insurance Commissioner, prepared "A Shopper's Guide to Surgery: Fourteen Rules on How To Avoid Unnecessary Surgery." Denenberg's "Rules," in checklist form, follow:

1. Don't go directly to a surgeon for medical treatment; go to your regular family doctor, a general practitioner, or internist for any initial diagnosis.

2. Make sure any surgeon that is to perform surgery on you is Board Certified. This means his competence as a surgeon has been certified by one of the American Specialty Boards after a vigorous oral, written and clinical examination.

3. Make sure the surgeon you are to engage is a fellow of American College of Surgeons.

4. Even if your family doctor and surgeon agree that surgery is necessary, consider getting an independent consultation.

5. Make sure any surgery is performed in an accredited hospital and, if possible, select a hospital that gives staff privileges (i.e., the right to practice in the hospital) to both your doctor and surgeon.

6. Don't push a doctor to perform surgery on you. If you insist on surgery, even if it is unnecessary, you are likely to find a surgeon willing to perform it.

7. Make sure your doctor and surgeon explain both the alternatives to surgery and possible benefits and complications of surgery.

8. Frankly discuss the fee for surgery with your doctor.

9. Check the surgeon out with those who know him or have used him. This includes other patients as well as associates

10. Make sure the surgeon knows and is willing to work with your general practitioner or internist. If they can't work as a team, you may be the loser.

11. Consider a surgeon who is a part of a group practice and preferably a group that includes internists, surgeons and other specialists. With a group practice, you are more likely to have a doctor available at all times who is familiar with your case and you have the built-in benefits of consultation.

12. Select a surgeon who is not too busy to give patients enough time and attention.

13. Be especially on guard if some of the operations that are most often unnecessarily performed are proposed for you. These include hysterectomies, hemorrhoidectomies and tonsillectomies.

14. The patient, not the doctor or surgeon, is supposed to, and is entitled to make the decision on whether to have surgery. Listen to the experts. But it's still your decision.

Reprint from *National Health Federation Bulletin*

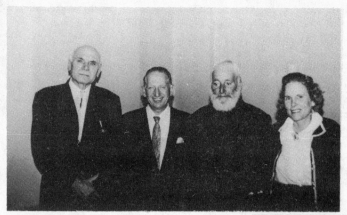

Peter Maloff, Dr. Jensen, Mr. Gasanov and Mrs. Jensen. We are visiting one of the oldest men in the world—Mr. Gasanov, 153 years of age—in Baku, Russia.

In this town in Turkey they find the men carry everything. I have seen men carry a piano on their back for 8 blocks and the man was 75 years of age. It is hard to believe the strength of these men in carrying the articles from one part of the city to another.

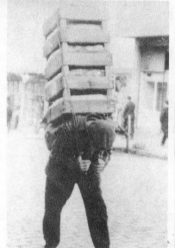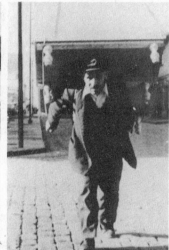

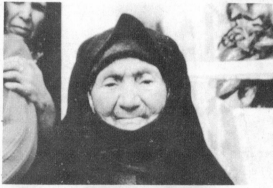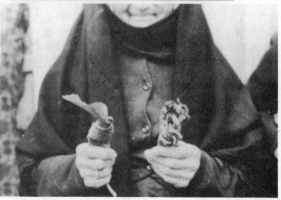

A lady 127 years of age in Armenia. She makes up dried foods for the winter months by putting away rose hips, dried comfrey, dried garlic, and learning how to dry all of her vegetables to survive the months when she is unable to grow vegetables.

Dr. Jensen Knighted For His Life Efforts

CEREMONIAL ADDRESS . . .

For your consistent life efforts in study, travel and teaching, for your persistent continued efforts to raise health standards for nearly fifty years, we commend you for crusading a more healthful life to the people you have met. The acceptance wherever you have gone, the numerous books you have written that have reached so many people, are a testimony to your untiring efforts. Visiting the Hunzas of Pakistan, native studies in the South Seas, South America, and teachings in Australia, New Zealand, France, Italy, Russia and various cultures in the world, is commendable. Your human endeavors have been outstanding in the refinement of the knowledge of foods to families and homes, to the profession for the natural care of ill health, especially in teaching preventive methods and of the discernment in detecting of ill health as found in the philosophy and theory of Iridology.

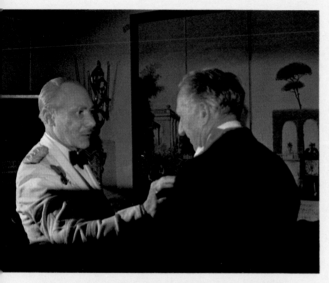

Dr. Jensen was knighted into the order of Saint John Knights of Malta founded in the Hague, Kingdom of the Netherlands June 26, 1978.

This is a picture of the Mir of Hunza whom we stayed with for 9 days in the Hunza Valley, the legendary Shangri-La. It is the wonderful philosophy of this most affable man that truly was the basis for the lovely Hunza Valley longevity as found in her people and wonderful philosophy as practiced by them. No jails, no crime, no police force and we find that the basis for this as the King has said in the many letters he has sent me is all that I have I wouldlike to share with you.

Lecturing in my Choga Coat that was given to me while in the Hunza Valley. This is a typical dress used on special occasions.

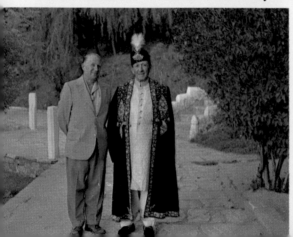

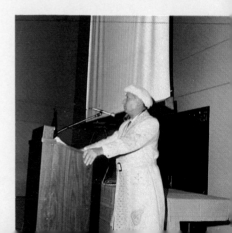

A World of Beauty and Health

Coloful Guatemala. Ripley has said in his books that Guatemala is the most colorful country in the world and I certainly believe it after going through the many different states in Guatemala and seeing their picturesque blouses, clothing and colored dresses that they use.

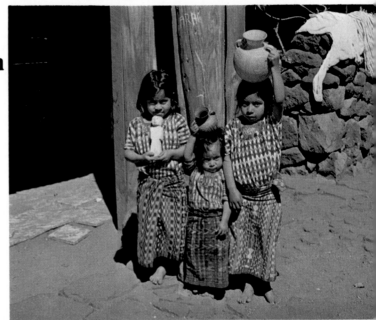

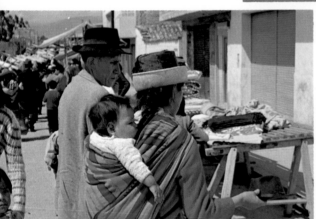
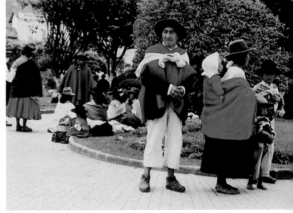

Children always steal the show. It is to them that we owe the next generation; we must influence the children so they learn to carry forward that which is good.

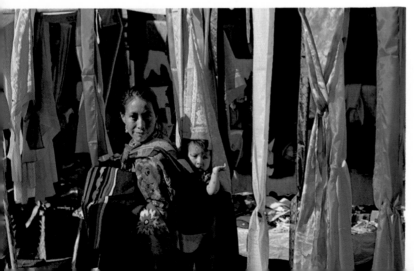

Whatever we do, whatever we eat, however we live, has it's influence in the next generation, and while they may be a burden that we carry on our backs for the moment, we have a great responsibility to see that the next generation has the finest body possible and the finest training that they may keep healthy and well.

Each Country Contributes Something of Value

Australia — In certain parts of Australia you will see these attractive windmills which conserve energy by using the wind as an energy source to bring water forth from deep within the earth.

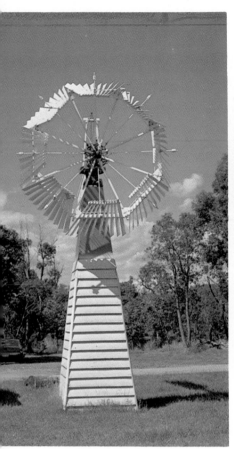

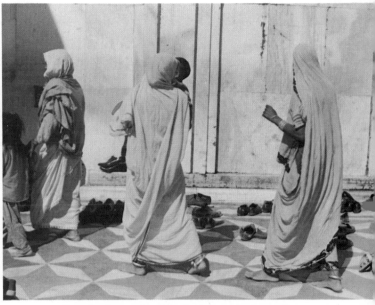

Free-flowing garbs of the Indian people are much healthier for a person than those that are tight and made of nylon as we have in our civilization today. Cotton and silk are the best of all the wearing apparel that we can use.

One of the greatest visits I've ever made was with Mr. Peter Maloff of Canada who traveled with me through Turkey and Russia. Here he is before a Turkish market where we were able to see that no matter where we visited in the world, fundamentally what came out of the soil was for man's use, God-given, and the thing we have to stay close to in order to be well. Mr. Peter Maloff is a confirmed vegetarian believing that the future world belongs to the vegetarians.

In going into the Amazon we see how many people live in their natural state. Many times we thought we would find the healthiest people living close to nature but we find that nature can be cruel by giving us a washed out soil from constant rain. These people many times can have a lack of calcium, building abnormal bodies, such as we found when they had curvatures of the spine, pronated ankles, pigeon chest, and so forth.

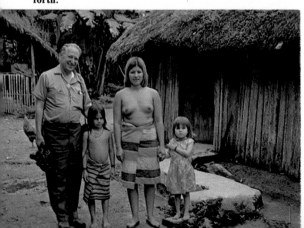

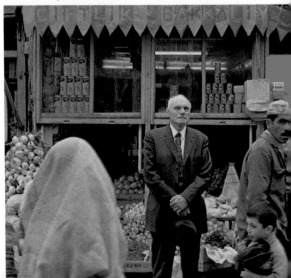

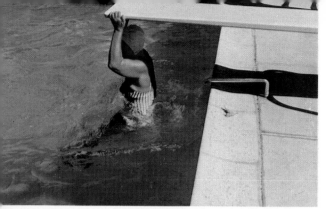

Exercises in swimming pool

Swimming is one of the most complete exercises we have. Here are 3 photos showing one of the exercises we developed which can be done in the swimming pool.

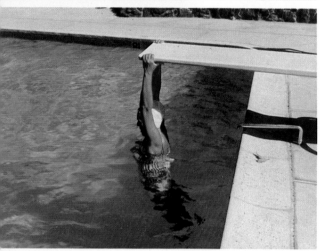

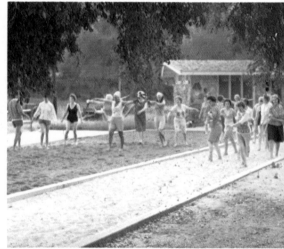

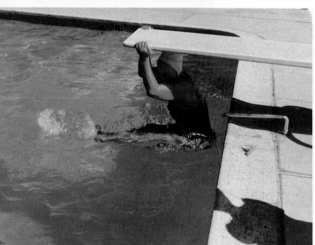

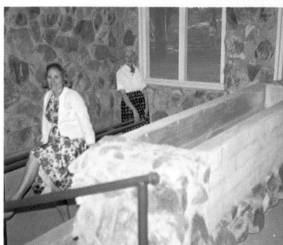

Sandwalking

Kneipp Baths, grass walking and sand walking at ranch. Photo of interior of Kneipp House has cold water arm baths and cold water leg baths for developing a good circulation for whole body. See section on sand and grass walking for good circulation and building leg muscles.

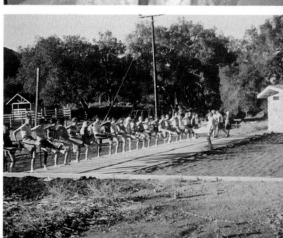

Student on the Extreme Slantboard

Student under close supervision on the extreme slantboard to stretch the cartilage in joints where tiredness and gravity have created disc problems, especially in spine. (See section on slantboard. Consult with your doctor before using any of extreme slantboard exercises.)

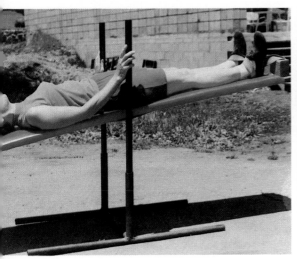 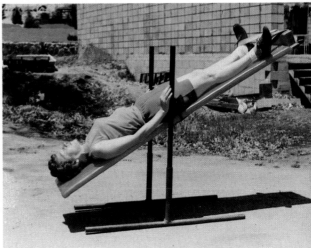

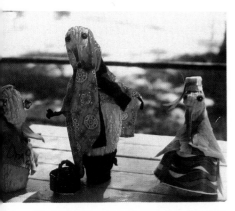

Much beauty can be created from the vegetables in decorating the table which we have used so many times at the ranch.

Squash is very good for the intestinal tract. You can see the black soil which is the basis for all good vegetation. Long life people always lived where the black soil existed.

Dr. Jensen has spent over 50 years with Ranch Style living helping 350,000 patients through nutrition, exercise and right living teachings.

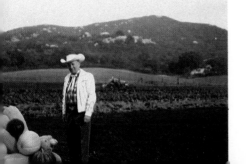

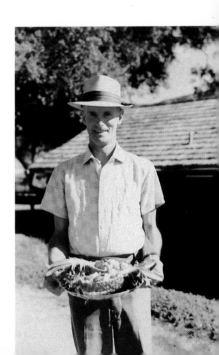

The World's Market Places..

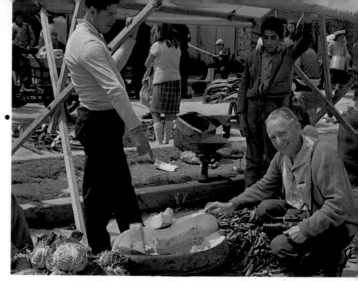

In the market in Peru we found they had so many squashes and natural food. Many people do not realize that Peru is the center or the breadbasket of the world. In many of their visits the Spanish carried these foods in their ships to many countries and established them as part of the food routine of other countries.

The markets in Armenia have wonderful grapes which are weighed out by a lovely person wanting to serve you and make you happy through the life of foods,

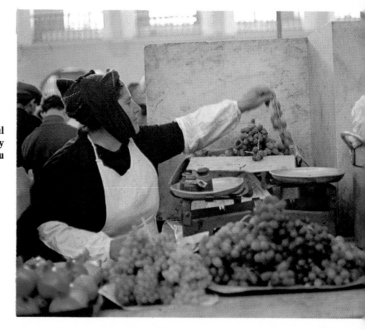

Huancaya Indians in Ecuador have their own herb drug store with no overhead. The herbs are very inexpensive and everybody use herbs as part of their living habits.

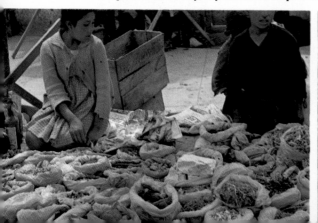
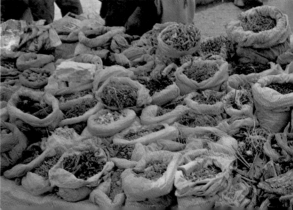

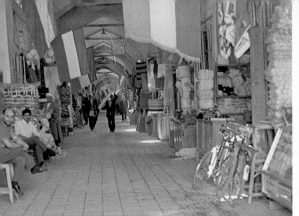

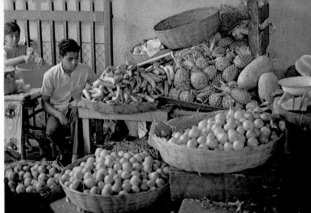

The interior of a market in Turkey where you can buy practically anything you wish.

This man is specializing in citrus fruit, melons, pineapples and bananas. A wonderful foundation for a good fruit salad.

Strawberries of New Zealand that are being shipped all over the world.

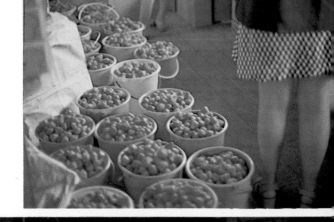

JAPAN—Fish is a brain food having a more highly evolved material for higher evolved electronic force than in the animal proteins or vegetables.

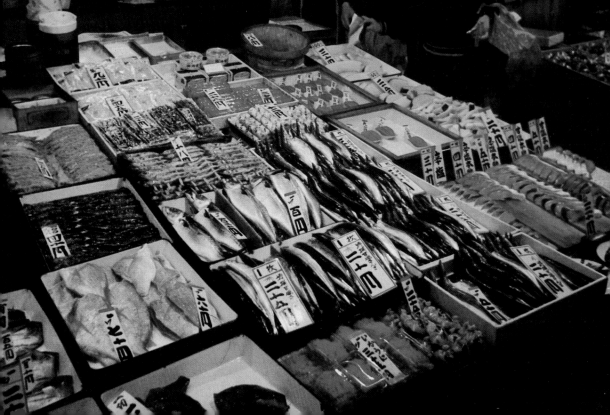

Good Foods from the Markets of the World

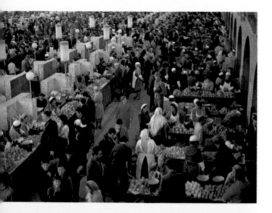

AN ARMENIAN MARKET where people bring the most natural foods, although inexpensive, and exchange or sell their products to the public.

Seeds from melons, pumpkins and squashes are the most valuable seeds we can have. It is to transfer the hormone values of seeds to the glands in our body which, of course, contribute to our own life force.

Here we have four ears of corn, all of different colors and different mixtures. This is showing where the little kernels of corn have an affinity for certain chemical elements to produce these various colors. The difference in color indicates a different chemical makeup. Color works with all the chemicals in nature and we find the day may come when a black corn may be used for certain conditions in the body because of chemical makeup . . . as well as the yellow corn, etc. The American Indians know the difference between these ears of corn, using them for different purposes, as well as medicine in the past. They were able to accomplish things that might even seem like miracles today. We should study more of what the Indian had to offer in his natural abode.

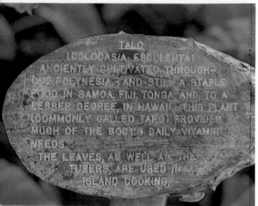

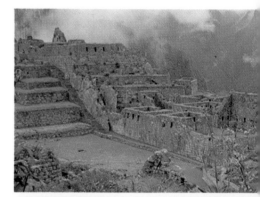

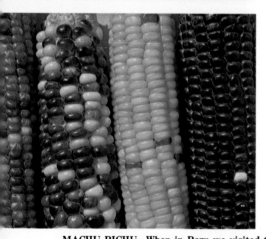

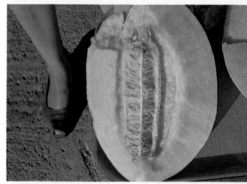

MACHU PICHU—When in Peru we visited the ruins of this amazing structure where ancient architects placed boulders together with perfect precision. No one knows why the people left. Agriculture was their main activity with terraces built right to the top of the mountains but how they got water there, no one knows. It is claimed that past civilizations have suffered because of the lack of water.

TARO ROOT is probably the most soothing of all the bulks that can be used in the intestinal tract. It can be baked or steamed. The South Sea Islanders use it so much in their Luaus. The young tender leaves are really tasty when cooked in coconut milk and very rich in vitamins and minerals.

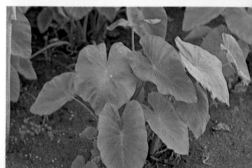

Nature knows a remedy

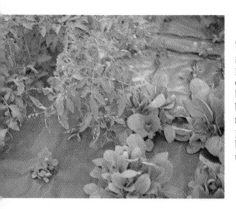

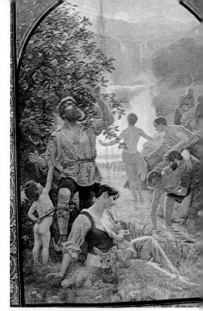

These are plants growing in a little greenhouse where we used a black plastic over the ground. We found we did not have to irrigate or water because water gathered under this black plastic and fed the plants naturally without irrigation. The plants were green, developed beautiful vegetation and fruits for our use.

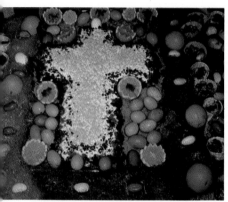

Papaya in the South Seas . . . a quick growing food and one of the great foods in aiding the digestion of protein. Right next to the papaya was the coconut, a high protein food. Papaya aids in the digestion of coconut. A wonderful combination growing side by side in Nature's Garden.

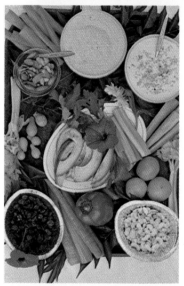

We must recognize that the food going into our bodies gives us the strength and energy to create a greater spiritual life . . . it is in this way that foods have a spiritual purpose.

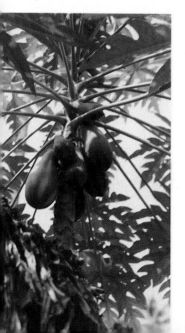

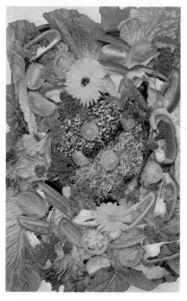

The lovely salads and vegetables as served at Hidden Valley Health Ranch. It is with the idea that we must return to nature and serve what God has given us in a ripe true state.

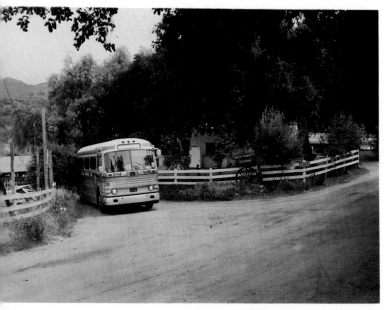

Happy folks who have learned a new pathway of life are returning home to live according to the new principles they have learned in living more closely to Nature and the natural way.

Chartered bus coming to the ranch health building activities.

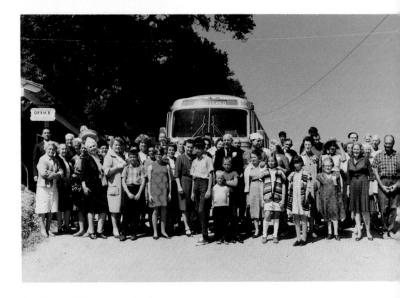

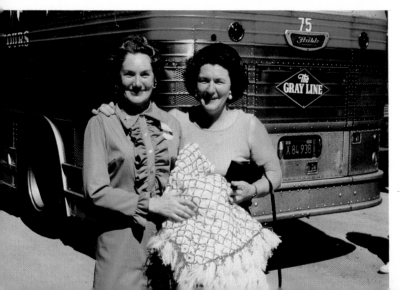

A happy and a more contented group going home to Seattle.

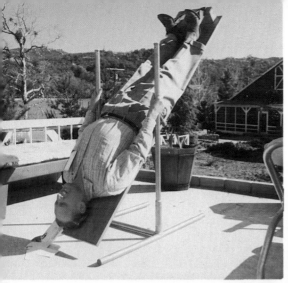

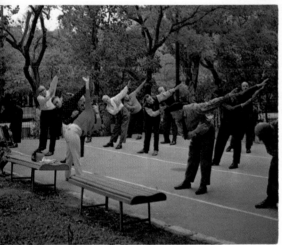

Extreme Slantboard I developed where intravertebrate disc can be stretched in this extreme slant position. Many cases of a slipped disc have been helped; however, read section on slantboard and consult your doctor because there are definite precautions to be taken in using the slantboard.

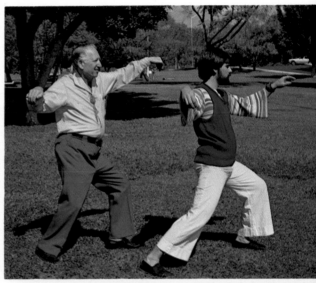

RUSSIA—8:00-9:00 AM—150,000 people exercising every morning in Russia. Also, most of the people go on a little cruise or a voyage on the Black Sea as a part of keeping themselves well.

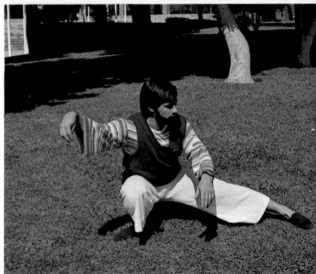

While visiting in Mexico I met David F. Sloane of St. Louis , Missouri, who is one of the most skilled men I have met in his understanding and demonstration of Tai Chi. Here I am demonstrating and exercising with him.

Chinese Tai Chi classes at the ranch. This is one of the greatest systems of physical exercises I have found for emotional stabilization.

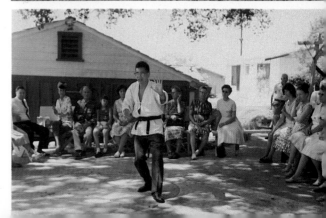

Dr. Jensen at entrance of his office at House of 7th Happiness. In his semi-retirement his future work will be in lecturing, teaching and conducting special seminars in other states and countries around the world in addition to his special Rejuvenation Week Programs one week each month.

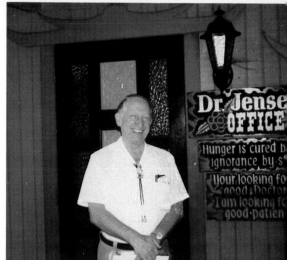

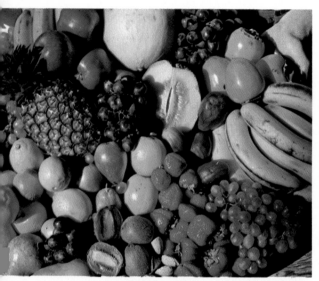

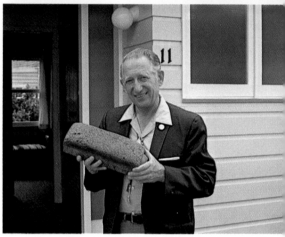

A loaf of bread slow-baked with lovely whole, fresh stone-ground flours gives us the ultimate.

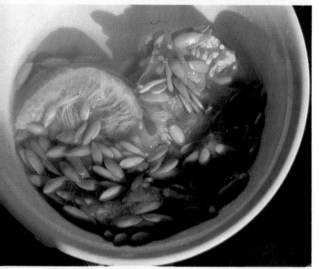

Nature gives so richly if we can only accept this abundance.

Cantaloupe, musk melons are wonderful for their seeds as well as for the meat therin. We find that the seeds can be made into lovely seek milk drinks.

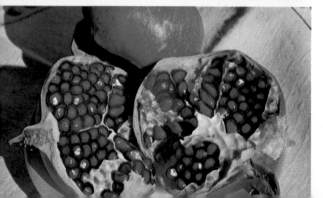

The Pomegranate can be used for genito-urinary purposes; prostrate gland disorders & bladder disturbances respond to pomegranate juice. Use the seeds as well as the juice. Put it in a liquifier and if it is too bitter, honey can be added.

Cold water is live water.

KNEIPP SANITARIUM in Woerschofen, Germany. This is where they say that cold water is live water . . . it really moves you . . . it moves the blood in the body! Old Father Kneipp introduced the benefits of cold water baths to humanity for its ailments. Today sanitariums throughout the world continue the work of the Kneipp Baths.

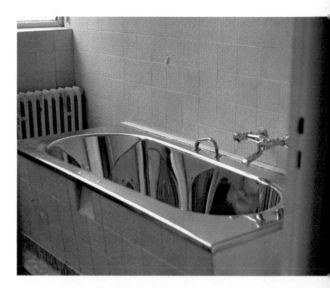

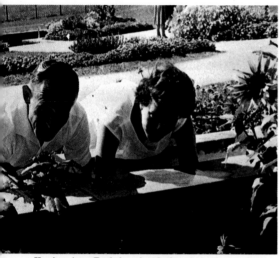

Kneipp Arm Bath for circulation through the chest area. (Woerschofen, Germany)

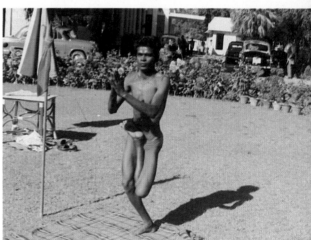

HATHA YOGA Exercises—This man from India spent 16 years developing a series of these exercises and using them perfectly.

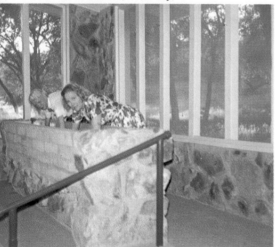

Reproduction of the Kneipp Arm Bath at our ranch.

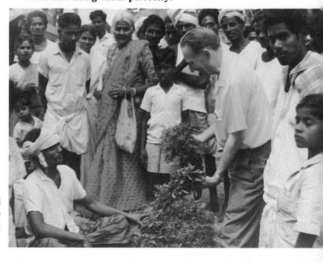

INDIA—Here we are interested in the types of food they are eating . . . they realize the greens are necessary and include them in their vegetable food program.

Frying of foods was so prevalent wherever we visited. We find that every country seems to heat their foods in oil . . . it seems this is a part of civilization which was brought to these simple people who did not have concentrated oils in the past. Heated oils are responsible for our high blood pressure, cholesterol, hardening of the arteries and many other problems.

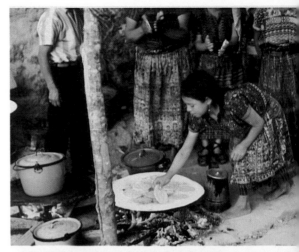

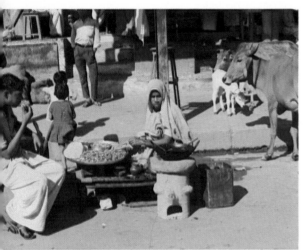

It was one of the greatest lessons to me in seeing in India how these boiled oils were used over and over again in preparation of their foods. Of course, there is protection from the flies but the repeated use of the boiled oils has its effect on the body later.

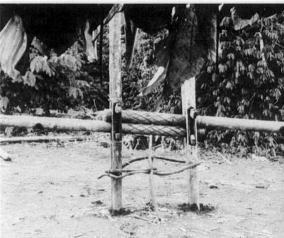

Here is a crude way of squeezing out the sugar cane from the stalk. Man is quite inventive and with vast modern equipment and methods creates a devitalized product.

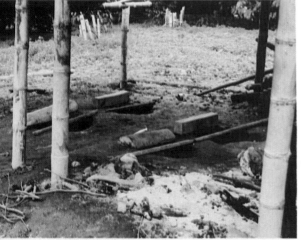

In the Amazon area of South America we saw these primitive forms of a Sitz Bath where people would come to take care of their leg problems. They would have either cold or hot water in these holes, place their feet in them and get relief from various leg disorders.

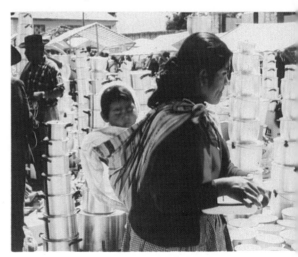

Civilization is sending aluminum cooking utensils to the Indians in Peru, South America. How life changes!

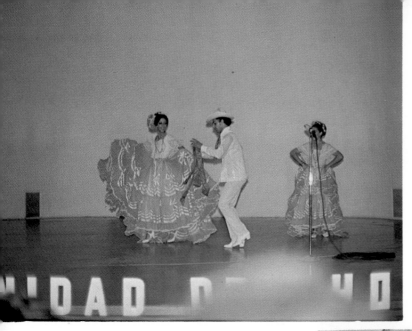

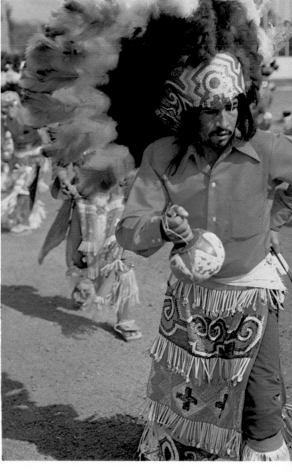

We always enjoy seeing the colorful festivities and dances of Mexico. Here we show the Baile Jarocho of Veracruz on stage and the parade and dance at the Fiesta Guadalupana. The people enjoy! and participate in the dancing and festival occasions with great enthusiasm which is wonderful to see. Enjoyment of happy social activities is very important for balanced good health.

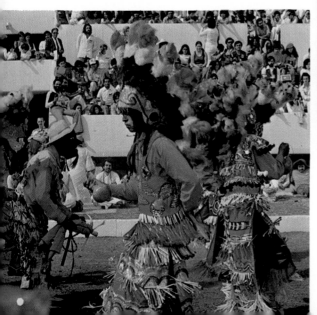

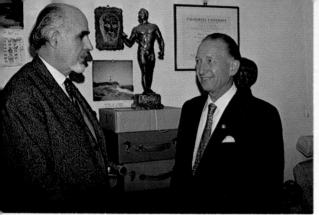

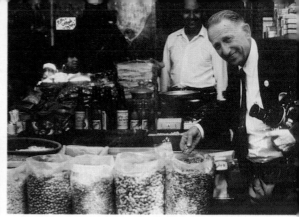

Dr. Marchesseau has a healing center in Paris where I taught some of my work in natural healing to his college students.

IRAN—The nuts and seeds eaten by the people of Iran furnish the hormones and the long life principle for them.

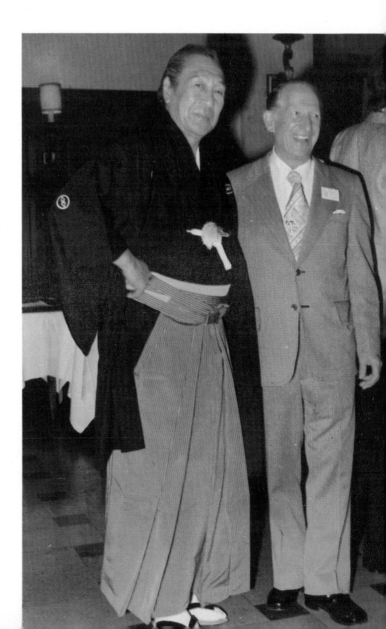

Standing beside me is Dr. Asai of Japan. We are in Aux Province, France, giving our work at a doctor's convention. Dr. Asai has been acclaimed for his great work in the discovery of Organic Germanium which we discuss in Chapter 4. It was here that I received the recognition and an award for my work in the natural Healing Arts.

FIVE

We are in a new age

THIS is the age of the atomic and hydrogen bomb, and of Strontium 90, through which tremendously powerful forces have been released. We are coming into a new day of culture. We have an entirely different outlook on life.

In his social behavior, man is just a child. We throw rocks at each other, just as childish pranksters do. It has been said that never has a wise old man been known to declare war. The wise avoid fighting. But the human race has not learned to solve its problems peaceably. So far man has gotten away without destroying himself. But I think it is necessary for us to consider the principles of survival.

I am interested in the nutritional side of survival more than the political or financial. However, the nutritional also embodies the religious side. Just what is going to survive? Our businesses, our homes, our money? What do we want to save? What is really most important? I am sure that if people really thought about survival and what it means, they would be more interested in nutrition than ever before. Nutrition and health are the survival principle; even a rich or powerful man may not survive certain adverse conditions if he is not healthy. Survival means keeping the best body- one that will overcome disease and rejuvenate and repair properly. This is the thing man has neglected. It is only those who have lost their health who are seeking and crying for the vital life they had. It is the survival principle they are looking for. We have been pranksters and it is time we woke up, all of us!

Good nutrition. Anything that does not nourish the body is taking away from the survival principle. A stomach full of nutritionless food has nothing to do with survival. It just means temporary existence. That person who doesn't realize the laws of nutrition is ignorant of the survival principle. Unpolluted air, unpolluted water, sunshine, good food- these make up survival. We have to get closer to these things. But we have to do it correctly. If we eat too little, we starve; if we eat too much, we kill ourselves. We have to have a certain amount of bulk, vegetables, fruit, proteins, and starches every day; we need variety in good proportion.

We have to know this; it means survival. We need to learn how to prolong life, how to get strength and energy, how to get vitality. If there is one way better than another, it is the way of nature. We will all have to go back to nature, to "the beginning," eventually. Man's inventions provide a lot of comfort, internally and externally, but they also too often work negatively. When man turns a food that could be nourishing to the body into one that is disease-forming, lacking in vital materials that are needed to build a good body, he has gone too far.

Because of what we too often do to our food, thinking is very necessary to survival. To go to a popular supermarket and buy indiscriminately may not even be safe! Though foods may be made of the best ingredients, they could be improperly prepared and could hinder the body in its attempts to repair, rebuild, or regain health once it has been lost. You have to be careful in what you buy. The survival principle demands that we *think*.

This way of looking at survival requires a change in consciousness. We need to look at things in a new way. A short time ago a newspaper reporter going through India noticed that the women had a lot of back trouble because of curves in their upper spines. He made the suggestion that they use longer-handled brooms so they would not have to bend over. Many did so, with the expected results.

We need to make similar changes in our way of thinking if we hope to survive. But many of us refuse to do so. Our thinking has deteriorated, we are not thinking about

23

what is best for our own bodies, we are looking for bargains.

When you go camping, what do you take along with you? Frankfurters? Marshmallows? When you stop and think about the bread we buy, puffed up, white spongy stuff, do you imagine that is good bread? Is that the bread that is the "staff of life?" No! We've traded survival for a bargain. And that bargain destroys rather than builds our health. And if you lose your good health, you are going to lose your family and your job and be no good to yourself or your husband or wife. It all comes back to principle in foods. Health isn't everything, but without health, nothing else counts.

It is still a matter of the survival of the fittest.Who is the "fittest"? The one with big muscles, the massive fellow who lives on hot cakes and prepared cereals? Or is it the man who is wise enough to do the right thing? The "fittest" is the man who knows the right thing to be done and does it. He is fit in every way: moral, mental, spiritual- *and* physical.

We need to develop ourselves in all these areas. I think we have to be much more conscious of what we are doing or we will be lost. Most of us are on a "sentimental journey." We are not using our intelligence to have the best life possible. We are having "too little, too late." Ultimately, the only thing that counts is the growth of our souls and our minds. A good life lived should be long enough. A long life lived is not necessarily good enough. Life must be earned from the inside rather than the outside. We are told that we die for a lack of knowledge, that without vision we perish. I even saw a sign outside a church offering candy to children to attend Sunday School. Do we have to be bribed to do the finer things in life? Do we have to be frightened into wisdom? How long will it be before we recognize what has to be done?

Foods for Survival

Some people have become very interested in putting food away. What should we put away and how much? Suppose you had to store food supplies for two years, how would you do it? The storage place must be dry. It must be cool. It must be safe from atomic radiation and light waves. The food should be stored in cans or airtight vessels where it cannot oxidize or break down. Concentrated foods are best. We might put away ten loaves of bread, but in the space we could store enough wheat to bake fifty loaves of bread. This wheat must be "alive" for our survival. You cannot afford to have any other kind of wheat. The importance of concentrated foods is one of the first principles we need to recognize.

In preparing for survival we must assume the worst- an utter devastation of all our crops and foods. Again, wheat is one thing we'll need to put away. Others are oats, millet, brown rice, yellow cornmeal, and some legumes- lentils, garbanzos.

Though we need to think first of an immediate food supply, we also need to prepare for our future food. Nature gives us a 300 percent return on whatever seed we choose to plant. We should therefore think of seeds to grow a garden. Have a variety of some fifteen vegetable seeds- beet, carrot, green kale, and lettuce, for instance.

For immediate food, we can store perishable vegetables in a dehydrated form. Celery and okra powders are available. Green kale is one of the foods highest in calcium, which is especially needed when we are under strain and stress. One who anticipates extreme stresses should also consider putting away a definite amount of rice polishings, which are very high in vitamin B, one of the stress vitamins.

We should use vegetable broth powder for seasoning, as this will supply the salt we should have. Some people want to have real salt. If so, they should use the earth salt, taken from the ground without any heat whatsoever. We should never have anything that has gone through extreme heat. This is another survival principle.

Then we have to have a certain amount of sweets on hand. Honey is a concentrated sweet; also pure maple sugar can be put away and used very well. Date sugar is fine. Dates are one of the highest foods in sugar content. Dried fruit must be sealed air-tight.

Have on hand powdered whole milk, soy milk powder, dandelion root coffee, herb teas and sunflower and sesame seeds left in their hulls to prevent deterioration. Alfalfa seeds are excellent — be sure you know how to sprout them. Keep nuts in the shell. It might be well to have a few liquid concentrates of both vegetable and fruit juices; also have concentrated fruit powder that can be stored well.

Make sure that any foods you store are nourishing. Remember to consider the protein and starch content. Vegetables may be in sprouts; and fruits can be dried. This will give you the proper variety. We should also have herbs. Different herbs take care of various parts of the body. If you anticipate struggling with any atomic radiation, consider herbs for the kidneys, digestive system, and muscular system. We should have a variety of herb extracts to take care of all parts of the body in case of stress. Some food supplements, such as vitamins A and C, and especially vitamin B, are needed. It might be well to have a green vegetable powder, which you can obtain at health food stores. Have a good source of bulk, such as flaxseed, which is high in vitamin F and can be used for any skin disturbances; it may also be used in making tea. For any kinds of burns, perhaps from radiation, consider peanut oil. Peanut oil also is high in vitamin F and is good for the outside of the body.

Another thing to consider is water. It should be distilled water. Any water containing minerals could attract some atomic radiation and become contaminated. Use what liquids you have stored until you're able to establish a good water supply. If you plan to dig a well, obtain a unit that will treat water to make it fresh and remove any contamination.

Finally, be sure you have a set menu plan (for 30 days), and directions and recipes for using all the food you've stored. Also have details on how many each can or container will feed (a given weight will feed a given number of people for a certain number of days). Have matches, a few extra polyethylene bags for storage, a first aid kit, and soap.

Atomic Radiation Problems

If a disaster occurs that forces us to use our food supply, it might well bring with it the problems of atomic radiation. It may be wise, therefore, to have foods that give the body the greatest resistance and rebuild it most effectively. Bone marrow has been used with animals that were exposed to atomic radiation, and it proved to be one of the greatest foods for preventing malignancies. In case of emergency it might be one of the things that will help us through an atomic radiation. Blue violet tea has great powers for ridding the body of toxic materials. I stress these foods, realizing that at the moment of any critical action you want the very best there is available. It is possible that if you don't have them, you may not survive.

We should be applying the survival principle to our *everyday* living and eating. If you are sick, you are not surviving well. The U. S. government tells us that 92 percent of all Americans are sick now. Illness is the

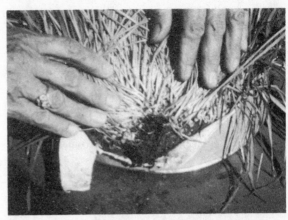

Sprouts as they grow from the soil. The first five days are so important because the grass comes from the seed and the seed offers so much. Green grass juice has been so wonderful in helping people back to health.

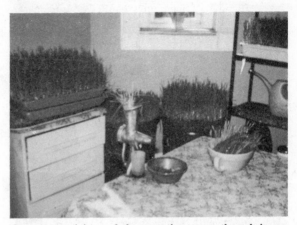

Green grass juice and the operation we go through in our laboratory where we have fed many people, bringing their blood count to one of less toxicity and to greater health.

result of not using the survival principles.

Inventory of Supplies for Emergency Storage

Following is a summary of foods to be stored in preparation for emergencies. For protection against atomic radiation supplies can be stored in steel boxes, completely airtight and waterproof, and buried ten feet below the surface of the ground.

1. Water. Preferably distilled, since water containing minerals could attract some atomic radiation and become contaminated.

2. Seeds for planting. Include a variety of vegetable seeds, including those of shortest growth period; grains (for those who may have use of land); herbs; nuts; fruit stones (begin to save a variety of these from ripe fruits—from year to year—it could be the means of starting trees bearing fruits and nuts); and seeds of different varieties of melons and squashes.

25

3. Seeds for food. May be ground or lique-fied. Include sunflower (with some unhulled to avoid deterioration in case of oxydation), sesame, flaxseed, pumpkin, and peptoria (a variety of squash).

4. Seeds for Sprouting. Especially alfalfa seed. In the absence of fresh vegetables, sprouts are our best source of the chlorphyll, which is essential to life. (Store the items of equip-ment which you would expect to use for sprouting. Also, have complete instructions for the making of sprouts).

5. Whole Grains. Whole grains can be stored indefinitely without spoiling. Good grains are wheat, oats, millet, corn, brown rice, barley, rye. If possible, store a mill for grinding- a hand mill could be used in the absence of electric power (some mills work both electrically and by hand); also have thermos bottles for use in preparation of grains, either whole or ground.

6. Nuts. Unshelled- almonds and other varieties.

7. Legumes. Lentils, garbanzos, beans of all kinds, peas- these may be used in sprouted form, especially for persons in whom digestive disturbance is occasioned by the dry form.

8. Root Vegetables. May be kept for some time if properly buried in the earth (supply should be renewed periodically, if these are to be available for emergency use).

9. Dehydrated vegetables.

10. Vegetable broth powder. Very essential in case of scarcity of fresh vegetables.

11. Dried herbs. For nutritional and medic-inal needs, especially to take care of the vital organs of the body, the kidneys, digestive system, and muscular system, in particular.

12. Dried fruits. Every possible variety. Store in airtight containers.

13. Extracts. Vegetable and fruit juice concentrates (these are especially valuable and practical for storing).

14. Supplements. Mineral and vitamin, especially vitamins A, B, and C.

15. Intestinal lubricants. Especially flax-seed (high in vitamin F, beneficial in cases of skin disturbances). May be ground, or use whole seed in tea.

16. Oil. Peanut oil (one of the highest foods in vitamin F, it may be used on the outside of the body).

17. Rice polishings. These are particularly beneficial under stress conditions.

18. Anti-radioactive factor foods. Bone marrow; blue violet tea (good for ridding the body of toxic material).

19. Powdered whole and skim milk and soy powder.

20. Sweets. Honey (a concentrated sweet), dates, pure maple sugar.

21. Salt (if desired). Use earth salt, which has not been subjected to any heat process.

Find a Philosophy

One thing that helps in survival is to have something larger than yourself to look to. One source of my strength is a belief in a Supreme Being. I believe he gives us our all and will help us in times of trouble — emotionally and spiritually, at least, if not physically.

The eighth chapter of Deuteronomy in the Bible in some ways summarizes this belief:

All the commandments which I com-mand you this day you shall be careful to do, that you may live and multiply, and go in and possess the land which the Lord swore to give to your fathers.

And you shall remember all the ways which the Lord your God has led you these forty years in the wilderness, that He might humble you, testing you to know what was in your heart, whether you would keep His commandments or not.

And He humbled you and let you hun-ger and fed you with manna, which you did not know, nor did your fathers know; that He might make you know that man does not live by bread alone, but that man lives by everything that proceeds out of the mouth of the Lord.

Your clothing did not wear out upon you, and your feet did not swell these forty years.

Know then, in your heart that, as a man disciplines his son, the Lord, your God, disciplines you.

So you shall keep the commandments of the Lord, your God, by walking in His ways and by fearing him.

For the Lord, your God, is bringing you into a good land, a land of brooks of water, of fountains and springs, flowing forth in valleys and hills.

A land of wheat and barley, of vines and fig trees and pomegranates, a land of olive trees and honey.

A land in which you will eat bread without scarcity, in which you will lack nothing, a land whose stones are iron, and out of whose hills you can dig copper.

And you shall eat and be full, and you shall bless the Lord your God for the good land He has given you.

Take heed, lest you forget the Lord your God by not keeping His commandments and His ordinances and His statutes, which I command you this day.

Lest, when you have eaten and are full, and have built goodly houses and live in them, and when your herds and flocks multiply, and your silver and gold is multiplied, and all that you have is multiplied, then your heart be lifted up and you forget the Lord your God, who brought you out of the land of Egypt, out of the house of bondage,

Who led you through the great and terrible wilderness, with its fiery serpents and scorpions and thirsty ground where there was not water, Who brought you out of the flinty rock,

Who fed you in the wilderness with manna which your fathers did not know, that He might humble you and test you, to do you good in the end.

Beware lest you say in your heart, 'My power and the might of my hand have gotten me this wealth.'

You shall remember the Lord your God, for it is He Who gives you power to get wealth; that He may confirm His covenant which He swore to your fathers, as at this day.

And if you forget the Lord your God and go after other gods and serve them and worship them, I solemnly warn you this day that you shall surely perish.

Like the nations that the Lord makes to perish before you, so shall you perish because you would not obey the voice of the Lord your God.

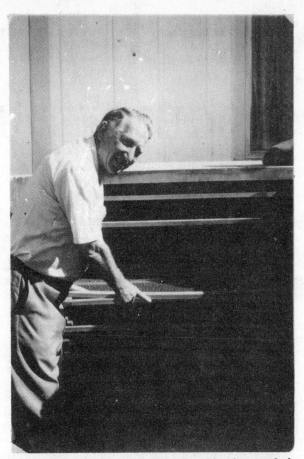

Dehydrating cherries and drying olives with a dryer we had made. It has a fan below and an infrared light in the lower levels where the heated air was transferred through the screens made up into shelves. Get ready for the winter by developing the natural foods for the winter. Dried foods are a boon to mankind if they only realized that we can avoid canned foods, additives and preservatives.

Another way – another direction

WHEREVER there is disease, God has put a remedy right next to it. We have remedies that will help us in every illness; but we cannot depend on just a remedy to get our problems solved; we have to take care of the whole man first.

We must recognize that the whole body's health is not to be found in any one remedy. You may take a remedy, but it will give you only temporary results. Some remedies are stimulating and some have a sedative effect; some cease to have an effect if they are used constantly. Remedies are only part of good health. They are unbalanced, like part of a diet. Good remedies have to work hand in hand with correcting the body, building new tissue to replace the old while the old body undergoes changes.

Caring for the Whole Man

It takes a year to convert broken down organs into new ones. It is a gradual thing, like putting clean water into dirty water: finally you have a good body. A person who does not take into consideration the whole person— body, mind, and spirit, using both fruits, vegetables, and nuts— is not doing the right thing for his body.

The Value of Natural Remedies

Natural remedies do not mask symptoms while the cause is still there. Symptoms such as discharges and ulcers are natural processes for the elimination of acquired and hereditary disease matter. If a poisonous drug is used as a remedy and suppresses the initial lesion, the disease matter will be diffused throughout the system, and the problem will show up in the next weakest organ. Suppression may go on for months or years, resulting in a chronic disease condition; the disease does not heal because the life force is so polluted it can no longer produce an acute reaction. As the disease dries up, it sets up a cumulative reaction that acts as a time bomb, and you are on your way to an abnormal growth. If the initial disease is not taken care of through the elimination organs, it may appear again either in the patient or in his offspring.

It's often a rule that one operation leads to another. The cause of the trouble was not taken care of in the first place, and it was bound to show up some other place in the body. When people come to me, I always make a record of the surgical operations they have had. They invariably had enlarged tonsils as a child. Why were they enlarged? Because catarrh, toxic materials, phlegm, and mucous were overtaxing the lymph glands.

These patients had too much white flour and white sugar products. This produced an overload on the tonsils. The tonsils are lymph glands; they become enlarged when they are overworked. The problem was that they were not cared for before they were overworked, and that is where the remedy should start!

We must move the whole body into good health; then the symptoms will begin to leave. Nature has stored away foods for our bodies and put certain chemicals in these foods. When our body chemistries are balanced, we rid ourselves of most of these symptoms. I don't know of anyone who doesn't need a healthy change in his body.

If we eat what nature has supplied we begin to follow the natural preventive laws. That means we eat pure, whole food; use the right proportions of six vegetables, two fruits, one starch, and one protein every day; and include variety in our diets.

One of the most important preventive remedies is to avoid overeating. Overeating will kill you. When you find how much you need to eat, eat no more. You will find this is the successful way of living.

You are endowed this moment with a

certain amount of energy to do a specific amount of work. That energy helps digest the food you put into your body. It heats your food. It absorbs, distributes, eliminates your food. If you use more energy than you have stored in your body, you will become depleted. And one of the quickest roads to depletion is to overeat, which causes your body to expend energy-processing food it doesn't want.

You can also starve from the food you eat. Malnutrition often accompanies the eating of devitalized, demineralized, processed food.

Find Out What Is Right

The first step in taking care of ourselves is to find out what is right. How did God intend for us to live? What foods are approved by God? How should we live physically, mentally, and spiritually so that all things will be put into their proper places? Pain and discomfort are nature's warning that we are not doing the right thing; we haven't been doing the right thing and the coffee and doughnut habit is catching up with us.

Something is wrong and you must awaken! It's a matter of toxic blood, overacidity, a growth stagnation pressing you on the shoulder, squeezing you, bending you, pulling, producing acute sharp pains, muscle weakness, memory loss, nerve exhaustion, decline in vision, anything to stop you in your tracks. Think for a moment! Take care of yourself. It's not time to carry on, go on, look outside, chase a cure, or replace this old body for a new body with a pill or any other cure. If it did cure you, you would be sick again tomorrow if you didn't learn to live correctly and maintain good health.

All species of animals live on foods they should have for their particular bodies. We find that horses and sheep in the pasture will pick out different grasses for their particular kind of body. The horse nor the sheep has ever studied what to select for a good life and for various levels of his development. It's all done by a basic wisdom they never lose. We should apply more wisdom and selectivity in foods for our good health. This has been neglected in our basic education and perhaps even because of a wrong education guiding our selections.

Health Power

Cilvilization is late in taking care of this, and if something isn't done now, it may become too late. There should be a definition of health given to people so they can sort these problems out. We have a health department in our government where everybody is working on solutions and nobody is working on the basic problems.

We are using up the resources of earth, wearing it down, burning it up, and we are also doing the same thing to our human systems. Our body is self-rejuvenating, self-repairing, self-building, yet we do not supply proper fuel for our bodies to repair and rebuild properly. Health education is sorely neglected with regard to building a good body.

Health is an important part of our life. In fact, it is *the* most important factor in our life. I will say that while health is not everything, without health, everything is nothing. We should get on a good nutritional program *now*. Then if it turns out you need a constructive operation a year from now, and there is such a thing as constructive surgery, you will be ready for it.

My interest in nutrition lies mainly in the healing art. To say a person needs help, or needs one element especially, is not enough. To be able to properly feed the whole body and see to it that food is contributing the essential chemicals to that body is truly an art. It is also an art to look into the eyes of a patient and see the causes that are brought on by a nutritional depletion in the body, and then determine what is necessary to build this body back toward physical and mental health.

The Magic of Foods

If I were going to recommend one particular food to cleanse and rebuild the body, it would be greens. If you are green inside, you are clean inside. Greens control the calcium in the body and are high in iron and potassium. The more bitter they are, the more potassium they contain. Greens are one of the finest things known for neutralizing the acids in the body. The chlorophyll in greens is high in vitamin K, the antihemorrhagic vitamin. Also, there is a lot of vitamins C and A in any of the green vegetables.

We can absorb greens into the digestive system faster than any other food. Less digestion is necessary for getting chlorophyll into the blood than any other form of food. There is nothing more wonderful to use than greens to sweeten the body, to clean the mouth, sweeten the breath, and take away ordors.

The individual who does a lot of physical work should have plenty of iron, calcium, and

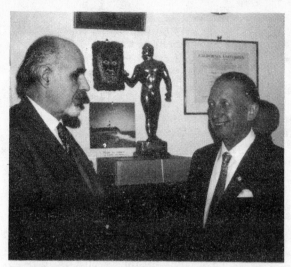

Dr. Marchesseau has a healing center where I taught and gave some of my work in Natural Healing to the students of his college while we were in Paris.

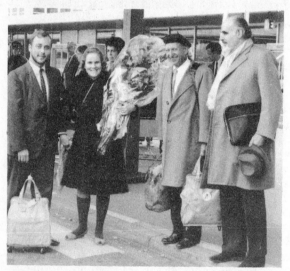

Here we are with Dr. Marchesseau and another doctor ready to depart from Aux Province, France. It was here that I was given the Gold Medal Award for my work in Iridology and in Nutrition. Dr. Asai of Japan was also honored at this doctor's convention for his development of Organic Germanium.

silicon. He needs a lot of sodium if he perspires a lot. I can look at anyone and tell if they are lacking in at least four chemicals- namely, iron, calcium, silicon, and sodium. I will watch him walk, watch his facial expressions, and take a look at his hair. Nearly everyone of us is lacking in these four elements to some degree, many of us gravely so. We must do something about it or lose our health. We need these elements for future health insurance. It is every man's job to give attention and serious consideration to the business of maintaining good health. Isn't it better to pay the cost of keeping well *(prevention)* rather than pay costly bills trying to cure yourself until you die? Think about that!

Changes We Can Make with Foods

London, England - "Can Diet Cut Juvenile Delinquency? A survey of 17 maladjusted or delinquent girls between the ages of 11 and 15 in a Salvation Army hostel seems to prove that diet makes good girls from bad ones. Previously the girls lived on the poorest possible types of meals, white bread and margarine, cheap jam, lots of sweet tea, canned and processed meats. Fish and chips had been one of their most nutritious meals. A year later their diet was changed to raw fruits, nuts, vegetables, salads, whole wheat bread, dates, prunes, figs, honey, cheese, meat, fish, eggs, oatmeal, crushed wheat. This is what happened: The girls quickly became less aggressive and less quarrelsome, bad habits seemed to disappear, 'problem children' became less of a problem and the bored ones lost their boredom. Physically they improved almost beyond recognition. A spokesman said, "It is amazing to see the difference in their complexions, general brightness and poise, but the difference in their behavior is the most significant. The part the diet played in their personalities is undeniable.' "

In another instance, similarly related, two doctors in charge of a mental insitution in Oklahoma changed the diet of problem patients and the patients stopped screaming at night. They also stopped fighting at the tables, skin conditions improved, thyroid disturbances were improved, and women patients became quiet and complacent, permitting their hair to be managed.

I did a study at the penitentiary at San Quentin, California. We found that lack of iodine brought these men to the brink of their brute tendencies- kill the other fellow before he gets a chance to kill you! Yet when they got iodine they changed completely. Without iodine we cannot think properly; we cannot be level-headed. Many of the subnormal expressions of our thinking can be cleaned up if we take care of the deficiencies of food elements that the body needs. Whether it is the 27,000 strings that are found just behind the eardrums or the 3,000 layers that make up the lens we look through, we need to feed every part of our bodies. If it's the heart pumping 115 barrels of blood everyday, it has to be fed. If it is the 215 bones in the body that carry our weight all of our standing hours, they have to be nourished. When they become broken down, they have to be mended. Our muscles must be fed. Our entire body must be nourished adequately for its many needs.

Use What We've Been Given for Health

With the wonderously created body we possess, do you think we have missed out on some of the natural things that we require? Do you think that we have a Creator who has put his children here and forgotten the means to sustain life?

Everything we need is here. From the very highest plane it gives the Father great pleasure to give from his kingdom. The power that He has is ours. From the grass on the hills to the iron in the hills, it is there for man's consumption. It is up to us. If we leave out what God has given us, we end up with a lack of our total needs or one of the deficiency diseases of today.

There is something about "doing the right thing" that is good for your health. Try doing the wrong thing and see what it does to your mind. What does it do to your thinking? How does your conscience feel, especially when you know better? It's true—you know better!

If you're interested in natural remedies, you're not going to get rid of a headache right now. You are going to start following a natural way of living so that those headaches diminish and leave.

Find a good, healthy way to live. If you don't live right and set the body up properly, you can take a remedy and no matter how good it is, it will never work. You will never get anything good out of a natural remedy if you do not live a wholesome life.

Go with clean living; eat good clean foods; have a right pattern for right living. The main thing in life is to find the right path, a path

that God would approve of, because the body molds to that path. It molds a little bit to the mind; a little bit to the spiritual; Some to good companionship, good climate, good air. These are remedies for people who are on the right path.

I am sure that when you get closer to the garden, closer to nature and further away from pills that sedate, stimulate, tranquilize, you are going to be in much better health.

But you are not going to get well overnight; you will never get well from anything in less than a year. You need two summers in a row for this healing. Climate and altitude may be your answer. Remedies that work overnight can be detrimental, because they put you under their control.

And a person who is living on constant resistance and resentment cannot ever be well. This person cannot digest his food. He will be chasing remedies for an acid stomach, rheumatic joints, and a host of other ailments. correct his present condition and prevent further troubles.

About the Healing Crisis

As part of the reversal process we must go through the healing crisis. This is a process the body goes through to eliminate accumulated toxic waste. At the time of the healing crisis we have new tissue replacing old tissue, and this is responsible for the elimination. The new tissue is strong, virile, young, and active; it is able to cope with any of the disease processes that have been built up through wrong living habits. In a chronic state of affairs, you will always find toxic-laden old tissue.

Correction of Body Tissue

Disease is when a degeneration of tissue has taken place, when toxic materials have accumulated and you are not capable of getting rid of them and there is a manifestation, or symptoms developed in the body such as boils, rheumatism, joint disturbances, or a headache, foot troubles, etc. A correction is brought about only when the condition is reversed. In other words, we have to have better functioning tissue than we had before. We have to have cleaner tissue than we had before. This brings about correction. When there is more vitality in the tissues to get rid of toxic material, we are working toward cleansing.

Old Ailments Come Back

Now if we are becoming younger as we become older, by reversing the process of tissue repair, many times we go back over the old diseases we have had in the past. The healing crisis always gives you symptoms of some of your past diseases. Anyone who can bring on a healing crisis, or who develops a healing crisis, is going through a reversal process as expressed in Dr. Constantine Hering's *Law of Cure.*

Rheumatic conditions, discharges, pains, and aches in various parts of the body are brought back, but they last only a very short time. The average healing crisis lasts three days, although it can last longer in elderly people. The average person develops a healing crisis during the third month of coming onto a good strict nature regimen. With children, it comes on much quicker, for children have not built up a chronic form of disease.

To bring on the healing crisis. Be sure the diet is proper. It may be that a fast is indicated for the first few days to ensure that the body is rested enough to have the vital energy to work on the foods. We must have quiet. We must also have rest, phychologically and physically. The more rest we have, preferably in bed, the better the cure.

A lot of liquids and juices in the diet are indicated, especially vegetable broths. Potato peeling broth is one of the best to use. Water treatments are important in reversing any disease. There is a water treatment that can be used for every part of the body, for every condition. We should learn which water treatments are indicated for our particular problem. The next thing indicated is to find the herbs most suited for a specific condition that you may be expressing or for any one organ that is not functioning properly. As my old professor said years ago, water can be used internally, externally, and eternally.

When you love, you recuperate. You do not recuperate in misery, depression, and resentment- only in love, understanding, and agreement.

We must eliminate all negative influences from our lives. Pick up all positive things and thoughts. "Neglect the weeds and nourish the roses." Organize your life. Reorganize your mind. Healing is impossible when the mind is in turmoil.

Pursuit of the ideal is another remedy for mental health. The only thing that will keep you young and youthful is an interest in life. If you have lost an interest in life, you're dying. If you have something to accomplish, to do, finish, or overcome, you have youth.

I make a hobby of collecting spoons from around the world. When I look at the thousands of spoons I have, I notice that every handle is different, and each represents a man's imagination and inspiration. It is in man's mind that we look for creation. Each creator was in pursuit of an ideal when he fashioned his spoon. In India they say a man should go through life giving to the world something of his own. That's what creation is all about.

If you are stopped at every opportunity, you will never be well. If you have no activity in the brain, you will have no activity in the body either, because the brain leads the body.

Watch Your Daily Habits

If you want to learn one of the big secrets in life, look closely at what you do every day and see if you are spending your time wisely. If it is the least bit wrong, or less than it should be for perfection, or for your best health, you will find that eventually it will break you down. I do not believe that one cigarette ever hurt anybody, but I think a cigarette every day for eighteen years will finally get you. I don't think one cup of coffee will hurt anybody, but one cup of coffee every day for eighteen years will give you a weak liver. So watch your daily habits. If there is one thing you do every day, watch it! This is one of the greatest remedies that I can tell you.

Be Big—Lengthen Your Steps!

Few occupations give us all the health essentials we need for a strong virile body. Working indoors, sitting, or standing all day in one position, commuting in poorly ventilated buses and street cars, grabbing quick lunches, working under tension of noise and time, all tend to jeopardize our health. We coddle our comforts and forget that we need fresh air, sunshine, exercise, and good wholesome food.

Most people huddle into themselves when walking along the street. Their heads are down, their hands are in their pockets and their toughts are dwelling on the worrisome events of the day. Be big- lengthen the circle of your step, throw out your chest, breathe in fresh air, look upward to the sky, and think outwardly on bigger things. The blood will surge through your body, feeding it and making it warm. You will be happier and healthier.

Fresh Air Heals Wounds

Never neglect the value of fresh air in healing. As Dr. Rollier says, "It is a well-known fact that wounds exposed to sunshine and fresh air heal more rapidly than when bandaged. In fact, no wound will heal *without air*. In order for wounds to heal quickly, it is most important that they be exposed to a constant supply of pure, fresh air."

What if you live in a smog-ridden city, and there is no fresh air? Use a combination of these foods and vitamins: Vitamin C, 500 mgs. daily; vitamin A, 30,000 units daily; green alfalfa- juice or tablet form; or any green juices (these attract oxygen from the air). Also, take more of the oxygen-giving foods. Sprouts are the best of all! And, of course, all the green vegetables. Eat lots of salads, all the water-bearing fruits and those that have a lot of iron in them. You must have iron to attract the oxygen from the air. Drink a lot of black cherry juice. Use black-cherries. This is necessary to regenerate the lung supply and to prevent many of the catarrhal conditions we develop in the wintertime and/or in the polluted air of the city.

Where Is The Cure?

Many people feel everything is just in the physical body. Actually the whole man is at stake when we treat the body to make it better. No part of the physical body or cell in the body can be divorced from the spirit, that life force that flows through us. Too many people have the idea that all we have to look for is a chemical reaction in order to find the cure. The more highly evolved man becomes, the more he recognizes that changes in consciousness rid him of sickness and make him "whole" once again. We have to return to nature and intelligent living. The physical in most cases cannot see what is going on in the spiritual realm. It takes a lot of studying to recognize the value of friendship, the destruction of emotion, or the involvement of what money can do to the heart, kidneys, and stomach. It seems we are involved more in *solutions* than taking care of *causes*.

We must follow the proper path for corrections to be made and true health to manifest itself. It must be an upward path, a better way of living; otherwise, whatever correction we make won't last. We cannot continually go against God and nature and expect this violation to maintain good health.

The Law of Reversing

Everyone wants a quick cure, "Get rid of the problem immediately!" They want to get back to work, to be able to walk or run again. They never seem to realize·that most quick cures will keep people from having lasting health. It is better to take the slow way of improvement over a year's time and develop good tissues and better functioning. At the end of the year you'll look back and say, "I am better today than I was five years ago." This is the true way of healing.

Dr. Constantine Hering gave us the law that we must reverse and atone for our sins and go back over our problems and troubles no matter what has been built into the body; then we can have good health once again. Whatever has been built into the body can be replaced by doing better things in its place. How could you expect a person who constantly does wrong in his life to have a good body? We have said many times, you *earn* your health, and *learn* your health. Hering's Law of Cure is that all cure comes from within, out, and from above, down. The symptoms disappear in reverse order of their original development. That is why the doctor must work with and teach his patient. The patient has the obligation of learning to undo what he has done. He must weave into his body (the rug of life) new threads, giving him the healthy body he wants. (I have gone into considerable detail on this in my book *Doctor-Patient Handbook.)*

We must have the desire to live a better life; otherwise, there would be no reason to improve, no reason for us to go on. We must recognize that there *is* a better way. In the dictionary the doctor is rightfully called a teacher. A person should learn from his doctor the proper way of living so he can correct his present condition and prevent further troubles.

Collecting spoons from all around the world is one of my hobbies. Have a hobby, develop, create, live, travel and do pleasurable things.

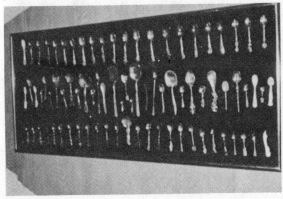

The Disease vs. the Healing Crisis

People, as a rule, will die in a disease crisis, but not in a *healing* crisis. When we think of a crisis, we think of something that is for the better or the worse. Usually, a healing crisis comes after we feel best. Nature tries to show us how good we can feel, and then a healing crisis comes to us. A healing crisis comes when we have developed enough of the vital energies in our body to throw off the toxic materials. Hippocrates, the father of medicine, has said, "Give me a fever and I will cure any disease." I believe that in the reversal process we bring a higher temperature in these crises and burn out much of the toxic conditions in our bodies.

The healing crisis should be studied by everyone who is interested in perfecting his body and having good health. In the healing crisis, we eliminate this toxic material through discharges, extreme contractions, convulsions, pains, eliminations from various parts of the body. It can be of a catarrhal nature, such as mucus phelgm from the bronchial tubes, sinus, ears, and other orifices of the body.

My old professor used to say that to pollute is to impair. Now, I believe this is true about the air we breathe, the water we drink, and the foods we eat. This is also the same as far as our body is concerned. We pollute our body with heavy toxic materials, bad foods, soft drinks, fats, fried foods, etc., to the point that when cleansing takes place, it comes on in a violent reaction or a fever. This can be termed as healing crisis.

There is no foreign matter than can stay in your body during a healing crisis because the blood is making new tissue. New tissue takes the place of the old and in the vitality of that new tissue, the old has to go. Even in a disease crisis, it is an elimination of toxic material and we should favor it. We find that

---

Remember This. . .

A long fast should be under the supervision of a doctor. Detoxification is like tearing down the walls of an old building. There comes a time when you have to rebuild and that results from a new eating regime afterwards. **Eventually you have to get off this diet idea and go on to a healthy way of living.** It is good to go from the elimination diet to a healthy way of living, then after a month or so on an elimination diet, and then . . . back to a healthy way of living.

Important Crisis Note

A crisis comes usually after you feel your best. It is the will of nature. No doctor, no patient, no food, can bring a crisis on. It comes when your body is ready. It does it in its own time. It goes through slow or fast according to the patient's constitution, nervous system and what you have earned so that it will come on. You **earn** this crisis through hard work. It comes thnrough a sacrifice, giving up bad habits, taking a new path, cleaning up the act that you've been in when your life wasn't working with the laws of nature. A crisis can come harsh, small, violently, softly, according to what is possible for the body to control and take care of. Some crises come in backaches, skin rashes, teeth can become on edge, a diarrhea can develop, joint pains can come. I have seen people have all of these symptoms, however, they do not usually come at the same moment but move from one part of the body to another or wherever the body is placing its energy for cleaning, rejuvenation and getting rid of the old tissue and acids that probably have accumulated over a period of year.

most people suppress this, driving the cold back into the body, suppressing various eliminative processes. When we suppress a discharge in the body, we are on our way to a chronic disease.

Fasting

Fasting brings the crisis on more quickly. The crisis can occur either druing the fast or many months afterwards. Crises develop much faster in the summer than in the winter. There are times we need more than one crisis to have a complete body elimination. They may develop one after the other- first in the bronchial tubes, then later in the bowel, and still later in the knees or wherever our problem might have settled.

It is a very interesting thing to observe as the body reverses itself in the process of healing, picking up first the problem you had several years ago, then the one you had five or six years ago, and if you continue with proper living habits, even retracing troubles as far back as ten or fifteen years. Again, it shows the wonderful working of the body and proves that the body works according to law. Without a doubt, we earn the diseases we have, but the wonderful part is that we may also earn our way back to health.

Fasting can also bring other good results. Dr. George Weger of Redlands, California, who was one of my first teachers, showed me what fasting can do. I had a boy who had been scheduled for surgery. The doctors were going to amputate one of his legs because the circulation was so bad. He had ninety boils on his legs and I couldn't cure these boils with all the infection that had been set up there. He came into my office one Friday night and the following Monday he was going to have his leg amputated.

I called Dr. Weger (I didn't even know him at the time), and said, "Doctor, I have a young boy; they are going to amputate one of his legs. I'm wondering if it is possible to save this boy's leg." Well, we put him on a thirty-day fast, and I *did* see this boy's leg saved.

Fasting is like having a lifesaver thrown to you, something to pull you out of danger. I have fasted no fewer than 25,000 people, so I do know the effects of fasting. But we should always seek the counsel of a doctor if we wish to fast for more than a few days.

There is one thing about fasting that may be a little foolish to some of you. Fasting is only squeezing your body like a sponge. You get rid of toxemia, but you must have a building job along with it, or following it.

Nature Does Have a Remedy

Scientists are looking for a pill to eat instead of a meal; they are looking for an injection to take instead of giving up coffee and doughnuts. They are not interested in changing their habits. If your wife can't cook, eat "TUMS." It's an unnatural life today. But if you want to go this unnatural way, you will be following the majority of people today.

The government tells us that 92 percent of the people in this country are sick, even though they are still working. I am convinced that the masses are messes. I am convinced that these 92 percent who are sick do not know the value of nature, the value of living a good life. There is an old saying that man's extremity is God's opportunity. It is possible that when we have increased our sickness to about 98 percent and have broken down to the place where the prevention of virus disease by injection doesn't work anymore, we will have to look for another way out. Did you know that they are now using antibiotics to take care of the antibiotics they used in the past? Flies get so used to the DDT spray that something else has to be found to kill them. One of these days we also might get hardened to all of the injections we have taken in the past.

Fly from the Artificial

We have to find another way out. I think there is going to be a flight from the city— a flight from the artificial. There is going to be a "back to nature" movement. People will find places in the country to enjoy. There will be communal places where they can live a natural life. I don't mean a nude life or an extreme life, with a carrot in one hand and a cabbage in the other. I don't mean a place where we can't use a typewriter or enjoy all the nice things that are found in civilization, but some nice place to get away from the artificiality that is found in smoking, drinking, hamburgers, hot dogs, and the type of lunches that are being served our children in the schools today.

Back to God

I think we are going to have many more surprises one of these days when we deal with the more natural things. When I said that man's extremity is God's opportunity, I think we will see this in positive operation when man reaches the extreme with these foodless foods, and then he will have to come back to the natural way. That's when God can serve us. I am utterly convinced that He is always ready to serve; He has never left us; He is the Almighty Healer, the Everlasting Healer. He will never leave His children. It is we, the children, who are going to have to recognize the fact that we must come back to God and nature before we can be completely well. This idea of straying away and leading an artificial life has taken us from the Garden of Eden, away from nature, away from God. I know that the Healer is ready to do His job; I know that He does not need a cook stove, He does not need an injection. There are no vacations in His plan. His plan requires us to balance our lives and to live normally, to learn how to get along with one another and to live without fear, recognizing that there is no death, but only life. In the New Testament you will not find any place where it says to be afraid of death. Instead, resurrection, a life of eternity, and a life more abundant are promised to us.

How can all these things be realized when we're taking this abundance and devitalizing and diluting it? We are taking the kingdom that has been given us and expecting to reap the promise of the abundant life by living by artificial standards. This cannot be done. Life and death do not live in the same place. Disease and health cannot coexist. Fear and courage cannot live together. Happiness and depression are mutually exclusive.

Nature's Way

The wonders we find in nature are something to be studied. We have to work closely with her in order to be well. In fact, my old professor used to say that we must pick the vegetables right out of the garden to be well. I was not brought up like that. I had to come to this like most people. I haven't met many who can sit down to spinach and say, "This tastes good." None of these things tasted good to me! I don't know about other people, but I came from a family that really sugared everything and fried things to a nice golden brown, that really sold you the sizzle in the steak. It was wonderful, too. Then you come into this health work, and they talk about coffee substitutes. There is no substitute for coffee— that's the real stuff!

The idea of studying this natural way, although wonderful, has been difficult for me. But the more I become aware of how wonderful and bountiful nature has been to my body, the more I go along with her. Nature is wonderful both to our minds and our memories. Our hearing depends upon our assimilation. Smell depends upon our

respiration; respiration depends entirely upon the muscle activity of the body; muscle activity depends upon potassium found in green leaves. We are inseparable from nature: her greens; her yellows, which have vitamin C; and her reds (e.g., tomatoes), which are high in vitamin D and fix the calcium in our bodies, thus giving us tone, energy, and power to work. We can't get away from nature, as much as we strive to find a way to live without her.

So many of us are looking for the substitutes. I have a letter from a lady who said "I find I can't drink coffee anymore, my stomach can't take it. What should I do?" Do you know what she should do? Quit!

This "Psycho" World

I am convinced that today, more than ever before, we live in a "psycho" world, in a psychological, subjective world. I feel that the individual has to be more balanced today than ever before. You have to "stand" more because of today's pressures, today's competition, today's communications, which are constantly bombarding us. We have gone back to a kind of "caveman-like" existence with our weatherproof, air-conditioned houses and penthouses, our automobiles and subways, huge offices and factories, and our inside living that often removes the necessity of ever going out into the fresh air. We hang landscape pictures on our walls and fill our vases with imitation flowers. But nature brings us entirely different suggestions, and when you live out in nature, the ever changing scenery is a complete wonderment, beyond all imagination. If you have ever lived near the Grand Canyon, you know that there is never any day or any moment when you look at the Canyon that you see the same scene. The lighting effects present you with an ever changing view.

Ministry of Healing

The physician needs more than human wisdom and power that he may know how to minister to the many perplexing cases of disease of the mind and heart which he is called to deal with. If you are suffering with poor health, there is a remedy for you.

Young children can grow into almost any shape by habits of proper exercise and positions of the body obtain healthy forms.

The living organism is God's property. God is the owner of the whole man.

The physical organism should have special care that the powers of the body may not be dwarfed, but developed to their full extent.

(Ellen G. White)

Heads up!

SEVEN

THE EYES and teeth are nature's barometer of health. They are the two things in your body that first begin to diminish when the rest of your body is going downhill. When your eyes or teeth start getting bad, that is an indication that something more general might be wrong with your health.

The head itself also tells us much about our health. Do you have headaches? How about dandruff? We can find remedies in nature for all these problems.

Eyes

Circles under the Eyes. Circles under the eyes are caused when the veins fail to get rid of the sludge blood, because the blood is lacking in iron.

Our bodies have their poorest circulation under the eyes because the underlids seldom move. When we blink, we use only the upper lids.

Here is a nice exercise to increase the circulation under the eyes and thereby help fight those circles: While facing straight ahead, with head level, roll the eyes upward as far as possible without undue strain. Then blink your eyes. Repeat three times; then close your eyes and rest them, covering them with the palms of your hands.

Infection of the Eye

Carrot juice is good for infection in the eyes. Vitamin A is good for getting rid of infection, and every glass of carrot juice contains up to 15,000 units of vitamin A.

Irritated Eyes

Honey: A drop of honey in the eyes is said to be beneficial. It must be running honey that has not been heated. If the full-strength honey is too strong, mix it half and half with distilled water.

Linseed oil: Linseed oil is one of the finest things we can use on our eyes. Putting a drop in the eyes is the best thing for eyes irritated by smog from the cities. We find that linseed oil has been used many times in the past, even for cataracts. (Sterilized linseed oil from Drug Store).

Milk Pack: A warm milk pack is a fine remedy for the eyes.

Potato Pack: A grated potato pack is good for irritated eyes. Leave on for twenty minutes. Select a potato that has not been treated with chemicals in growing or storage.

Sinus

Horseradish: Put a little horseradish on the tongue and take a deep breath.

Sage: Sage is a wonderful thing for the sinus. Rub it through the hands and breathe in. It stimulates sinus drainage.

Bay Leaf: The bay leaf is a wonderful stimulus for the sinus. Just rub it in your hands and breathe. Also, you can do the same with mint and eucalyptus leaves.

Throat

For sore throat, use ½ teaspoon of liquid chlorophyll in ½ cup water three times a day.

Mouth

Do you chew tobacco? How about gum? Both of these have a definite adverse effect on the digestion. Constant chewing causes excessive salivation, and the prolonged stimulation of the salivary glands results in an inactive juice with little ferment.

The activity of the saliva in various people shows tremendous differences. Tests indicate that in some cases it is capable of digesting all the starch eaten; in others scarcely one-tenth, or even one-twentieth, is broken down. In the average person only about half the starch liquefied in the mouth and stomach is completely digested by the saliva.

When the saliva is not doing its job properly, stomach digestion is interfered with. The food arrives in the stomach in an inadequately processed form; also the undigested starch absorbs the pepsin of the gastric juice, giving rise to gastric spasm, pain, and other discomforts. It is therefore imperative that we chew our food well to at least give the saliva a chance.

While fruit acids, such as malic and tartaric, exert very little effect on the saliva, citric acid stimulates its flow greatly, aiding protein digestion. Acetic and oxalic acids (rhubarb and spinach) interfere with digestion. One to two teaspoons of vinegar or one part oxalic acid in 10,000 are sufficient to entirely stop the action of saliva. Tannic acid has a similar reaction. This is another reason why tea and coffee, which are high in tannic acid, are not healthful.

The saliva possesses valuable antiseptic properties. Although typhoid fever, tetanus bacilli, colon bacilli, or pus-producing organisms are not destroyed, many other pathogenic bacteria cannot survive in human saliva. The saliva of goats and other ruminants, especially parotoid saliva, has been found to have distinct bactericidal properties. Clairmont of Vienna, who conducted many experiments, concluded that saliva maintains the mouth conditions unfavorable for the growth of micro-organisms which might otherwise remain there, and cause decay or ulceration. It is well known that wounds in the mouth heal rapidly. Pickerill and Gies urge the use of salivatory stimulants as an excellent way to preserve the teeth.

Disease can affect the reaction of the saliva. In cases of diabetes, cancer of the stomach, leukemia, pernicious anemia, jaundice, and sometimes chlorsis, Fleckseder discloses that the saliva becomes acid. Certain diseases can increase the chlorides; others diminish them. A reduction of chlorides in the urine is usually accompanied by their diminution in the saliva. If diabetes is severe, there may be sugar in the saliva.

The quantity of saliva is also affected by disease. It may be very scant when profuse sweating, insistent vomiting, dropsy, diabetes, anemia, cachexia accompanying carcinoma of the stomach, fever, uremia, and cirrhosis of the liver are present. The saliva in such cases is usually cloudy and acid, with a peculiar sweetish odor. In pytalism the saliva is clear, thin, and alkaline. Pregnancy is accompanied by a marked increase in saliva. This is also the case in many painful stomach ailments such as stomatitis, nausea, and gastric ulcer-ation; while in facial neuralgia, gastric crises of locomotor ataxia, and neurasthenia, the flow is frequently intermittent.

The taste of food does much to aid digestion. The pleasure of food in the mouth stimulates the stomach, pancreas, liver, and other organs of digestion to secrete their juices. This is accomplished by the nerves of taste, sending messages to the reflex centers of the brain. The longer food stays in the mouth, the more gastric juice will be in the stomach to receive it. Where the taste has not been perverted, it also acts as an automatic control on the body's needs, governing our desire for a type of food according to our nutritional requirements of the moment. Thorough chewing is another prerequisite to the effectiveness of our built-in regulator, especially with regard to quantities. The uvula, or soft palate, at the back of the mouth is sensitive to solid food, rejecting any such particles and routing them back to the teeth for further breaking down. It also protects the mouth of the esophagus from the entrance of any foreign or injurious articles.

Tongue

Why is it that a visit to the doctor invariably involves a look at the tongue? Well, as the eminent French physician Laseque said, "The tongue does not indicate the disease, but the state of the patient."

The mouth and the nose are vulnerable parts of the body, coming constantly into contact with microorganisms. It is only the action of the saliva that prevents the tongue and all mouth surfaces from being continually coated with molds and other organisms.

In the average sized healthy individual, about 30 billion leucocytes (white blood cells) are constantly active, destroying bacteria. Freshly secreted saliva contains many white blood cells, as well as opsonins and alexins (other agents hindering the growth of bacteria), which help to keep the mouth clean. If the mouth becomes dry due to fever, disease, or sleeping with it open, the tongue gets thickly coated with molds, yeasts, and bacteria.

But a much more common cause of coated tongue is autointoxication. The saliva is incapable of supplying its normal protection of the mouth against uneven odds. So when putrefactive products and virulent bacterias are present in greater numbers than its germicidal action or that of the blood can handle, the tongue becomes thickly coated and the breath has a bad odor.

Most often the colon is at fault. With intestinal sluggishness the body wastes are retained in the bowel sometimes for days and are not properly eliminated. Thus, quantities of toxins find their way into the bloodstream. Invariably, the coated tongue is a sure sign of a toxic condition of the body and a lowered resistance to bacteria; it is practically always coated in fever, whatever the cause of infection.

Gums and Teeth

Bleeding Gums. The herb calendula can have a wonderful effect on the most chronic cases of bleeding gums. Calendula should be used in a tincture and can be held in the mouth for two or three minutes upon arising and before retiring. A teaspoonful is enough, mixed with a small quantity of water.

Liquid chlorophyll is another fine thing for bleeding gums. Use it as a mouthwash, holding it in the mouth two or three minutes until the effect of chlorophyll can come about through the absorption of this fluid.

Other remedies are bonemeal, taken in four tablets, twice a day, and vitamin C, taken in 1,000 milligram doses every three hours for one week.

Breakdown of Gum Tissues. Many people have pyorrhea, gum disorders, and mouth disorders. The teeth are only as good as the gums.

A papaya tablet is recommended where there is a breakdown of gum tissues. Immediately following a meal, place a papaya tablet on each side of the mouth and let it soak for ten or fifteen minutes or until completely dissolved. This will rid the bacteria and dead tissue that have gathered around the teeth. Papaya eats dead tissue but does not hurt live tissue. It is a digestant and a wonderful remedy for getting rid of old structure which most of us have in our mouths. This same method of using papaya is good for people who find that tartar forms easily on their teeth.

Loose Teeth. Loose teeth are a problem today because people do not chew any hard foods. If you cannot chew hard foods and cannot take care of the salads we use today, the teeth become loose. It is recommended that you chew a carrot before breakfast, before lunch, and before dinner. It will not only tighten the teeth, but it will also strengthen the gums so that the teeth will harden. It is hard to believe that we can set our teeth in the gums by chewing that carrot before meals, but this is absolutely true. Spit out the pulp, you do not have to eat the pulp. You can then eat your regular meals, but be sure to chew your food well.

The dentist wanted to put braces on my son's teeth at the age of ten. However, I told my son to chew a carrot before each meal, and it actually straightened out his teeth so that braces were not required. You can expand the jaw on some children, who are born with narrow jaws by making them chew a carrot before meals.

Canker Sores. For canker sores, use calcium lactate. Also it is recommended that you care for the stomach.

Toothache. When you have a toothache you can use cotton wool saturated with oil of cloves. There are packs we can get from the drug store to use alongside the gum for an abscess. Sometimes using flaxseed meal packs

Statue of Morelos in Morelia, Mexico. He is always pictured with a cloth around his head. It has been claimed he wore this tight and wet to control a migraine headache.

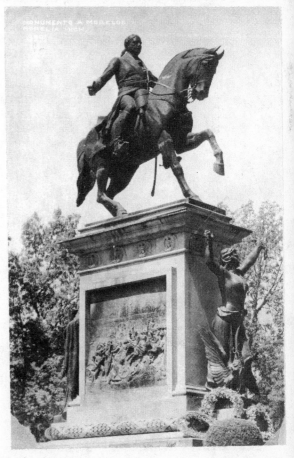

will help a toothache. Put it into a little bag inside the mouth, alongside the tooth.

Tooth Surgery. To speed recovery following tooth surgery and to lessen the pain, use one teaspoon liquid chlorophyll, straight or diluted in one half cup water, about five times a day. Work the liquid around the teeth and hold in the mouth for two or three minutes. This is very soothing as a mouthwash.

America's Dietary Deficiencies
Show in Its Citizen's Teeth

The problem of tooth decay is one of the major problems of the dental and medical professions today, to say nothing of the expense that must be added on to the family budget to take care of the family's deteriorating teeth. A recent survey by the Public Health Service shows that more than 21 million Americans have lost all their teeth. While teeth compose only one percent of the body, there are about 100,000 dentists in the United States today— compared to 250,000 physicians for the other 99 percent of the body.

There are innumerable research programs being conducted in laboratories all over the world with just one idea in mind— the prevention of tooth decay. Most of these research programs have recognized that the most glaring fact discovered to date is that decay is caused by faulty diets and nutritional deficiencies.

Dr. Michael J. Walsh, director of clinical nutrition courses at the University of California Dental Extension in San Francisco, say, "Americans are waterlogged and are

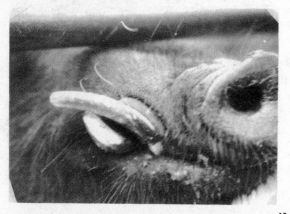

A wild boar that runts and razes his food, roots for his food out of the ground, has to have teeth that rub together like pinchers, to cut off these roots.

suffering from dietary deficiencies— but don't know it. What the public must look upon as three square meals a day is likely to be a starvation diet and one that will decay the toughest tooth." Instead of calling up your neighbor and inviting her children to come over and have ice cream and cake with yours, you should ask her to send them over so that you can drill holes in their teeth! The result *is* the same. Chinchilla breeders, dog fanciers, and even poultry breeders give more thought and attention and pay more money to learn how to feed their animals than the average American does to learn how to feed his own family.

False Living— False Teeth

One of my own recent experiences brought this home to me. An eleven-year-old boy was sent to me by another doctor. The boy had a complete set of dentures. When we have to face the fact that a boy of eleven has to have dentures, it is time to start doing something about this horrible scourge! Every sincere and thinking medical man or healer today should be giving a great deal of his time and energy to this problem.

Another dentist sent a young chap to our office with most of his teeth gone. He was only twelve years old. The dentist claimed he could not do anything with his teeth; that it was a body condition. What a shame to see these teeth, the beautiful pearls of the mouth, broken down when, after all, good food could be taking care of them.

And good food *can* take care of teeth. Dr. George W. Heard worked as a dentist in Hereford, Texas, for over thirty years. During that period his patients had such healthy teeth that he did not have to pull a single one. The reason? Their diets protected their teeth.

We know that teeth are broken down and deteriorated when a person does not live right and follow a proper diet. In our diet, greens are most important; they control the calcium in the body. The Hunzas, who had such beautiful teeth and kept them until they died at over 100 years of age, followed a diet in which they ate a lot of greens and the tops of vegetables. We should eat more parsley, beet greens, watercress, spinach, and the many different greens that we can get for salads daily. These will help to keep our teeth in tiptop condiiton.

Chlorophyll

We have also found chlorophyll effective

in halting tooth decay. Chlorophyll is best known for its mysterious action in the process known as photosynthesis, which is the complicated chemical process in which a green plant converts the energy of the sun's rays into stored food energy. Science has never been able to break down this process and discover exactly how it works, but it has long been known that without chlorophyll neither plants nor animals, including humans, could live. Chlorophyll is the substance that gives plants their green color. We can get chlorophyll by making juice drinks from the tops of vegetables. The liquefier comes in very handy for this purpose. Green kale, turnip tops, carrot tops, beet tops, and other green vegetables run through the liquefier and made into a drink should be a part of your program for the entire family. It is much easier to do this than to suffer with an aching tooth or to pay the dentist's bill.

Take Time To Learn: Save Money

We cannot give the best to our job if we are suffering from an aching tooth. This, of course, goes for all dietary deficiencies as well. It has been stated by health authorities that billions of dollars could be saved by employers each year if the employees were better fed through improved nutritional programs. Better fed people work more efficiently. Americans can be better fed if they will only take time to learn how to use better foods.

The physiological symptoms of malnutrition come in the forms of headache, burning sensations in the eyes, apprehension, pessimism, nausea, or bloodshot eyes.

We know that millions of dollars are spent each year to improve personal appearance by having teeth straightened or a cap put on a discolored tooth; mental attitude is much better when we are satisfied with our personal appearance. Is it not smarter, then, to learn how to produce these beautiful teeth we so earnestly desire by finding out which chemical elements and vitamins are required in our diet to make them what we desire?

Vigorous Chewing

The average person does not chew his food thoroughly enough. He does not have the habit of chewing in the first place. Many children's jaws have not been developed fully and the teeth are crowded because they have not had hard foods to chew. Give the child nuts to chew, or a raw carrot every day, while his teeth are growing and developing.

To make gums well, hard, and to keep them from bleeding easily, chew hard, crisp foods. Eat dry starches and keep away from mushy, soft foods.

Ears

General Remedies. Proper diet balance will help when the blood is the cause of deafness: improve the blood and circulation in the brain by hot applications, strong light, neck exercises, massage, and strict attention to the liver, blood, and eliminative organs. Strong garlic juice dropped into the ear a few times overcomes colds and catarrh. Remove natural gases from the bowel system, because this has a tendency to disturb the auditory nerves and the basal membranes of the ears.

Ear Drum Hardening. The ears change gradually and many times we do not even realize that changes are taking place. This is not uncommon in the body. For instance, when a hardening occurs in the tissues of the body it sometimes takes twenty years to develop. It may be twenty years before a handicap in the ears shows up in a lack of response. Twenty years may pass before hardening develops in the arteries, or even cholesterol settles in our bodies.

When the ear drum has a hardening set in, it usually has a long-standing cause. Some causes are the eating of too much salt, a lack of sodium in the diet, poor circulation of blood to the ear structure, a lack of nerve supply from the spinal cord, or complete tiredness, resulting in not having the proper blood circulating to the upper extremities. A tired body cannot force blood up hill. Whenever we are sick or tired nature always wants us to lie down. I am sure that is to rejuvenates the brain tissues.

Catarrhal Conditions and the Ears. Lymph drainage is important. Whenever a catarrhal condition is dominant in the body, especially in the bronchial tubes, a certain amount of this catarrh will be backed up into the lymph glands, which are numerous along the spine and the neck. A sedentary occupation sometimes does not provide enough activity for normal emptying of these glands, which leads to a congestion that backs up into the smaller tissues nearby. The ear drum is one such tissue.

Also, when things are not working properly within the abdominal region, toxemias develop, resulting in an excessive elimination of catarrh. This catarrhal elimination can spread to all the orifices of the body. In this case, the ears in many cases develop into what is called mastoids, a running ear, and over a period of time this catarrh can cause a deafening effect in the ear.

Symptoms such as buzzing in the ears may come from an anemic condition in the head and can come also from high blood pressure. It can come from emotional strain, from indigestion, and from excessive gas pressures in the bowel.

In taking care of these problems, the first thing we should think about is the law of exercise that helps to get the blood into the ears (making sure first, of course, that the blood is high in quality and quantity). An extra rush of blood can be brought about by getting as nearly as possible in an upside-down position, so that the blood can flow easily into these upper areas. The slant board exercise, with the feet above the head, the feet and legs performing "bicyling," will help to get extra blood in the head. While in this position on the slant board, pull the knees down to the chest and hold for five minutes. This also helps to get extra blood into the head areas and the ears, which in turn stimulates the lymph drainage in the neck, helping to drain this area of any heavy catarrhal conditions and in time helps the ears.

Using vitamin B and especially a heavy amount of nicotinic acid will also drive the blood into the extremities of the body. For instance, taking rice bran syrup, a product high in nicotinic acid, on an empty stomach causes the ears to become red. Use the rice bran syrup directly after a meal to enjoy the benefit while avoiding symptoms of local manifestation.

There are ways of entering the mouth to drain the catarrhal settlements in the back of the uvula. From there drainage of the sinuses can be forced— especially if any excessive tissue has developed there and adhesions are keeping the catarrh from flowing freely from the sinuses. This is done through the manipulation called finger surgery.

Cleansing and eliminating foods, such as those found in vegetable juices, are best for the ears. The "Eleven Day Elimination Diet" as found in my *Vital Foods for Total Health* is an excellent start, then follow up with my *Healthy Way to Live* for the best results. Parsley and shave grass teas work miracles on the kidneys, and that has real benefits for the ears. Cucumber juice and whey are

good foods for dissolving processes. A combination of these two helps tremendously in dissolving any hardness of the ear drum. Okra and celery are also very good for hardness in the ear drum. And they have the added effect of helping those with high blood pressure conditions.

Neck exercises, thyroid exercises, lymph gland drainage exercises, and tension and relaxation exercises that deal with the head and neck are important when we have any ear trouble. The best nerve foods for taking care of the ears are found in desiccated liver, powdered yeast, wheat germ, amino acids, lecithin, and gelatin.

Whenever we treat one part of the body we must treat the whole body. A lack of vitamin C can lead to hearing problems, especially during the winter months, when the body's reserve is limited because of a lowered intake of fresh vegetables and fruits. And that same dietary deficiency in vitamin C can often produce the *common cold.* So, as we build up the liver, the stomach, the digestive powers, the elimination ability, we find that the ears will improve. Always take care of the whole body when you take care of any one of its organs.

Hearing Problems. Hearing problems can come from clogging of the Eustachian tubes; too much blood in the brain; pressure on the nerves, basil membranes, or some other part of the inner ear; thickening growth around the ear; stiffness or ossification of the three ear bones; and a mind that is too abstract, so that the external world is forgotten and the man never listens to sound. When we have a weak development of the faculties that pay attention to sound, music, melody, and speech, the hearing depreciates. We should learn to imitate people, to imitate languages, tones, and sounds enough to pay conscious attention to the air vibration and the bone vibration and the vibration that falls on the ears through the bones of the body. Holding a tuning fork in the mouth and paying attention to the vibration or to the types of music played, or to sing and hum along with it, helps cultivate the consciousness one needs to maintain excellent hearing.

Boxing the ears also many times causes injury to the nerves of the ears; deafness is the result. Putting hair pins into the ears to clean them can also injure the ear mechanism.

The tendencies toward flu and catarrhal discharges in any part of the body will no doubt harm the ears, for the ears are an organ of catarrhal discharge, and settlement of catarrah in this area could in time affect the hearing. Catarrhal conditions settled in the throat can migrate into the Eustachian tubes.

A lot of vitamin C should be used at all times to help the ears. Vitamin C takes care of infections and all the catarrhal conditions that may settle in the ears. Dr. William Evans has shown that when vitamin C level is high, bacteria are less likely to be found in the nose, throat, and ears, and, if present, seldom become virulent. Experiments conducted abroad demonstrate a direct relationship between vitamin C and infection of the middle ear, which is often a factor in loss of hearing. Eighteen cases of middle ear infections examined showed a high vitamin C deficiency with chronic pus secretion. Administration of vitamin C stopped the secretion completely.

Dr. Edmund Prince Fowler, in examining school children in slum areas, found their percentage of ear troubles much higher than that of children in private schools. The children in slums had repeatedly suffered from infectious diseases, due in part to insufficient diet, especially nonvariety of food and lack of vitamin content, which reduced resistance to infection. Vitamin A is also found to be lacking in many of the people who have ear disturbances. It is also needed in nasal discharges and many abcesses of the middle ear. Surveys show large doses of vitamin A to be effective during the duration of colds.

In checking some people, it has been found that intake of vitamins A, B, and C has been short a good part of their lives. In one case, for instance, subjects were given treatment of these vitamins along with some endocrine substances for one year; the result was complete relief from fatigue and marked improvement of nervous condition. The women's audiograms showed a definite change, and whispered voices that could not previously be heard at all were audible at a distance of six feet after the treatment.

Based on these findings, it may be necessary to add vitamin concentrates to your regular diet. These should be given to you by a well qualified doctor.

Dr. Fowler also found that excessive sweets and starches may bring about a lowered resistance of the nasal membranes and in turn aggravate existing ear conditions. Clear up your nervousness; do not hurry through your meals. A highly nervous person very seldom eats properly; they eat too fast; they eat

under stress and in the long run this can bring on ear conditions.

A small tribe of Sudanese, 20,000 strong, called the Madhians live in a swampy, steamy, primitive, mud-hut village in the jungles of northeast Africa. The Madhians are possibly the healthiest people in the entire world. Despite the extremes of climate and circumstances, and a diet of sour pasty bread, the Madhians are a tall, muscular people who remain extraordinarily youthful into old age.

Dr. Samuel Rosen, a New York ear specialist, led an expedition into the Madhi country and learned that the average Madhian of seventy-five years can hear as the average twenty-five year old American. Another report of Dr. Rosen's was that the Madian simply does not die until his body completely wears out.

The Madhian speaks softly, and the loudest sound heard in the village is the cry of a bird. The average Madhian tested could hear a soft murmur across the length of a football field. Loss of hearing from old age was virtually unknown. Scientists hope to learn the secret of the slow aging process of these people. Dr. Rosen feels that an alleviation of the pressures of modern existence might increase our life span considerably.

When any one of this tribe moves to Khartoum, the nearest outpost of civilization, he falls prey to heart attacks, ulcers, and other civilized ailments.

Headaches

Causes of Headaches. There are many causes of headaches. President Theodore Roosevelt once said, "We have to be very careful going to a surgeon with a pain in a toe because the surgeon might want to cut it off." The same goes for a pain in your head—you could lose it! It is possible that many headaches are caused by troubles quite remote from the head.

A headache that is twisting, boring, burning, or jumping is caused by aching nerves. We must rebuild the nervous system in order to get rid of this kind of headache. Headaches that are dull, heavy, and persistent are either of the brain, skull bones, blood pockets of the brain, periosteum, scalp, base of the brain, or cerebellum.

Headaches that are depressing, confusing, dull, interfering with the eyesight and hearing, and accompanied by chills, nausea, vomiting, fevers, confusion of ideas, third tongue, buzzing, ringing, roaring in the ears, bad dreams, temper, sleeplessness, indifference, dislike for food, and fear are usually from a food source either improperly combined foods or overeating. They are caused by gastric disturbances in the digestive system.

Headaches can come directly from an acid stomach when the hydrochloric balance is off. Whenever we have heartburn, it can cause reflex conditions, including a headache throughout the upper part of the head; a dull headache at the upper portion of the forehead, with tired eye muscles, drowsiness, dislike of using the brain, study, and talking. There are also people who have pain from abnormal sounds and who dislike other people's voices or talking, which is usually caused from an overworked brain. They are at the end of their rope, so to speak.

There may be toxic causes for headaches that are accompanied by severe coughing, moisture in the skin, colds, catarrh, night sweats, flushes of heat and cold, temperature change, or a breeze that is cooling the skin.

When we have starved our nerves and brain cells over a period of time, we may have headaches that are tingling, jumping, mashing, or even creeping. These headaches are caused by poor drainage of the lymph system. Too much blood in the head can cause this trouble also, as can indigestible foods; loss of sleep; excessive studies, poisonous medicine; too much thinking, talking, noise, or rattles; or germs and gas in the intestinal tract.

Disappointments in love, excessive bile, a bad liver, pressures from excess gases on the pheumogastric nerve, splenic nerve, and diseases of the scalp can also cause headaches. Other causes are lack of blood, excessive use of the eyes in reading and studying, poor glasses, improperly fitted glasses, constipation, diarrhea, a diseased womb, malfunctioning ovaries, menstraul disorders, or a poorly nourished spinal cord.

Many people have headaches when giving up coffee, tea, and poisonous foods, because the food goes through retracing processes. This throwing off process can be the cause of a headache.

Prolapsus, a dropped transverse colon, pressure on the kidneys, lack of magnesium salts in the blood, the excessive use of starches and proteins, or too many fruits that stir up the acids all cause headaches.

Too many liquids can thin the blood and cause ringing disturbances in the ears. Eating too many starches, which causes too heavy blood, and too hot blood in the summer time, can cause headache.

Remedies for Headaches. If there is an anemic condition in the body, it may cause a headache. Turn to the iron foods and get plenty of oxygen by living outside in a cool, invigorating atmosphere. Use more of the iron foods: blackberries, strawberries, cherry juice, and spinach.

If your headache is caused by a disturbance in the liver, use beets in the diet: shredded beets, shredded raw beets, cooked beets, beet juice. Have beets in the diet every day.

If a headache is from the intestinal tract, make sure you get the proper diet, use a lot of the acidophilous culture, get the proper exercise to develop the tone of the intestinal tract, take internal baths, and use enemas made with baking soda or lemon juice and water. If the bowel is irritated, use flaxseed tea enemas.

Physical work helps nervous headaches; good activities are swimming, outdoor exercise, morning walks, bending exercises, and skipping rope.

Some headaches are caused by climatic conditions. Seek those parts of the country that are conducive to healthful living. An altitude of about 1,700 to 3,000 feet is usually best. Hot, humid weather can be the cause of headaches. Seek a dry, breezy-cool climate.

In many cases, the elimination of a headache will come when we improve our marriage relations, our relations with our children, our relations with our occupation. If you live in grief, sorrow, fear, disappointment, depression, get a new outlook on life. If you have lost a lover, find another. If you have had a disappointment, find another avenue of growth. Every experience will turn out to be a blessing, though you may not see it at the moment. Do not live in grief; do not live in resentment. You may have to change your environment, change your philosophy. Develop a set of controlled exercises, breathing exercises, get into games, learn to play, forget your troubles.

Hot teas (lemon grass and camomile) are exceptionally good for headache distress. Some of these teas can be taken every hour; we can have quarts of them every day. Use this for elimination purposes, to clean the bloodstream and eliminate the toxic gases and materials from the body. Get away from heavy catharsis.

What should we do in general? Lots of sleep, lots of rest, getting to bed before midnight, developing the faculties of control, and living a peaceful, serene life will help most headaches that are constant and recur over a period of years.

Cool applications to the head, hot foot baths, manipulation, massage, working on the spinal nerves, warm applications to the body, a warm sulfur bath, lots of fresh air, foot exercises, sand walks, and early morning grass walks will develop the circulation and also help in most cases of headache.

Sleep with your head to the north; sleep on pine needles; sleep on the ground; sun bathe, but do not overdo it. Use the leg bath in cool water up to the knees for one minute at a time. Skipping a meal once in a while will help with a headache.

Take on new associates in your job, in your home; seek new companions—whatever you do, balance your day to live well.

Migraine. Migraine is one of those increasingly prevalent maladies of our day. Distressingly painful and crippling, it is often shrugged off as being incurable. But there is much help for the migraine sufferer.

Evidence shows that it could be psychosomatic. That is, it has a basis in nervous and emotional stress and strain as well as physical causes. It is just this correlation which enables us to achieve good results by raising the physical level of fitness.

Diet has tremendous implications to the migraine victim. With a stronger, less fatigued body, his anxieties automatically fall into proper perspective. The basic regular daily diet is essential for his well-being. It may be advisable to take a short fast, in spite of the natural cleansing action of the vomiting and abstinence from food usually accompanying migraine attack. Juices are excellent for cleansing. The carrot, beet, and apple combination should be tried, along with liquid chlorophyll drinks.

Manipulative therapies also help. They tend to relax the nervous system as well as correct the functional organs of the body. Adjustments to vertebrae out of alignment may be necessary.

Stretch and turn the head and neck from left to right, gently. The use of the neck stretcher is very valuable to relieve the body and head from severe pain. I have found in my practice over a period of years that the neck stretcher is the one thing that helps the migraine sufferer most. The neck stretcher is an apparatus that pulls the head straight up while you are sitting on a chair. It is best not to twist the head while you are in this apparatus; instead, use a straight pull on the

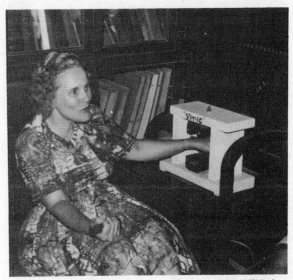

Marie Jensen having a treatment with magnetism. This is a force that man is trying to harness and maybe use in our treatments in the future.

head. If there is anyone in the family who can pull your head in this manner, it would be helpful.

All efforts to improve the circulation will help. Sand and grass walking, plus regular use of the slant board, should be an integral part of the daily routine. Immersing hands or feet in a bowl of hot water gives relief and reduces the severity of an attack.

Stretching the abdominal area, drawing in at the upper solar plexus, helps release all the tensions in the digestive tract. Moderate exercise, including plenty of walking (out in fresh air and sunshine if possible) without overdoing it, helps raise the health level and thus helps the migraine sufferer.

Besides building bodily strength, the careful avoidance of exhaustive reactions such as worry and tensions, will hasten the recovery. Get an interesting hobby to relieve the strain of work. Then change your diet: drop bready and baked goods for your head's sake.

Crazy "Cures" for Migraines. Want to get rid of a migraine headache? Just drill a hole in your skull or put a hot iron to your head. These are two of the more drastic "cures" prescribed in ancient times for this most painful of all headaches, says Dr. Seymour Diamond, president of the National Migraine Foundation, a Chicago organization formed in 1970 to help headache sufferers.

"Migraine headaches are nothing new," he said. "They have been around as long as man himself."

"The medicine men of Jericho around 2000 B.C. favored drilling holes in the head to allow evil spirits to escape to cure ailments of the head. Variations of this same treatment continued throughout recorded history. In the tenth century an Arab doctor advised applying a hot iron to the site of the headache or making an incision in the temple and inserting pieces of garlic sharpened to a point on each end."

Dr. Diamond, a prominent Chicago physician, said other old "remedies" included spreading a salve made of poppies on the forehead, chewing cashews, and plastering a live fish to the head. But migraines are a serious problem, he said. "They cause throbbing, pulsating pain that may last for several days, and people have been known to attempt suicide under the influence of a migraine headache."

"Many famous people have been migraine sufferers," he said. They include writers Alexander Pope, Rudyard Kipling, Edgar Allan Poe, Leo Tolstoy, and Lewis Carroll; composers Frederic Chopin, Peter Tchaikovsky, and Richard Wagner; scientists Sigmund Freud and Charles Darwin; and such political figures as Julius Caesar, Peter the Great, Thomas Jefferson, Ulysses S. Grant, and Karl Marx.

"Migraine sufferers tend to be hard-driving, hard-working individuals," said Dr. Diamond. "Some modern day sufferers who fit that category are comedian Woody Allen, movie producer Frank Capra, and basketball star Kareem Abdul-Jabbar."

Hair

Hair Culture. In taking care of the hair, we have to recognize that the hair is part of the bloodstream. It belongs to our body, just the same as our eyes. It must be fed by the digestive system. It lives. It has its roots right in the blood, as well as in the scalp. In order to get a good plant to grow, we must nourish it, care for it and see that it has a balanced ration of sunshine and water. This is also true of the hair. It has to be nourished and cared for.

There are many things we neglect in our body and in our daily habits. And there is good evidence that hair is one of them: people are losing their hair because they do not take care of it in the way they should. Hair must have more care than just a daily combing or brushing.

As we consider care of the hair, let us remember that the hair is functional as well as ornamental. It is a receptor, it helps to keep us magnetically balanced. It holds the greatest amount of silicon in our body, and silicon is the "feeling" element of our body; silicon is the magnetic element in the body.

I believe we would have a better-balanced nervous system if we had longer hair. Our hair is an extension of the nervous system, and we cut off part of what gives us balance when we cut off our hair.

I know of many doctors who take care of hair, and they all have the same idea: the hair must be taken care of the same as the teeth. When the hair begins to deteriorate, the whole body is also deteriorating. Anything that interferes with the blood getting to the head can be considered one the the first things that prevents the proper development of good hair. When we are tired, it is difficult to get fresh blood to the head. Tired tissue cannot force the blood against gravity, maining it cannot force the blood away from the earth very well.

Baldness. If we went to Mexico, we would find very few Mexican workers who are bald-headed. They are people who do not work hard when they are tired. "Mañana" is their favorite word.

Whenever there is baldness or the hair starts to turn gray or gets brittle, it is a definite sign that the person is not eating enough of the proper chemical elements—or that he is burning them up too fast. A breakdown of the nervous system will cause thinning of the hair. Fevers often produce an extreme thinning of the hair. Breakdown of the cerebellum of the brain is one of the main causes of thinning of the hair. When hair roots have been destroyed entirely, there is no way of growing new hair; just as when teeth are gone or when a leg has been cut off, a new one cannot take its place. We must hold on to what we have. People who eat properly and have proper circulation can do much to rejuvenate their hair.

There is much research going on these days showing that the pituitary gland is largely responsible for growth of the hair, and for baldness. Scientists are finding out that the men who have masculine tendencies are the ones who are bald-headed; while those who have more female hormones in their bodies and are more physically feminine— small stature, small bones, etc.- are the ones who have a full head of hair. Dr. V.G. Rocine, a Norwegian homeopath, used to say, "The cerebellum is responsible for the growth of hair." The cerebellum is a brain center, and I believe it is very closely related to the pituitary gland function.

Every hair has a hair-bed in the skin, with a bulb at the end of the hair root, through which the hair draws its nutrition from the blood. The hair contains a food substance called keratin, which contains great quantities of sulphur. The scalp, which is made up of muscular material, should be relaxed so blood will circulate well beneath it. A tight scalp keeps the blood from circulating to the hair root. Many people find in old age that the top of the head is not properly nourished because their tissues have become flabby and do not allow proper circulation of the blood.

We also neglect the hair and the scalp when we do not sleep enough. Sleeplessness is one of the causes for a lack of hair growth as are overstudy, worry, and insufficient oils and nutrition in the blood. Baldness can come from a lack of lecithin, which is a brain and nerve fat. When we lack sulphur, silicon, and iron in our food, the hair shoots will not develop and grow properly. Typhoid fever and many of the diseases found in childhood can bring on loss of hair.

The thyroid gland has a lot to do with hair also for when the thyroid becomes underactive, the circulation is slow and the tissue is flabby. An extra amount of iodine in the diet can help this condition, and that in turn will help the hair.

Strong acids and alkalines, when applied to it, can destroy the hair. Germ poisons, diseases, lack of nerve force, or certain parasites, which generate poisonous gases and gnaw at the hair roots or infect the sabaceous glands, can use up the oil and vitality of the hair roots. Dandruff can smother the hair shoots and the scalp in general. This is causes by a lack of skin fat in the sabaceous glands.

Beautiful Hair. To have a beautiful head of hair one must give it care and attention. Learn what diets are good for the body and find out how to feed the weaknesses in the body that prevent it from circulating good blood. Live on nutritionally balanced foods: stay away from devitalized foods, especially demineralized starches. The demineralized starches take away the outside layer (or silicon layer) of the grain, which is specifically needed for hair growth. The finest foods to get into the body and into the bloodstream, and thereby to the hair, are found in the following: oatstraw tea, rice polishings, rice bran syrup, wheat bran tea, shavegrass tea, radishes, horseradish, sprouts, sole, black fish, smoked blue fish, white fish, shad roe, bran bread, strawberries, avocados, cucumbers, steel cut oatmeal, graham bread, seaweed, the shell of grain, nuts, fruits, dandelion, leeks, romaine lettuce, parsnips, whole barley meal, tender raw carrots, marjoram, collards, caraway, whole rice, and wheat or oat straw broth cooked slowly for one hour.

It is best not to use a nylon brush on the hair. One hair in the head is worth two in the brush. For brushing, a natural bristle brush helps in keeping the hair clean and shining.

Graying and Thinning Hair. There are many things we can use in the diet to help the hair, but the one thing that seems to get the best results is Nova Scotia dulse tablets. Also good are three or four parsley tablets taken three and four times a day, or one-half glass of parsley juice taken daily.

Alfalfa tablets and alfalfa tea are especially good for helping the hair regain its original color.

These things, along with a massage on the slant board, will change the hair considerably in a period of six months. You will find that you will bring a good supply of blood to the hair if you massage your scalp while lying on the slant board, head down. Massaging the scalp with the tops of the fingers about twenty minutes three times a week helps tremendously.

One shampoo that is very stimulating to the hair and to the scalp is made of an egg yolk combined with a quarter teaspoon of sea salt. Rub this well into the scalp and let it set for some ten or fifteen minutes, then wash it out with castile soap. This can be done twice a week.

Watch your elimination; make sure that the kidneys and the bowels are functioning well.

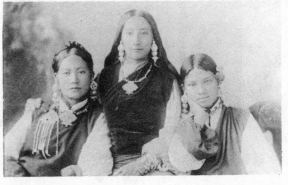

In Nepal and in Darjeeling we saw such beautiful hair, with oils. Living on natural foods, high in silicon, gave beautiful hair to these maidens.

Be sure that the skin is cared for by brushing it. It might be well to stimulate the circulation in the head areas at times by using hot and cold packs while lying on the slant board. Use the packs one-half minute hot, one-fourth minute cold. Make about six or eight changes while on the board. Do this once a day.

To revitalize our hair we must conserve our energy, control our imagination, stop working when we are tired and use a lot of silicon foods. Give your scalp a thirty-minute massage twice a week for at least six to eight weeks, and a noticeable result will be observed; however, scalps that are put under extremely hot hair dryers and subjected to the use of some of the dandruff cure-all remedies available are having much of the hair growth destroyed. The itching of dandruff can also be relieved through the use of the above methods.

If there is a fungus growth on the scalp, a good remedy is to use sheep fat and a little garlic oil. Leave it on the hair for a period of twenty minutes, then shampoo. Washing the hair in soft water and castile soap is wonderful. The gently friction of the massage as we mentioned, will bring the proper heat and blood to the surface and help the hair shoots to develop and to grow in the proper head of hair.

Hair Tonics. An egg yolk in grape juice is a great tonic to help the glands and to help the circulation. Whenever there is any hardening of the arteries, it is advisable to use whey and as do grapevine root and leaf tea, although the coloring is poor.

We had a nice experience at one time with a man who was billed as the strongest "upside-down-man" in the world. His name is Joe Tonti, and he lives in Oklahoma City. He told me that years ago when he was a child he had a severe fever and lost his hair. He also had blemishes on his face, an eczema that was very difficult to get rid of. As he grew older he went into weight lifting work and athletic activities. He did a good deal of his work upside-down and found that in getting more blood to his head in these upside-down activities, the blemishes on his face left and his hair returned. Onions, horseradish, and the sulphur foods will help to drive the blood to the brain areas and to the scalp.

Dr. Rocine used a wash made of the roots of the ordinary grapevine once a week. He believed that drinks made of honey and tonics made of celery with Concord grape juice were good for the hair. Weak tea made of the roots of the grapevine should be taken occasionally.

Remember that hair is like a vegetable growth. It resists dyes and colors of every kind. You can take the color out of hair, but you cannot put color back into it. Gray hair is not a hair color; it is aged hair and it indicates that the hair is dead to pigments. Hair can be dyed, but the dyeing will never be finished. Sage tea washes darken the hair,

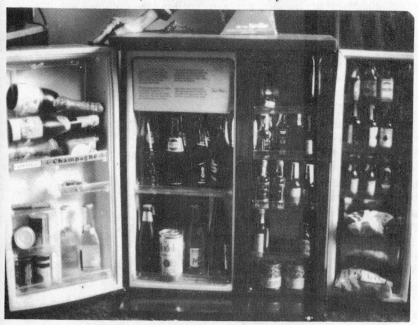

In one of the international cities we visited we snapped this photo of an icebox filled with liquor, drinks and snacks in the hotel room where we were staying. We are getting so evolved and developed today that they will not even allow you to make an effort to go out and get your drinks . . . the drinks are waiting for you and making it very easy for you to run down your body.

Brain and nerve force

EIGHT

I LEARNED from one of my greatest teachers that for vitality of the body we have to depend upon the brain force. The brain does its work through the nerve system.

To take care of this nerve system we have to consider the right direction in life, happy surroundings, pleasurable friendships, the proper climate, pleasurable exercises, and the proper balance of natural foods. All these are necessary for the repair and rebuilding of the nerve system in order to have the brain force we need.

The trophic brain has charge of hunger, as well as the digestion and the assimilation and elimination of the foods. The sex brain is in charge of the sexual system—the secretion of the life principles of growth, cell building, and reproduction. The hydric brain has charge of the lymphatic glands, the liver, the kidneys, and the urinary mechanism—the organs of absorption and hydric elimination.

So to get rid of toxic materials in the body we have to look to building the brain force. The brain controls activities throughout the body. Included among its many functions are mastication, insalivation, swallowing, digestion, and the many-sided activities of absorption, secretion, excretion, appetite, internal secretions, cell building, growth, vital life, defecation, and diffusion of heat. The brain also controls assimilation, circulation, and respiration.

The brain controls the five physical senses, sexation, perspiration, enervation, the sensory parts of the nervous system, hunger and thirst sensations, the distribution of the blood and the general vital metabolism, hydration or the distribution of water in the body.

After looking over the above list, you can see why when we are working with healing a person and bringing in new tissue, the first thing we do in our program is to take care of the nerve supply, the brain.

The second thing we do is help them get good blood through foods. The third concern is exercise. And then the fourth remedy is rest. When we have all of these things put together, we start a good healing job.

Some of the vital functions are automatic—circulation, heart action, respiration, and vasomotor functioning. These functions are closely associated with and mainly under the direct supervision of the "chest brain," where the vagus nerve and all its branches originate. There is a centralization in the chest brain in the head, the medulla.

Develop the chest brain in order to save or increase the nerve force. Sit still for a-while—for an hour every evening—when everything is quiet and the air is fresh. Pay attention to nothing but the breath as it moves up and down the chest. *Enjoy your breath*. This is one of the very best methods for developing circulation, the heart, and the chest brain.

Easy vital action in the open air will accomplish the same thing. The one great principle that should be remembered in regard to vital development is easy, vital, and joyous motion.

Attitude and Brain Force. Our feelings about life can strengthen or drain our brain force. It is important that we enjoy kindly feelings, sensations of hunger and thirst, wholesome sexual desires, pleasure in the circulatory system, the actions of parental faculties, love feelings, hope and working in hopeful plans, cheerful aciton, laughter, prudence, easy changes, reading, and studying. Talk to people and associate with the people who leave you with good feelings.

Other important life-giving tonics are playing with pets, admiring the opposite sex, taking a special interest in the growing vegetation around you, music, songs, speech, easy memorizing, politeness of manners, social ethics, games, home love, home pleasure, public and private speaking, pleasing environment, beautiful paintings, artistic surroundings, easy breathing exercises, easy walks, recreation, social work, rural sports, fishing picnicing, a relaxed social life, a sociable church life, lovemaking, travel, scenery, boatriding, horseback riding, automobile riding, evening walks. All sorts of physical enjoyment and pleasures develop the vital man—the vital functions and the vital faculties in the brain of man.

Remember the pleasure that is felt during eating, drinking, exercising, baths, recreation, song, music, or in looking at food, or admiring growing vegetation, animals, or the beauty of nature. This pleasure is the developing agent of vitality building.

Anything that is playful develops the vitality necessary for life. Warmth favors vitality and sexual life. Relishing and enjoying food and drink favors cell building in the vital system.

Make your foods and surroundings attractive. Place flowers on the table, green plants around the walls in the dining area, wallpaper showing vines, beautiful fruits and delicacies and pleasing food articles on the table—all these stimulate appetitie and vital spirits. Arouse the food appetite and gastric secretions and improve digestion with pleasing aromas of foods, fruits, liquids.

Look at the food, listen to food talk, think of food, dream of delicacies. This is the most wonderful thing you can do to stimulate cell building in the vital organs.

Easy and pleasing conversation about everyday affairs and about physical wants is another vital factor in building the cells of vital organs.

Joyful and hopeful feelings and states of mind that make you pleasing, affectionate, sympathetic, kind, friendly, sociable, agreeable, genial, mirthful, and loving are a form of nourishment in themsleves.

Turn your attention to easy expressions of life, easy emotion, pleasing exercises, good sound sleep, good-naturedness, laughter, recuperative exercises, entertainment, sports, fishing, banquets, and relaxed diversions.

To create a joy for living a person must do that which he loves and takes great delight in doing. When you exercise, don't feel that you're persecuting yourself, but exercise with easy, smooth movements, motions, and actions. Tai Chi is a study that helps you develop this approach to exercising.

We have gone over the building aspects of creating vitality. We should also recognize the agents that destroy the vitality of the body and the mind. The bad-tempered person is a seething volcano of depressed emotions, disappointments, worry, hatred—all the things that eat at the vitals and the vitality.

One of the first things an angry person should develop is a feeling of gratitude, no matter what the situation is. Gratitude is a development agent for happiness. Soon there will be friendships, love, pleasant associations, optimistic feelings, pleasurable activities. Be thankful. Be grateful. And the rest will follow.

Health follows calmness, self-composure, and a happy mind. Anybody who has pleasure in his body and mind will develop a strong will to live and enjoy life, to help others to enjoy life, too.

There are certian types of people we have to get away from if health is to be regained. The cynical, the nervous, the hysterical, the angry—all disturb the magnetic aura and the inner man. If you are in the company of a friend, or a foe, or a stranger, and you suddenly feel weaker, find some way to excuse yourself and leave at once.

Your sleeping arrangements are very important, too. While you may have great compassion for elderly people, or people with low vitality, or people with diseased conditions, it is necessary for your own strength and vitality not to sleep near them. The healthy one loses brain force, and the old or sick person does not gain. This is outraging nature and must be avoided.

Sickness is destructive to vitality and health and life. Pain is destructive to vitality because it uses up the nerve force and sends nerve energy to the surface of the body, where it escapes.

Terror, panic, fright, and alarm are all destructive for vitality. Again, the nerve force travels to the surface of the body and escapes. A person can be so terrified that he may perspire blood. He becomes like an empty bag after the nervous struggle is over and the vital principles are lowered to a dangerous degree. This is when sickness comes in.

For this reason we have to develop the brain centers, we have to strengthen the inner self so that we are not terrified or alarmed about anything. Without these protective faculties a person is too weak and it's not easy for him to build up the necessary vitality and nerve force. He can look healthy but be sick. The protective forces must be developed to make a healthy, happy, sane, and successful man or woman.

Timidity and a nervous disposition cause a person to lose his nerve force every minute of the day through this uncontrolled sensitiveness, restless action, fear, fussiness, temper, and intensity of emotion. Without the protective force of a sane and balanced philosophy toward life, he cannot build. He may look strong but he is weak. He may appear calm but inside he's like an aspen leaf shaken by strong wind. He needs nerve force and must learn how to conserve what he has in order to build more. Spend time each day to calm and build the brain cells and the nervous system.

Waste material is retained in the body when the nerve force is depleted, and healthy cell building cannot be done. Then a person becomes heavy and restless, suffers from sleeplessness, finds thinking difficult, loses his ability to remember well. In a surprisingly short time he can be built up by drinking warm water in great quantities, by doing soothing breathing exercises, and by taking long relaxing walks.

The brain and nerve force are probably the most important elements of the entire body. We should learn to understand the part they play in our lives, and learn to provide well for them. Very few people go to the cause and the beginning of their problem. Usually they treat only some symptom. That symptom could be changed by changing the life pattern, the daily thoughts; by caring for the brain through proper nourishment, exercise, climate, friendships, and all the other things that nourish and strengthen the vitality of body and mind.

Think about these things. They are so important.

There are many other things we can do to build the brain and nerve force. Following are a few of the most important.

Building Brain and Nerve Force

Self-esteem. Each person needs a self-introduction. Self-recognition is imperative. Man does not know himself; he is more than he realizes. Exalt people in their own eyes and you become popular and influential whether you want to be or not. They find your own higher qualities and you become great in your own eyes. It all depends on how you feel. Feel great and you become greater; feel exalted and you become more exalted; feel noble and you enoble yourself; feel honest and you grow into honesty; feel bashful and

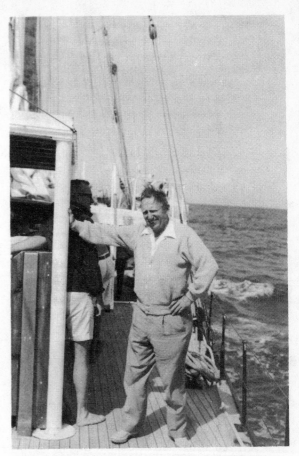

A moment of relaxation, sailing with the ocean breeze off the Australian coast. Relaxation is part of a good life.

you look like a sheep, act like a sheep, and talk and look like a sheep. But dwell upon your heavenly birth, your great mission in life, and exalt yourself in your own eyes and bashfulness will evaporate like smoke.

Sentiments and thoughts are cell builders, brain builders, and soul builders. You may just as well dwell on your own greatness as upon your own littleness. Imagination is one of the greatest forces we have. It is a great constructive force to be used and to use as one of our faculties. You will find that imagination helps to develop the greatness within you.

If you lack courage, imagine a few times a day that you are a courageous person, that you can meet anyone—the devil included. In about a year you will feel a remarkable change.

Save your nerve force until you need it. Tempers, arguments, dissipation, dances, cinemas, talk, worries, strife, anxieties, jumpiness—each and all of these are mental and physical energies. When nerve forces are not used nobly and usefully, they should be stored away in the nerve batteries. This will make you greater, more useful, more popular, more composed, mightier, and nobler. If you ever feel unable to use your own forces, you are controlled by hidden forces. That is the time you should dwell on your own greatness, fill your lungs with air, tense your fists, nerves, and muscles, call up exalted thoughts, commune with your own God that dwells within you. Then no power on or under the earth can overcome you, no devil can influence you, no schemer can intimidate you or coerce you. Learn to be your own company, learn to value your own sacred selfhood. It is the highest, noblest power you possess. Never stay too long with others. Be your own companion as long as you are building brain cells within. All have genius slumbering within. To discover it is your greatest mission.

Learn to live with Change. There is nothing permanent in life but change! It is unfortunate to get into a groove and be unable to get out. Be flexible enough to take on the new practice and become new.

As soon as we realize we cannot go through life with everything always the same, we will find that things begin to work out better.

I have reached the point where my days are completely full of change. Extra responsibilities are often forced upon me, and I have to do them. One of the finest things I have learned is to anticipate the unannounced, the unexpected. Many people are looking for business; business is looking for me. Some people are looking for complaints; complaints are looking for me. Of course we should be immersed in a regular round of activity, but it is also good to be able to deal with the unexpected.

Work with Joy. Another thing that will help to give us more vitality is to learn to enjoy our work. There is no such thing as getting out of doing your work. You will always have work to do, and you might just as well accept that fact now. So, work we shall do. But, we can work with joy. Joy makes time go by swiftly. Many persons say they have time on their hands; they say they don't know what to do with all the time they have. Well, any job which causes you to feel there is time on your hands is not an enjoyable one. For the happy man, there is no time.

Then, along with our work, we should learn to enjoy our leisure activities. When I went on a business visit to Hawaii recently, I took an hour off and went swimming. A hobby that will overtake you and thus replace some of your already busy hours is valuable. Some creative hobbies can literally steal you away from your work.

Find Joy in Color and Music. Besides a pleasurable job and a good hobby, two other things contribute to happiness: color and music. Wherever there is color, wherever there is music, you will find happy people. Color can put some people into ecstacy; music delights others.

When certain music is playing, look around and you will see toes tapping. It does something magical to the body. We are carried along with it; there is spirit in music.

There is also spirit in color. We find some colors stimulating just as we find certain music stimulating. Other colors are sedating and tranquilizing to the body.

We have all witnessed the effect of a band playing a stirring march. Men have come under the influence of martial music and have done amazing things. I had a friend in the English Army, Captian Murdo McDonald Baine. He told of seeing men practically dead come alive suddenly and stand up on their feet at the sound of Scotch bagpipes playing their national anthem. These boys, with their energies miraculously restored, would pick themsleves up and start marching to this music. It gave them a surge of spirit that nothing else could have mustered into their depleted bodies. We find that music can bring tears, joy, and laughter. It can affect the entire gamut of man's feelings.

We select our clothes as much for the color as we do for the style. I've had some suits of my own that I liked and others that I just didn't like, yet, they were all practically the same style. A brown suit, for instance, I wore only two or three times and then gave away. I didn't feel good in it. Many people go through life at home in a spectrum of colors, but they don't realize it. We have what we call "colorful moods." We talk about being green with envy and red-hot mamas. We know some people who sing the blues, and there are those people who look at the world through rose-colored glasses. Just think about it. We all live in color.

Color affects our Emotions. There are cold and warm colors. There are exciting colors and subduing colors. A lot of work can be done in a room painted red by some people, but by the end of the day they could very easily be fighting with each other. Red is a stimulating color. When a matador enters the bull ring you do not see him wearing a blue cape; he enters in a red cape. He is arousing the lowest emotions in that animal. Red also can be used in breeding. Flies that do not breed in a blue box will quite readily breed in a red box. We are all guided by the red light that means "stop." It draws attention. There is never a lethargic response to the color red.

In certain religious faiths, the believers are not allowed to wear red. In Spain, all the Catholic pomp and ceremony is found in very bright colors. In Scotland, Presbyterians and Lutherans use only the cold, quiet colors.

Different colors call forth different responses in people.

We find entirely different colors are worn in different climatic regions. The same colors are never used when it is warm as when it is cold. The gay, wild colors children wear disappear as they become adults. Perhaps grownups grow up too much.

Remedies with color. There is a lot we could see and use in nature if we knew the value of color and its effect on the body:
1. All yellow-colored foods have a laxative effect. Yellow apricots, yellow peaches, yellow castor oil, and eggs are all laxative. Senna leaves and senna flowers are yellow, and so are all the other laxatives in nature.
2. We should know not only the laxative foods but also the constipating foods. For instance, blackberrries are one of the foods that can be used when a person has diarrhea. When we understand nature, we can use this knowledge for a good purpose.

Music affects every mood. Music can do the glands a lot of good. Within music there are so many variations of consciousness that everybody can be reached. Music works through various levels of feeling, and this feeling is sparked in the glands more than in any other part of the body.

We have all heard music that makes us want to cry, and we have felt joyous with gay music. We find that in drawing us close or inspiring us, music plays on the full gamut of senses in the body, from the lowest to the highest. Fish and other animals turn away from certain kinds of music, yet those same fish and animals will turn toward other types of music.

Music has an effect upon the human body, just as it has on fish, animals, and even plant life. Certain plants will turn away from jazz but will actually bend toward such music as a Strauss Waltz. There is something about music that either repels you or draws you to it.

Music is a level of consciousness, a level of response, a level of feeling, a level of doing and growing and working. Of course, music is not the only way we get a response from the body. We get a reaction from words and color, just through their associations. There are some people we like to be around; there are others we just can't seem to stand being near. We have all experienced that—it is only human.

We usually pick the type music we like. Classical music has a soothing effect. When a person is tired, music can be quite pleasing and uplifting to him, just as some people enjoy music that makes them want to dance.

Energies in Sexual Union. We know that sex is used for procreation and the continuance of the races, but there are many more values that the average person does not know about. Recreational sex is used too much by men and women as a mere physical expression. It could become an uplifting experience. One of the greatest regeneration factors come when the unclothed body is in contact with another without overindulgence. There are some people who take energy from the other; others give energy to one another. The energies can be rebuilt in each other this way. The powers of life flowing through the body can be increased. All the physical powers as well as mental powers can grow and develop in proportion to the feeling and contentment that a person has in this contact.

Pure Fragrance—Food for the Soul. There is much talk today of the healing value of color, music, and fragrance. These three are all related in their harmonics, but perfume is the higher octave of the spectrum. Roland Hunt of California wrote a book on the subject entitled Fragrant and Radiant Healing Symphony. Many people believe fragrance is vital in promoting health, claiming it is "food for the soul," just as beauty is. They say without it the visible body will follow the spiritual into a decline. Strengthening aromas, however, must be genuine. No artificial perfumes can replace the scents of nature in building a happy old age. There is healing value in a garden, its greens and perfumes.

Bring fragrances inside. Put them in your window boxes and planters; decorate with cut flowers. Use sachets of dried lavender in your closets and thyme in your kitchen. Their fragrance will delight you, and they act as insect repellents, too. For your evenings out, buy exquisite natural perfumes made from essential oils.

Sleeping to Rest the Brain. Many people do not understand sleeping. Everybody is looking for an insomnia remedy; hundreds of gadgets have been made; hundreds of drugs have been developed. People tell me that if they could only sleep, they could relax. The secret is that if you relax, you will sleep. You learn to relax through eating warm foods, having warm feet when going to bed, drinking a little warm milk, and doing isometric exercises. A cup of valerian tea always helps, too.

But if you still can't sleep, don't despair: it has been found that 90 percent of good resting is equal to sleep. So if you are in wonderful contemplation, free of anxiety, living in joyful thinking, and allowing harmonious thoughts to pass through the mind while your eyes are closed and completely relaxed, 90 percent of that time is equal to good sleep. Just remember that sleeping is mainly for resting the brain.

Music before sleeping helps a person to relax. Dr. Fournier Pescay used the music of a flute for insomnia in the case of his own son.

See that hypersensitive children have rest in the afternoon by lying in a dark room with no disturbances. Whether they are asleep or not makes no difference. Do this in the afternoon when they come home from school. Some moments of quiet rest will give their metabolism a chance to slow down after all the mental and physical activity of the day. Then allow them to go out and play. Slow music is also very good for a hypersensitive child.

We should try to get a hard mattress for our sleep. If necessary, put a board between the mattress and the springs. There are some people who sleep better in the presence of a different atmosphere and even with a perfumed atmosphere.

I remember while in Austria that when we pulled down the covers of the bed one night to go to bed, there was a lavender sachet bag in the bed. The sachet added a very pleasant feeling to the atmosphere, and we fell asleep very quickly.

Make sure your bedroom is painted in a pastel color, using greens and blues. They are cooling colors and do not stimulate the mental or nervous system.

Warm feet are very important to sleep. Walking ten minutes in sand or grass to build up the circulation in the legs will help you to have warm feet. Warm feet allow for perfect relaxation when we go to bed.

Insomnia can sometimes be caused more from bowel troubles than anything else. Other causes are late hours, excessive mental labor, close study and figuring, sluggish liver, dull spleen, insufficient secretions, low blood temperature, coffee, tea, tobacco, too much blood in the brain, neuralgia, pain, anemia, an excessive sex desire, a wrong climate or altitude, the improper diet, or having too much protein (especially meat) late at night. Remedies include hot foot baths, hot mustard foot baths, changes in your work, sleep between sundown and midnight, a vacation, warm drinks, a light supper, quietness, pleasurable evening walks, hot tea in the evening, letting the world die, easy breathing, non-use of the brain in the evening, cultivation of uplifting thoughts in the evening.

Nightmares or hallucinations are caused by too much food at suppertime. Night sweating indicates an iron deficiency. Insomnia sometimes indicates a calcium deficiency, magnesium, or phosphorus deficiency.

Some good herb teas for sleeping include valerian, hops, catnip, and black cohosh. A combination herb tea that helps to promote natural and refreshing sleep can be made from hops, valerian root, and scullcap.

A good juice tonic is a combination of celery and lettuce.

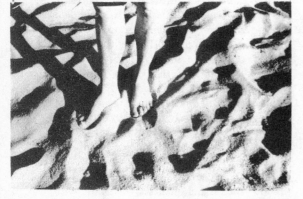

Walking in the sand is one of the greatest circulation builders for the whole body, bringing blood to the brain and preventing senility to settle in the brain areas.

Sleeping Nude. People should sleep in the nude. We get into clothes in the morning to hold ourselves together; we jump out of our clothes at night and before we can hardly drop them to the floor, we jump into pajamas and more clothing.

Our bodies should be kept loose and free at night so that we can turn and move in any direction without any restrictions. You will get more rest. You will better restore the brain force for the next day. It's impossible for the body to rest properly with corsets, garments or bras in the way.

Snoring. Sometimes snoring hinders good sleeping. A good remedy is to place a small quantity of sesame seed oil or peanut oil in each nostril before retiring. This prevents drying out of the nose. Drying automatically opens the mouth, and snoring begins. It is claimed that this oil treatment is as effective as the sledge hammer or rolling-pin.

Do not sleep on the back. Have polyps in the nose broken down through massage. Stop using heavy starches. Taking the time to be sure that you have peaceful and restful sleep will make a new person out of you. Avoid negative and destructive thoughts at all times, but especially before going to sleep. You should pack up such thoughts and send them off into the purifying light of exalted thinking.

A Mental Formula That Works. To increase serenity for sleeping, on going to bed, relieve yourself of the day's problems and accept the last thoughts you have at night as the thoughts you want to ring through your subconscious mind all night. Say to yourself, "My nerves are strong and calmer. I feel in harmony with myself, with the universe, and with everything around me. I am rich with inner powers that give me harmony, security, and serenity. No one—nothing—can separate me from unity with Higher Powers which protect me from all evils. The Higher Powers make me invincible."

New Vitality to Start Your Day. You can bring vitality and energy into the body through your mind. For new vitality say this at the beginning of the day, repeat it three times, say it consciously, think it deeply each time you repeat:

"I am filled with health and the joy of Living.
There is sunshine in my soul today.
The clouds have rolled away and I feel
Confident, reassured—ever so confident.

I feel young, ever so young.
Every day in every way I feel younger and younger.
I feel like a new and wonderful personality, and I can overcome everything
With the greatest of ease. I feel Wonderful—Truly Wonderful!"

Building the Nerves

Feeding the Nerves. Nerves must be fed—mentally as well as physically. Behind every function of the body, nerve action is needed. Your eyes are an extension of the brain. They are nerves. Many times eyes are broken down because the nervous system has been used too much. Many people have nervous breakdowns because their eyes are being used too much, possibly they are reading too much. Doctors' records of people who see a lot of motion pictures show that the constant flickering of the film can produce epilepsy. Some people develop a tendency to have convulsions from looking at motion pictures. Many people develop epilepsy from looking at television. Doctors know this from hospital reports. I also have these reports.

Many things can harm the nervous system. It is affected through the eyes, through the mind; you are always thinking. You can wear out the best flint in the world with a little water. Remember this if you let "flickering thoughts" affect your mind.

Outdoor Activity. Dr. Rickly, one of the greatest naturopaths of the past, found that he could normalize the thyroid gland by putting a person out in the air. Putting a person with either an overactive or underactive thyroid out into the air normalizes the metabolism quicker than anything else. We need air, and to a nervous person it is the most soothing massage to give to the nervous system. Get air and wind to the body.

Warm Baths. Sarah Bernhardt, a famous French actress (1844-1923), said she never could have carried on her wonderful work without warm baths. Sometimes I think warm baths are overdone, but when we work under tension, we need relaxation. Napoleon, in order to carry on his work, always carried a bathtub with him. He felt the need to have a warm bath during his campaigns.

Skin Brushing. Massage is also wonderful for the nerves. A good massage bath is the skin brushing bath. Use a dry brush and brush the entire body. Do it every morning before you put on your clothes. It will do more for the nerves and the body than anything else I can tell you. Use a natural bristle brush. Never nylon.

Egg Yolks Feed the Nerves. I want to tell you of a tonic which is splendid for the nerves. Dr. Alexis Carrel (a French surgeon and biologist, 1873-1944) at one time worked with a chicken's heart. He put it in blood plasma, thinking that blood was a complete food and that he could keep this heart alive. In two weeks time it started to degenerate to such an extent it could not regenerate itself. Before the heart died completely, he started feeding egg yolk to the chicken's heart tissue, and it revived, living over thirty years.

I consider egg yolk one of the finest foods for the nervous system. You don't have to have it raw. You can have it cooked, but I don't believe it should be fried. There are many ways to cook eggs. The part of the egg yolk which is so good for the nervous system is called vitellin. Vitellin goes along with lecithin. Lecithin is a brain and nerve fat, and it is also found in egg yolk. Egg yolk is a far richer source of lecithin than any other food, although soy beans, avocado, and olives also contain liberal amounts of lecithin.

We must recognize that egg yolk is one of our fattiest foods. The liver and gall bladder must take care of that fat. Whenever you serve egg yolk, be sure to serve with it a food for the liver. The best liver and gall bladder food is greens. The most specific food is dandelion greens or dandelion tea. One of the finest nerve tonics is magnesium chlorophyll, available in your health food store. Another splendid tonic is a teaspoonful of chlorophyll in a little cherry concentrate or grape concentration base (foods high in iron and good for the liver). Put egg yolk in this for a complete nerve food. Don't overdo it. Have it only once a day. Just add it to your regular way of living.

In Italy many doctors use this tonic for treating patients going through the change of life. It helps to control hot flashes and other disorders caused by the change of life.

The egg yolk may be slightly cooked and eaten separately, but be sure to have something green at the same time. Do you remember how Grandmother served poached eggs on spinach? That was a good combination. Serve poached eggs on beet greens, Swiss chard or have it with a salad. Then when it is carried to the liver it will not cause trouble.

Sprouts. One of the finest sources of protein is the sprouted seed. Alfalfa seeds, wheat kernels, and even garbanzos are wonderful when sprouted. You can grind them or put them into various dishes. Have them in your salads. Sprouts are wonderful for the nerves.

In Germany a short time ago doctors experimented with about 100 patients who had multiple sclerosis, which is a degeneration of the nervous system and the spinal cord. Some of the patients were cases for which medical treatment could do nothing. They were given green juices and sprouts as the main part of their meals. Every one of them improved; 15 percent totally recovered. Food does affect the nervous system. Food affects our entire body.

Avoid Excessive Noise

Noise can break down the nerve force and leave a person weak and depleted. A recent news article, headlined "Nerve Ailments Linked to Airport," explained:

"Residents living near the Los Angeles International Airport suffer a higher rate of nervous breakdowns than people less exposed to constant jet noise, according to a University of California at Los Angeles study.

"Prof. William C. Meecham, a UCLA engineering professor who conducted the three-year study, found that mental hospital admissions for persons living within a three-mile radius of the airport ran 29 percent higher than for residents some six miles away.

"His findings closely supported earlier British statistics which showed a 31 percent increase in the nervous breakdown rate above the national norm for neighbors of London's busy Heathrow Airport, Meecham noted.

"The UCLA expert on aeroacoustics analyzed the geographical distribution of residents referred to mental hospitals by South Bay Mental Health Service in reaching his conclusions.

"He counted patients living in what he called the maximum noise area in Inglewood, where the jet noise level is at 90 decibels, and selected a control area in El Segundo some three miles to the south for comparison.

"Meecham said the two areas are similar in their social and economic makeup and since few of their residents could afford private physicians for mental problems most cases probably passed through the county-supported South Bay Center.

"The 90-decibel level in the maximum noise area is considered by acoustic experts as hazardous to mental and physical health and may trigger social tensions and a wide range of physical health problems," he explained.

Best Brain and Nerve Foods

How can we best strengthen our brain and nerve force through food?

We need lecithin and the nerve salts, both found in egg yolk and prune juice. We need phosphates as found in yellow corn meal. We need animal proteins, including cheese and dairy products. Animal phosphorus is necessary for building brain and nerve energies. Vegetable phosphorus builds mostly the physical organs and the bones.

We can get brain building material from all of our foods, but there are some mental faculties that use more of one kind of food for repair than another. Those mental faculties that are used for love, veneration, and similar feelings can use the phosphorus from apples and other fruit.

The best brain foods are silicon foods, as found in oat straw tea, barley gruel, shavegrass tea and bran tea, all used between meals. Manganese is found in high quantity in Missouri black walnuts and is wonderful for the memory centers. The high phosphorus content of North Atlantic fish is considered a wonderful brain food. Often use fish broths and clam broth or juice.

The finnan haddie and smoked black cod are the finest of all fish. I know there are some vegetarians who will disagree, but if you want to build nerve and brain structure, you have to have amino acids, which come only from animal products. We also can get these from eggs, cheese, milk, and soybeans.

Grape juice or whey with lemon juice is very good if the brain carries a lot of heat or if there is a lot of congestion in brain areas.

A good herb drink for the brain and nervous system can be made by stewing together one oz. each of vervain, mistletoe, and valerian steelcaps in two quarts of water for twenty minutes. Drink two or three glasses per day.

For poor memory use sodium and manganese foods and vitamin B complex with the RNA factor. Also good is a juice tonic of carrot, celery, and prune, with rice polishings; rosemary and sage teas; and slant board exercises.

An alert, quick mind needs phosphorus, calcium, and silicon foods. Heavy mental work needs selenium. Phosphorus and sulphur foods improve ability to make decisions.

Hysteria and crying spells often indicate an iron deficiency. Pronunciation difficulties indicate an iodine deficiency. Fits and migraine often indicate malnutrition of brain and glands. For a tendency to fainting spells, use rue tea and gentian tea.

The Goal of the Disciple

*The goal of the disciple is within himself—
it is God.
Many in the world seek outside of themselves;
That is why their lives are full of discontent.
Everything is within,
Be always content,
Then there are no obstacles on the way
to attainment.
Never desire more suffering or joy than
is necessary.
No one is measured by the number of
sufferings
He goes through,
But by what he has learned from them.
Have Peace internally, externally, and
eternally.
If love cannot give Peace, it is not Love.
He who lives in Love is always young,
Calling the powers of Heaven to his aid.
Go in Peace . . .
Then healing enters into the body.*
(Author Unknown)

The blood

A person can't be healthy without healthy blood. The blood distributes and stores food, collects waste throughout the body and helps eliminate it, regulates the heat in the body, kills germ life, and above all, carries its secretions to the various organs that are in need of it.

We respond immediately to the adrenal gland substance carried by the blood through the lymph stream to every cell in the body. Every bit of blood in the body travels through the thyroid glands every hour and a half. Silicon in the blood speeds through the body to reach the toe nails, the hair, and other extremities that require it. The same blood that is depositing the calcium in the bone will also deposit whatever calcium is needed in the transverse colon to keep it from developing a prolapsus.

The blood travels through the body at a rate of thirty feet per second, sterilizing wounds, distributing cell building chemicals of digested foods and taking away broken down cell wastes. It constitutes about one-twelfth of the body weight. When normal it resists all disease.

But chronic colds, pneumonia, bronchial troubles, and catarrhal disturbances lower the resistance of the body and take away the vital values of the blood. And those ailments get a foothold when the body is weakened by improper care. Bad food is one culprit: it takes away the good from our body. A pint of champagne will put twenty percent of the blood cells out of commission. Salt dries it out; and distilled vinegar and whiskey are literally embalming.

Remedies to Promote Healthy Blood

Higher Altitude — More Oxygen in Our Blood. High altitude is a great help in building a healthy body. It quickens the thyroid gland so that oxygen can enter the bloodstream. We must remember, that oxygen demands the chemical iron because iron attracts oxygen. You could breathe from now until infinity and never have oxygen in the body unless you have enough iron in the blood. The tissues will never be oxidized without iron.

The higher the altitude above sea level, the greater amount of oxygen we take in. At ocean level our blood count can go as high as five million. For example, those living on the shores of Norway average a blood count of five million. In Peru, where elevations reach about 12,000, the average blood count can run from seven to eight million. While we need a high count for good health, our body cannot respond to extremely high altitudes, especially if we have heart trouble. We would most likely end up panting, nauseated, and perhaps vomiting. We must therefore be careful in choosing our altitude. We should not overlook or ignore it.

Circulation

Venous Congestion. When the arteries or veins become clogged, high blood pressure can develop. Blood does not pass through the capillaries as fast as it should and anemia begins to develop in the brain. Proneness to strokes increases. This is why it is so important to keep the blood on the move. Soreness and pressure on the nerves of the legs can be a sign of venous congestion. Whenever we have cramps in the legs, we should look first to venous congestion. Look to the veins and see that they are draining the blood well.

Ways to Improve Circulation. There are many things we can do to help our circulation. It's always best to take care of the heart first. The heart is one of the strongest organs in the body. Many people develop fears about a weak heart. But there are many things you can do to make it strong again.

To begin with, start a program of slow

walking. I specifically prescribe slow walking, because overexertion can break down a weak heart. Build it up gradually each day.

There are also natural foods that help strengthen the heart. Try liquid chlorophyll, vitamin E, and hawthorne berry tea, for instance. Avoid beef.

A fast pulse is usually caused by a thyroid condition. Many times the thyroid controls the heartbeat, and if we would take care of our emotional system, many times we wouldn't have thyroid trouble which eventually leads to heart trouble. Our mind gets to the heart by way of the thyroid gland.

Breathing Outdoors. Breathing out in the fresh air is excellent for circulation. Massage of the body, massaging toward the heat, is good. Quick inhalations and slow exhalations are good. Make sure the peristaltic action in the bowel is good. When this action is slow, activity in the bowel and circulation of blood are also slow.

Cheerfulness. We must develop cheerfulness for good circulation. Cultivate your love emotions; they're a necessary function. This doesn't necessarily mean sexual love, but it does mean love for people, love for surroundings. Love has many connotations and we should try to see all the facets of life affected by love. Each of us knows that we love to be loved. Go where you are loved and live so that you love others. Love is important to all our lives. As my mother used to say, "Hate and fear only hurt the people who use them." You don't have to love your enemy for his sake; you don't have to love your neighbor for his sake; but you *must love for your own good.* Most of us are our own worst enemy. That's where love has to begin. Love is your best friend.

Exercise. Our circulation improves when we learn to contract the muscles in all parts of the body. There are many forms of exercise that are good for the whole body. I'm not recommending strenuous exercise that builds big muscles and strains the heart, but rational muscular activity that keeps the cells of the body alive and vigorous. Such an exercise is walking; but I think we should learn to hike, not just walk. Hiking is going into the hills, going up hills and down. Remember to avoid overexertion. Walking on ground that is not flat helps to develop the small muscles in the leg structure. We develop only the long muscle structure when we walk on sidewalks or the street. Anytime we are using the muscle structure in the arches of our feet on uneven ground, we develop the small muscles. That is why we have the sand and grass walk. There isn't anything finer to build up circulation in the body, especially the legs and lower extremities, than the sand and grass walks.

Swimming exercises every muscle in the body at one time. It is the finest exercise known, developing good circulation while we are in a prone position. Golfing is also an excellent exercise. It entails much walking and gives the mind needed relaxation. Not all of us are so situated that we can spend several afternoons a week on the golf links.

Walking, on the other hand, does not require expensive equipment or membership in a club. Everyone who is able to be up and around can get in some walking every day, even though it may be only walking to and from your work. Walk from two to five miles a day and at the end of three months you'll feel like a different person.

People who have sluggish circulation have to quicken it; this is done through quickening their thoughts and body through exercise and work. Some people have to slow down, to learn to rest, to be still and quiet. Being quiet sometimes is very important, too, and to breathe slowly controls emotional strain.

Kneipp Baths. The Kneipp bath is a wonderful water treatment for better circulation in the legs. It also relieves heart pressure. The bath consists of splashing through a 25 to 30 foot walk in cold water up to the knees, then a barefoot walk in grass or sand until you are dry. Do not wipe dry; if you do, you lose the value of the bath. The value is in warming your own circulation and working to make sure that the circulation takes care of that cold water. This builds up the resistance in the body to take care of ordinary drafts and ordinary problems.

Another way of taking the bath is with a common garden hose, without the sprinkler attachment. Run cold water starting at the farthest point from the heart, which would be the ankle of the right leg, move the water in a stream from the toes to the groin, then around and down the back of leg to the ankle. Spray first the right leg front and back, two or three times; then do the left leg in the same manner. You should be able to count to six while running water up and down each leg. This is very good for circulation of the entire body. Again, don't dry off. Run or walk until dry and warm. Do it once a day.

Grass Walk. In the early morning, while the dew is still on the grass, get out in your bare feet and shuffle up and down a few minutes. This will do wonders for the circulation, and, if begun in summer, can be carried through most of the winter in temperate climates; thus one can sleep with warm feet.

Sand Walk. Walking barefoot in sand is excellent for the feet and helps the circulation. Walk on the beach without shoes as a before breakfast exercise or set up a long "sand box" in your own yard to use as a "walk." If possible, walk in four or five inches of water while at the beach and walking in the sand.

Hot and Cold Water Baths. If you cannot take the Kneipp bath, you can take hot and cold water baths. Put your feet in hot water for one minute then into cold water for half a minute. Make this change five times. It helps the circulation tremendously.

Sitz Baths. Sitz baths or foot baths are very conducive to good circulation. They get the blood moving. We use hot and cold foot and sitz baths for moving blood along. Warm water brings the blood to the surface and cold water drives it away again. In this way good circulation is developed in the bloodstream.

Warm Feet. Cold feet affect the entire body and we cannot sleep, or for that matter, do anything comfortably. The entire circulation is dependent upon keeping the feet warm.

Kneipp Baths, Grass Walking, Sand Walking at ranch for building good leg circulation for a better bloodstream.

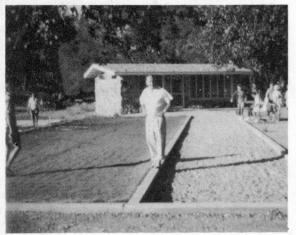

Living in the sunshine, breathing plenty of good fresh air, sleeping where the air is active, and in other ways getting close to nature are the life-building principles. Children especially should keep their feet warm. Particularly keep children's ankles warm, since the ankles are a very vital center in the body and definitely should be kept warm.

Breathing. There are various techniques for driving blood into different parts of the body. This can be accomplished through taking in a full breath and applying pressure to the specific organ or area you are trying to affect. Then relax while exhaling. Inhaling a full breath and holding drives blood into the liver area. Quick inhalations and slow exhalations are good for the body and help development of lungs. Rue herb tea helps with difficulty in breathing.

Sniff Breathing Exercise: Walk three steps sniffing deeper at each step. Exhale on the fourth step. Do not breathe for the next three steps. Then repeat.

Breathing benefits good circulation in many ways. The Valley Forge Heart Institute revealed that cholesterol and triglyceride levels of joggers and long distance runners were lower than those of the average man.

Foods and Circulation. There are a few foods that work well to increase the vitality of the circulation. Make sure that the liver is not overworked through the ingestion of too much coffee, sweets, and starches. Keep the liver clear and clean by taking iron foods; vegetable juices are best. Of course, herb teas are also good. If you know you have liver trouble, take dandelion tea, dandelion root coffee, liquid chlorophyll drinks, and cherry juice.

In the wintertime keep the venous congestion down — congestion evidenced by blue flesh, a blue discoloration under eyes, or blue fingernails. Get those cold feet and hands warm by drinking sage tea for this. Raw cucumber juice is wonderful for any venous congestion, and don't forget parsley juice.

There is a wonderful food for people called rice bran syrup. It's made from the polishings of rice. It's one of the foods highest in vitamin B content; it is also high in nicotinic acid. Doctors have found that the use of nicotinic acid can drive the blood into the ear structure and help those who have difficulty hearing. The same principle— and remedy—works with the eyes. Sometimes the eyes fail to function properly because the circulation in the head is poor. Through the use of nicotinic acid, doctors can quicken the circulation and drive the blood into the head, into the arms and hands, and down into the leg structure.

Vein Problems

Superficial Veins in Lower Extremities. The superficial veins of the lower extremities bear a heavier burden than any other vein in the body. They carry along a heavy column of blood extending almost perpendicularly from the sole of the foot to the heart.

In persons with weak connective tissue, the valves and the walls of these superficial veins yield to this heavy pressure. The valves become incompetent; the blood ceases to flow toward the heart and stagnates in the veins. Nodes form in tubes or veins with wide flocculations. These are known as varicose veins. The circulation is impaired when the blood stagnates. The surrounding tissues are damaged by the waste products that collect in the area (veins carry the toxic blood). The tissue around these areas breaks down many times faster and ulcers are produced. The best remedy for varicose veins is prevention.

If you have weak veins, pick out an occupation that does not require you to be on your feet continuously for hours. You should not be a baker, motorman, conductor, grocer, postman or laundry worker.

Gymnastic exercises help to strengthen these veins. The barefoot sand walk, barefoot grass walk and the Kneipp foot baths are exceptionally good. Leg baths, massage, slant board, leg exercises and wearing lower heels could also help greatly.

Remedy for Varicose Veins. In dealing with varicose veins, savoy cabbage can be used as packs. Take the cellulose structure from the center of these cabbage leaves and roll the leaves out flat with a bottle or rolling pin. After you have manipulated the leaves to make them soft, put them flat on the veins. You can walk around, leaving them on all day if you wish. If you are working in the daytime, put them on every night. It is a wonderful remedy for anyone with heavy varicose veins.

It would be helpful if you put your legs up at every opportunity, and if you took an exercise break every hour, if possible.

Another remedy for these veins uses 20 Mule Team Borax: take one tablespoon of Borax to about one gallon of hot water. Soak for approximately ten minutes or longer if possible. This mixture is also good for packs on the legs. Dip cloths into the mixture, wrap them around the legs and leave them on all night. When you use hot water packs on varicose veins, do not walk around—stay off your feet! Use cold water on legs if you are going to walk around after a hot bath.

Still another treatment is to keep your feet above the rest of the body at night. This doesn't mean to elevate the foot end of the bed, because we don't want all the soft organs of the abdomen pushing against the heart area all night. Simply elevate your feet by putting a pillow under them.

Remedies for Fragile Veins. One of the best ways to help veins that break is rutin, which is found in buckwheat and has what they call the antifatigue factor. Rutin, however, should always be taken with vitamin C. Vitamin E is also good in all muscular conditions, since the veins are part muscle. We must also use silicon to back up the treatment. This the chemical element that makes veins stronger. Oat straw tea and the daily use of rice polishings are also very necessary. (To make oat straw tea, cover ordinary clean oat hay, oat straw or chaff with cold water. Bring to a boil and boil gently for ten minutes. Strain carefully.) Use more vegetable broths and less fruits. Potato peeling broth is one of the best broths to use. Consider the liver and toxin in the blood and the elimination program. Using our elimination diet will also benefit.

It would also be wise to consider quick inhalation; slow exhalation; games; laughter; change of scenery; change of occupation; pleasing companionship; proper glandular release; developing a strong feeling of love and good will for one another; clearing the mind of worry, fretting, and stewing; and stopping the production of fatique acids.

Ulcerations Inside the Legs. Ulcerations can be formed on the inside of the blood vessels and calcium can deposit in the form of microscopically small granules and combine to form placks. In extreme cases the entire vascular wall may become cemented with calcium and various deposits.

Several things can interfere with the passage of blood through the legs and result in ulcerations and placks. Some possible causes are prolapsus of the bowel, prolonged crossing of the legs, wearing garters, constipation, the existence of spinal distortion bad arches in the feet, the wearing of poor shoes, pregnancy, overeating and prolonged sitting.

Understanding and Correcting Anemia

Anemia responds best to iron foods. Iron attracts oxygen—all the oxygen you could breathe would never do any good unless you had iron in the blood. We have breathing specialists going about telling you how to breathe, but we must have iron in the blood to attract the oxygen.

The food that we have to consider most is the food that will take care of and build a good bloodstream. If the blood is not healthy, it won't do an adequate job of taking remedies to other parts of the body. If a condition of anemia exists, therefore, it should always be handled first.

In treating anemia, the best iron food is black cherry juice and blackberry juice. These are two of the highest iron foods. (As a drink, blackberry juice is constipating, and as a drink, black cherry juice is a laxative.) Eat strawberries and wild cherries.

Remember, anything green always has a lot of iron in it. Anything grown above the ground has an abundance of iron. Use green and leafy vegetables, spinach, concentrated chlorophyll from alfalfa, wild clover honey, Concord grape juice, watercress, romaine lettuce, brown goat cheese, warm foaming goat's milk, eggs (either raw or cooked under

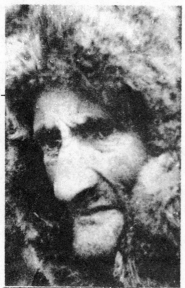

This is a man who was in a concentration camp practically starved to death and we find that he is only 27 years of age in this photo. Going home to his family, they did not know their own son. This is what starvation and malnourishment can do to the human body.

very low temperature), red pepper used in marrow soup, cod liver oil, and sweet cream.

Rocine is also recommended: one tablespoon of macerated calves' liver juice in Concord grape juice three times a day.

Chew all food well. Make sure the teeth are in good condition. Sometimes liquefied foods are necessary when digestion is low and poor.

Watercress is a powerful blood purifier. It is very delicious, although it is peppery. Watercress is now classified a vegetable. Whether eaten as a vegetable or made into a tea, you can get good results if it is eaten regularly over an extended period. Also good are pungent bitter salad greens.

Other tonics for blood building: foods that contain silicon, iron, sodium, and chlorine. Red cabbage, coconut, fish, fish roe, oat and barley preparations, beets in abundance, Chinese cabbage, and salads are especially good. Include in your diet parsley juice, dandelion juice, dandelion greens, wild lettuce, tomato juice, desiccated liver, tops of vegetables, sarsaparilla tea, nettles tea, and raw juice from onions, from cucumbers, and from lettuce.

In conditions of anemia, use no iced or cold foods or drinks.

Other things you should know to help anemic condition: protect the vital parts of the body, such as the brain, sex organs, eyes, and breast, from extreme temperatures, long exposure to the sun, and washing with harmful solutions. Short but adequate periods in the sunshine helps to control the calcium which comes from eating the iron foods, deep breathing and being in higher altitudes. Warm salt baths help to get rid of uric acid.

Get a brain change; get a new outlook on life; get plenty of rest and sleep in moving air. Sleep out of doors, on the ground if possible. Try sleeping on pine needle mattresses.

For tension-relaxing exercises try rowing, which is good for the lungs, too; mountain climbing in a breezy climate or forest air; going to the mountains, buying a goat, and living on the south side of the hill.

Cast out fear. Stop using the motor force of the brain, such as that which is used in leadership, driving in traffic, working with a high-pressure boss, antagonism, resistive feelings, lecturing, gossiping, and the heavy responsibilities of executive positions.

Anemia can be caused from an emotional soul, a weak will, and a lack of potassium salts, calcium salts, magnesium salts, chlorides and iron salts.

Anemic blood lacks iron, solid matter, and albumen, and instead is full of water. Anemic people need the mineral salts.

A sentimental mind can cause anemia. These people must have a change of scene, rest and sleep, development of the will faculties, nerve tension exercises, plenty of sunlight (never excessive), gymnastics, lots of oxygen and warm salt baths, horseback exercise, games, golf, warm baths with sudden cold showers at the close to stimulate circulation, mountain air, breezy climate, scenic surroundings.

Send the anemic to the mountians where the elements play havoc, where the air is alive and pure, and where nature develops the will faculties.

"Gravitosis"

A new disease will be identified in the future, and it will probably be called "Gravitosis." We recognize the condition when we become tired. The legs begin to give way, varicose veins begin to form, and the veins in the legs begin to break. Gravity is pulling the blood downhill, making it possible to become anemic in the head.

All sick people who come to us are anemic in the head. They have a lack of blood in the head. In this gravity pull, the heart does not have the energy to work the blood uphill against gravity. Tissues, expecially those in the arteries and the muscles of the legs, cannot contract properly to force the blood uphill. This is how the head becomes anemic.

Why do you suppose the tiredness center is in the topmost part of the brain? When this center becomes anemic, it tells you that it is time to rest. It tells you that the body should be lying out prone so that the blood can circulate properly.

Blood Pressure Problems

Low Blood Pressure. When the adrenal glands become low in hormone function, we find that the blood pressure is lowered. On the other hand, adrenalin coming from the adrenal gland raises the blood pressure. Adrenalin is one the most powerful bodily substances known to us. It is almost a poison when you stop to think of its immediate effects on the various parts of the body. It is present in the blood in dilutions ranging from one to two billion to one to one billion. The fantastic dilutions of this hormone through the body produces extreme reactions and does it very quickly. It acts like an oxidative ferment during nerve cell activity. It dilates the pupils, contracts the capillaries and seems to play a part in the formation of skin pigment.

When a person has a disease of the adrenals the skin becomes pigmented, ranging from light yellow to dark brown. While the adrenalin raises the blood pressure, it has the opposite effect on the bronchial tubes and the intestines. The bronchial tubes dilate, and the intestine relaxes under the influence of adrenalin. This is why they give adrenalin to the person who has bronchial congestion, especially in asthmatic attacks. The tone of the heart muscles is increased with the adrenalin hormone in the blood. Many allergies are taken care of with adrenalin when the effects are attacks of hives after eating strawberries, tomatoes, crabs, oysters, etc.

Bringing Up the Blood Pressure. We find that protein stimulation seems to quicken the body and will raise the blood pressure. In all cases of low blood pressure an extra amount of protein is indicated. This is one time when, if permitted, we add meat to our diet. On the other hand, if we need just extra protein we should use cheeses, milk, eggs, etc.

The Sun Raises Your Blood Pressure. The action of sunlight on the skin also produces a substance which contracts the blood vessels of the skin and thus raises the blood pressure. On this account persons who must avoid any rise in blood pressure, such as cardiac and pulmonary patients, should be very cautious when taking sun baths.

Lowering the Blood Pressure. Whey and other sodium foods can be used to bring blood pressure down if there are no heart complications. Sodium is one of the elements that is so necessary for relaxing the arteries, dissolving cholesterol, and any hardening of the arteries; however, we cannot use an excess of sodium in the diet if there are heart problems. When this hardening in the body must be dissolved by the slower process, we can resort to the extra amount of potassium found in our foods. The use of many of the herbs that help the kidneys to act and take out hard excretions from the body are buchu leaf tea, shavegrass, and cornsilk tea.

Fear Dilutes the Adrenal's Function. Fear and resentment will wear out the adrenal gland more than any other thing. The adrenal glands are responsible for the hair standing erect in time of fear and troubles. If a person lives in constant resentment and fear, his body will eventually dilute and break down the adrenal glands and hormones to such an extent that he will develop low blood pressure.

Low blood pressure can come from extreme enervation in the body or when our bodies are debilitated from overwork. It can come when the arteries are weak, the heartbeat skips, there is poor support of the heart elements, or we have an impoverished blood supply.

Things To Do for Low Blood Pressure.

1. Add protein to the body. Sometimes you need animal proteins to bring the blood pressure up.

2. Have enough hydrochloric acid.

3. Make sure you also take a good blood-builder.

4. Get into something you love to do.

5. Use cold water treatments which build up the blood pressure.

6. Get exercise and be with stimulating friends rather than those who are depressing.

High Blood Pressure

Many people have high blood pressure. How can it be dealt with?

1. Nine times out of ten, if you will get rid of your excess weight, high blood pressure comes right down.

2. High Blood pressure usually goes along with hypertension. It is usually found in a person who has an overactive mind, he's too ambitious, he's critical, too serious, driving himself, he is an extrovert. There are many factors that can produce high blood pressure, and we always check on the mental status first. It is important to know that a person has a good philosophy and uses his philosophy — that he lives a more placid life.

3. Blood pressure can be altered by glandular conditions; for instance, the pituitary gland can bring up a blood pressure. An aggressive person in many cases has an overactive thyroid, which can raise blood pressure. The adrenal glands can also be responsible for blood pressure disturbances.

4. Diet has a lot to do with blood pressure. Meat is one of the things that keeps blood pressure up. A meat meal stimulates the heart and circulation 26 percent while a vegetarian meal stimulates the heart 6 percent. When we have extreme high blood pressure a fast for a few days may help. But don't go longer than three days if you are not under a doctor's supervision. You can also go on either fruit or vegetable juices for a few days, making sure that the bowels are regulated. During a fast or juice regime, we must take enemas to make certain that the bowels are free of any toxic waste, if they're not moving.

Use carrot juice diets or the grape diet; they are both capable of bringing blood pressure down. Cut out citrus fruits also. At least one meal a day should consist of cooked brown rice and vegetables or rice with a stewed fruit. You could have this at lunch every day, then follow my regular diet.

In many cases, where blood pressure has been very high, we have two rice meals a day. If we want to bring the blood pressure down very quickly and still allow a person to eat, we give them as much as three rice meals a day.

5. We need to make sure that the environment is right. Make certain that your occupation is not too demanding, that the boss doesn't keep you under too much pressure. Make sure you are not overworking, putting in too many hours at work. Make sure you are living in harmony with your family, that your children are not disturbing you to the point where you need to have a watchful eye even when you are sleeping.

Get to the point where the body works under tranquility, serenity and calmness.

6. Above all, take care of the skin. Brushing the skin takes care of the kidneys, and many high blood pressure cases accompany weak kidneys. When we have this type of high blood pressure, we should be sure to seek the help of a doctor.

Wherever blood is needed in the body, the fibers relax and the vessels dilate. Actually the caliber of the vessel is determined by the degree of tonus or the state tension. We have a good example of the tension and relaxation of blood vessels in the blanching and the blushing of the face.

7. When the muscle fibers of the blood vessels underlying the skin of the face relax, the vessels dilate and the individual blushes. When the muscles contract, the vessels become narrow and the face becomes pale. When we have chronic spasms of the vascular muscles it not only causes high blood pressure but can also cause hypertension in parts of the body. When we have spasms of the cerebral arteries we can develop fainting spells. Spasms of the coronary arteries can cause angina pectoris. It is well to realize that our attitude of mind has a lot to do with the spasms, tensions and relaxation of the muscle structure of the body.

Angina Problems. For angina troubles, pains in the left arm, pains in the center of the chest, seek a doctor's care. Find out if you actually do have heart trouble, or if the pain is caused simply by gas pressures or other causes. You may have to take care of the cholesterol deposits.

Sexual System in Relation to Blood. The blood-making capacity of the system depends upon the strength and development of the sex brain and the conditon of the sexual system. The red corpuscles are very important for good health, sexuality, youthful appearance, and personal magnetism. There are many agents that increase the red corpuscles: a good married life, cultivation of the affections, a strong sexuality, a strong amativeness, outdoor exercises, cheerfulness, foods coming immediately from nature, spending some part of the day in the free and open air—in the sunshine where the vegetable kingdom is in a flourishing condition, living where there is an abundance of greens around you. (There is a life principle in the oxygen given off by the vegetable kingdom.)

Remedies for Blood Problems

There are certain remedies that have become standards for certain problems with the circulatory system. Here are a few.

For circulatory system and heart:
Green Drink
Liquefy a small handful of parsley and alfalfa sprouts in a cup of unsweetened pineapple juice. Sip slowly. This drink is excellent for the heart and circulatory system.

For the heart:
Potassium Cocktail
Mix
¼ cup celery juice
½ cup carrot juice
¼ cup of the following, combined in equal parts: spinach juice, beet top juice, and parsley juice

Honey Treat
1 teaspoon honey diluted in 1 glass of water. Drink two or three times a day.

For venous congestion:
Elder Flower Tea
1 teaspoon elder flower herb
1 cup boiling water
Steep three minutes, strain, sweeten with honey if desired. This tea brings on perspiration and is also good for the skin.

For varicose veins:
Oat Straw Packs
Make up your oat straw tea in the usual manner, strain it, but keep the straw. Make the straw into a warm pack and wrap it around the congested area, leaving it on all night long. Do this for a period of thirty days. Drink the tea, which is high in silicon.

Here are typical blood-related problems and their best remedies.

Hemorrhages: Increase iron intake. Use Vitamin K. Use burnett, comfrey, plantain, nettle tea, shepherd's purse.

Iron-poor blood: Use greens to build, as well as black cherries and strawberries.

Circulation problems: Spinach and celery juice with sulphur foods.

For cleanser: Use sage and watercress. Use bran tonic for one month.

Poor coagulation: Use chlorophyll.

Low blood count: Will increase with chlorophyll supplement and higher altitude.

Discharges; Increase manganese intake.

Clotting problems: Increase calcium intake. Use figwort.

Walk the Upright Man

That's the food side of it. But we can't neglect the mental and spiritual side. On the spiritual side, St. Paul put it very nicely when he said, "Set your mind and heart on higher talents and even higher paths. I will go on to show you." (See Colossians). In other words, allow no stagnation in your life. Life is eternal; it is forever; it never quits. You never die, but are born again. There is no sunset but that a sunrise follows!

We are meant to live and go on; yet, for the overactive and for those who are fighting themselves and their way through life, it is said, "Be still . . ." One of the greatest things for the person who wants to be quiet is to know and agree with a lot of what is going on in this world. It is truly an irrational world. It is a speedy world, and we eat that way also. It is an overactive world. It is an overpowering world.

So we have to face the fact that if we're going to be well physically, we must deal with this world from a spiritual standpoint, too. Don't forget you can't have sweet thoughts with a sour stomach. The physical body is a manifestation of the invisible. It is the end result. It is the effect of our thoughts. Thoughts are things. Our bodies are made by Divine thinking and broken down by humans. To get acquainted with it is to control it.

The nicest thing I can tell you is this: "Thou shalt have dominion over all that flies." And have we got the fussy and flighty things to take care of. "Thou shalt have dominion over all that swims." Ah, there are troubled waters to go through! "Thou shalt have dominion over all things that can get into your consciousness; all things that get into your mind; all things that get into your life." They can disturb and distort you to such an extent that you wake up a wreck — seven mornings a week.

Get out of the ruins! Lift up your head! Lift up your consciousness and walk, walk the upright man! Find the good life and live that life. Let life flow through you, don't *make* life happen. Then you will have no underactivity and no overactivity. Balance your activities and you won't live in misery, pain, depression, and false hopes, either physically, mentally, or spiritually!

A Doctor's Diagnosis

"No one can appreciate so fully as a doctor, the amazingly large percentage of human disease and suffering which is directly traceable to worry, fear, conflict, immorality, dissipation, and ignorance — to unwholesome thinking and unclean living. The sincere acceptance of the principles and teachings of Christ with respect to the life of mental peace and joy, the life of unselfish thought and clean living, would at once wipe out more than one-half the difficulties, diseases, and sorrows of the human race. In other words, more than one-half of the present afflictions of mankind could be prevented by the tremendous prophylactic power of actually living up to the personal and practical spirit of the real teachings of Christ."

—Dr. William S. Sadler, Director
Chicago Institute of Research and Diagnosis

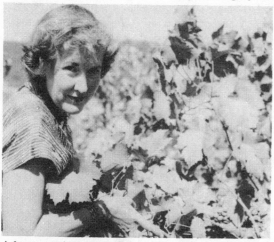

A former patient of ours lived on the grape diet and cured herself of one of the incurable diseases that man is plagued with so much today.

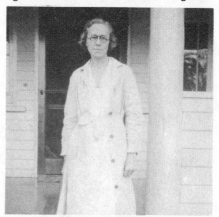

One of our former associates that corrected a condition of a so-called incurable disease through the natural Healing Art using mostly the grapes, fasting and so forth. These two women were both former nurses.

TEN

Your circle of life

You must keep the bloodstream and the blood system clean in order to keep your organs alive. The organs are only as clean as your bloodstream.

The blood is kept clean through the eliminative processes of four major organs—the skin, the kidneys, the lungs, and the bowel. These are generally the most neglected organs in the body. If too much attention is given to food and drink and not enough to the eliminative processes, we create an imbalance in the body that leads to disease.

The skin is treated at length elsewhere in this book. In this chapter we will deal with the kidneys, lungs, and bowel.

Help for the Kidneys

If you have kidney troubles, cut out citrus fruit. We stir up the acids in the rest of the body and the extra liquid of the citrus fruit has to go out through the kidneys. The kidneys are overworked with the extra toxic materials that we are breaking down in the body. We cannot expect a weakened, or many times diseased, kidney to take care of all that extra work. Move from fruits to vegetables.

Many times, in helping the kidneys and helping the skin, you have to have the vegetables in a cooked broth. Even raw vegetable juices can stir up the acids too fast. This irritates the skin and kidneys and makes them act too fast. Try to keep away from that irritability as much as possible.

For the kidneys we sometimes advise using extra water. A good remedy is to take two or three glasses of water every morning before breakfast. It might be good to use a little liquid chlorophyll in one of those glasses. Liquid chlorophyll does not cause kidney disturbances as do the fresh vegetable juices.

Care of the Lungs

<u>Catarrh Elimination</u>. The lung structure is a vital one to take care of because it is a great catch-point for catarrh, phlegm, and mucus which settle in the chest as part of the elimination process. This material is thrown off by the mucous membrane, where excessive acids are thrown off from the body.

Accumulated toxins in the bowel are thrown back into the body, absorbed by the blood, and finally go to the lung structure. This is where we have large amounts thrown off in a hurry. I have seen some people throw off teaspoons of catarrh through the bronchial tubes. This is something we do not try to stop. We try to bring more of it about, if possible, to cleanse that lung structure. How do we do that?

We must start eating noncatarrhal foods. One of the greatest remedies for getting rid of catarrh in the lung structure is to cut out milk and wheat. Cut out bread and citrus fruit. They stir up the acids and force all of this heavy toxic material into the lung structure to be eliminated. Use more from the vegetable kingdom and liquid chlorophyll.

<u>Chest Breathing</u>. Anytime you can put your mind on your chest, it will develop. Anytime you can do some of this while you are on the slant board, you will get more blood into the medulla, which is the part of the brain that helps you to breathe well. Chest breathing is dependent upon the brain. This is why a person gets tired and mentally fatigued. He is always yawning. He has depleted his nerve supply. The chest will breathe as much as you want if the nerves are good. Make sure you have enough iron to oxygenize the blood; then make sure you use your chest through exercise to get that oxygen to the brain. Laughter exercises the chest and recharges the medulla.

Plant life throws out oxygen, the very element we need to keep us alive. *Deep breathing; hiking in the mountains; and dry, warm air will help the lung structure the most.*

Take a hundred deep breaths before dinner and a hundred breaths afterwards. When you breathe out, flex your hands. This stimulates circulation throughout the system.

Foods for the lungs. Turnips are excellent for the lungs. I have also used garlic, or, in many cases, a garlic and onion combination, with considerable success. Like the turnip, these odorous vegetables are a wonderful thing for catarrhal problems. When taken along with a regular health diet, they can be used for packs on the chest and throat, or they can be chopped, mixed, and eaten.

Bowel Management

The bowel and the liver work together as a team. Detoxification of the whole body works through them. No matter what treatments, no matter what doctor, no matter what kind of special diet, be sure the bowel is clean. Nutrition is first among the healing arts, and healing takes place first through the bowel.

We can have a lazy bowel and not know it. The bowel is one of the softest tissues in the body, and it has the poorest nerve supply of any organ. It does not tell us when we have real problems. We can have gases and not know it. We can have obstructions, constrictions, spastic conditions, and still not know it. Feelings in the bowel are very poor.

There are certain things we can do, and should not do, to have healthy bowels. A few ideas follow:

Bowel Bacteria. Acidophilous bacilli create an acid medium in the intestine where unfriendly disease–producing bacteria do not thrive. In most people, the ratio of unfriendly bacteria is 80 percent to only 20 percent acidophilous. This ratio can be reversed by using an acidophilous culture to destroy the causes of constipation, auto-intoxification, and other intestinal disorders.

There are many brands of acidophilous culture available in most health food stores. There are brands made from broth if you do not want to use those made from milk products.

You can take the acidophilous by mouth the first thing in the morning and the last thing at night. You can also use it in enemas and in colonics. To get the best results, it should be used for two months straight without stopping. If you have bowel troubles, use it for two months, skip two or three months, then use it again for two months.

Do this three times a year until the bowels are under control.

Yogurt is a good protein food that builds the friendly bacteria in the bowels. They are also fed by using whey, high sodium foods, salads, greens, sprouts, and other natural foods. Raw foods help the bacteria to grow best.

Some foods break down the friendly bacteria. Coffee breaks down the friendly bacteria significantly, and it is a detriment to the bowel and the liver. Chocolate also is bad. Too much meat in the intestinal tract also destroys friendly bacteria. If you have a good intestinal tract, you can handle a little meat. People who have meat three times a day are building up too much putrefaction, and the friendly bacteria cannot take care of it. Even cooked food is not the best food for friendly bacteria; 60 percent of your daily diet should be raw.

Antihistamines, penicillin, and sulpha drugs all destroy the friendly bacteria in the bowel. This is of great concern to the gastrointestinal specialist these days. It is good to use kefir or several bottles of acidophilous milk to sweeten the intestinal tract and to give food to the friendly bacteria.

Formula for Feeding the Bowel. I had given to me an excellent formula that uses eight ounces of powdered buttermilk, eight ounces nonfat milk powder, and two ounces pure fruit pectin. Then add one quart of fresh buttermilk, and one quart of water, and sweeten each cup with one teaspoon of milk sugar. Take two tablespoons of acidophilous milk four times daily and drink two quarts or more of the formula for several days.

Clabber Milk. Many old men in the Balkan countries make this high protein, high enzyme, easily digestible food an important part of their diet. When prepared, clabber milk undergoes one of the enzyme actions that would naturally occur in the stomach when hydrochloric acid is present. Clabbering the milk before ingestion, therefore, gives the stomach an easy way to absorb the milk proteins. Most people over the age of fifty lack hydrochloric acid, so preparing clabbered milk is a good deed they can do for themselves.

To make clabber milk, all utensils should be clean. Heat two quarts of raw milk to lukewarm. Powdered milk (½ cup) may be added *before* the milk is heated, if desired. Blend the powdered milk well with one cup of raw milk to make a thicker clabber. After the milk is heated to lukewarm, take one cup of it and mix with one cup of yogurt or buttermilk. Stir well and add to the rest of the warm milk. Place in the oven with only the pilot light on, or in a warm place where it will go undisturbed until it sets. The time needed may vary from four to eight hours, depending upon the culture and the temperature (90 to 115 degrees). When ready, refrigerate in the same pan.

Alfalfa Tablets. Alfalfa tablets are one of the best remedies for bowel pockets (the small, weak spots in the bowel called diverticulae). These pockets fill with toxic materials and then interfere with the health of every organ in the body. Alfalfa tablets provide the bowel wall with a fibrous material which can get into these pockets. It gives the bowel muscles something to work against these settlements. Alfalfa tablets help get this stagnant, gas-forming toxic material moving along, and start developing tone in that part of the bowel that is not working right. The tablets are slightly laxative; and there are some people who cannot take them.

Take four to eight alfalfa tablets at each meal. Be sure to break each tablet before using. The tablets are pressed at 3,000 pounds, and should be broken so they will disintegrate.

Take a Good Digestant. Along with the alfalfa tablets, we add a digestant of some kind to take care of the gas. There are many digestants on the market that have a little pancreatic substance, hydrocloric acid, papain, bile salts, and probably a little stomach substance. This helps in the digestion of starches and proteins, and helps get rid of the gases. We do this until the bowel is well enough to take care of itself.

In some patients, it takes about a year for the bowel to be well enough to function properly. You can help take care of the bowel overnight by the food you eat. But the bowel will not be well overnight. You must develop tone in it over a period of time.

If Elimination Is Poor, Prefer Vegetables over Fruits. Fruits stir up the acids in the body and vegetables carry off the acids. Many people who are having discharges from the body, where elimination channels are not working properly, should use less fruit and add more vegetables to their diet. In this way acids are not stirred up so fast and are carried off a little slower.

There are some foods that should be avoided in cases of bowel disorders. For example, head lettuce is very gas-forming and slows down the digestion.

Aloe Vera. Aloe Vera is one of the oldest remedies known to man. It is the source of a well-known, drastic purgative drug, Barbados Aloe, which is a solid extract obtained by evaporating the plant juice. It is also one of the ingredients of the famous "Sacred Bitters" of ancient Egypt.

The Aloe Vera, or Barbados Aloe, comes from a rare old tropical plant. It is sensitive to cold and thrives in the tropics or adjacent subtropical areas. Referred to in the Bible, it was not until 1935 that it came into modern usage. Its popularity as a new "wonder drug" is spreading quickly. It is cultivated commercially in the southern part of Florida, and acreage is rapidly being increased to meet the growing demand. A surprise to strangers is to see its fresh leaves in almost every grocery store.

Aloe Vera is a succulent plant belonging to the lily family. It is decorative as well as medicinal, being effective as a center of floral designs for garden vases. Its leaves are long and narrow, fleshy with a spiny margin about two inches in thickness, four inches broad at the base and twelve to twenty inches long when fully grown. It grows particularly well in the dry beds of soil common to the Florida area and requires

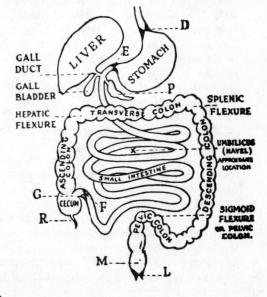

little or no care. It propagates primarily by means of the suckers or small plants growing out from the roots of the mother plant. These should be carefully removed and transplanted. From three to five years are required for plants to grow to marketable size and, when properly cared for, they may be productive for ten to twelve years.

Not being hardy except in the South, Aloe Vera is usually planted in tubs or flower pots, where it thrives for years without transplanting. To plant, fill a pot two inches from the top with garden soil. The top two inches should consist of loose gravel or small stones so there is perfect drainage at the crown of the plant. After a few weeks each plant sprouts many baby "shoots" which can be transplanted to other pots. A little manure and a very small amount of limestone should go into the potting soil. Water aloes very sparingly, never more than once a month. Plants will live months without water. They will rot quickly in soil kept too moist.

The Aloe Vera is the only true medical aloes referred to so often in magazine articles about the healing aloes used by native Indians in Florida. It is a mucilaginous plant. Most of its tissue does not contain any medicinally active substance, but when the leaf is peeled back, you find the crystal clear, jelly-like juice of the plant which is the reputed healing "gel." This aloe gel is soothing and rapidly relieves pain, burning, and itching. It acts quickly because it is speedily absorbed. It seems to reduce scar tissue formation, does not stain, and has no unpleasant odor. Its popular use ranges from treatment of ulcers, arthritis, constipation, boils, skin erruptions, chapped lips and hands, asthma, coughs, to body beautification. Many southern Floridians claim it is a "cure-all." The gel-like fresh juice is of a highly perishable nature after it is cut from the mother plant, but for home use it can be treated as an ointment for insect bites, barber's rash, burns, sores, and swellings by merely spreading it upon the afflicted part.

The juice can be taken and bandaged onto afflicted areas by slicing the leaves open and placing them over the wound. Unused portions of leaves may be laid aside for future use. It will keep for many weeks.

To obtain the juice, cut the matured leaves at the base, then place the cut end downward in an inclined trough or receptacle so that the juice, in trickling from the leaves, may be collected. The leaves may also be crushed to a pulp and the juice strained out through a closely woven thin cloth. The juice may then be dried by evaporating off the water at a low temperature. This produces the dried aloe of commerce.

The fresh juice is also used by incorporating it into an ointment and applying it locally, and also by diluting with water and administering by mouth as a liquid.

Aloe is good for any burn, especially X-ray burns, sunburn, and friction, electrical, chemical, hot fat, fire, and steam burns. Doctors have used Aloe Vera in the treatment of burns of all degrees of seriousness, and several large hospitals have tested the aloes in the treatment of X-ray and radiation reaction. The "Aloe Gel" is also used as a household remedy for burns, skin disturbances, sties, cysts and other external disorders.

The jelly can be used as a shampoo. It is also a good body lubrication for arthritis and crippled arms and legs. Recently, the healing properties of the Aloe Vera have been incorporated into medications, suntan preparations and cosmetics. To apply, use the gel liberally on the affected areas, or spread on waxed paper and bandage in place. Replace before it dries out.

The gel-like fresh juice of the leaves is also taken internally in place of the drastic concentrated Aloe pills, which often cause gripping pains. This juice is much milder in action. For stomach, liver, and kidneys, try this efficient method: cut up leaves into small pieces and place a cupful in a quart of cold water. Place in refrigerator and drink a small tumbler full on an empty stomach, morning and evening. Add more water as it is used until one cupful of the cut leaves makes two quarts of aloe water. Be careful not to take too much or you will experience a heavy dull feeling in the neck of the bladder. When this occurs, merely dilute the aloe with more water.

For stomach ulcers and constipation, wash well about three "prongs" or leaves and cut up the flesh into a quart-sized jar. Fill the jar with water and refrigerate. The water will blend with the mucilaginous substance and form a sort of syrup. Take a small glass half an hour before each meal. The quantity should be regulated according to the laxative effect on the user. An easier way is to put the fleshy cubes in an electric blender, add a small amount of water, and blend the mixture into a foamy liquid, which can be poured into a jar and refrigerated. Shake before using.

Hemorrhoids and Piles. Many people have developed rectal conditions as the result of sedentary occupations. Constipation, sitting on the "civilized" stool, eating too many foods that dehydrate before they eliminate, and eating the wrong combination of foods produce a pressure that results in prolapsed rectal tissue and can result in bleeding piles and bleeding hemorrhoids. The veins that surround the rectal opening can stand only so much pressure, then they will burst and cause bleeding.

These veins can enlarge and produce external nodules and tabs. Many times the tissue becomes so mutilated that it is advisable to have a doctor's care.

In trying to overcome these conditions and alleviate simple hemorrhoids and piles which may have developed, the following exercise routine and natural means can help:

Use a Potato Plug. One of the most important things to be accomplished in cases of enlarged veins in the rectal tissue is to shrink it back into place. For this purpose, we use what we call a "potato plug." This is cut from a raw potato, the size of a thumb, rounded on both ends, dipped in oil if you wish, and placed just inside of the rectum. This presses gently against the enlarged vein and puts it in its proper position, preventing its distention, while we try to correct the prolapsed condition from above. Insert one of these plugs into the rectum *after* each bowel movement. Leave it inserted. It will be eliminated automatically with the next bowel movement.

Assume a Squatting Posture. To assume a squatting position for evacuation of the lower bowel is very important. It is helpful when having elimination to keep the hands above the head. In this position the tissues cannot be forced out of the rectum and a more complete bowel elimination will be accomplished. The extensive use of the modern toilet seat, a contrivance of civilization, is responsible for most of these troubles: it is not conducive to elimination by Nature's method, the squatting position.

If you use the customary sitting position, place your hands palms up on your knees, incline the body forward and rest your forehead against your cupped palms. Then rest the forehead on the knees and bend the arms over the head and massage the neck area to relieve tension, which is beneficial and also accomplishes the purpose of raising the arms upward. This is generally helpful.

For Inflammation with Piles. In acute inflammation accompanying a condition of piles, a garlic oil capsule or clove may be placed in the rectum each night. In many cases, the use of an enema is an aid in the healing of damaged tissues.

A Healing Enema. The best enema for *lower rectal problems* of a simple nature is flaxseed tea with chlorophyll. This allays inflammation. Use one teaspoonful liquid chlorophyll in one-quarter cup of flaxseed tea, to be retained in the bowel.

Improve the Bowel Tone. These suggestions cannot be expected to bring much relief until the bowel tone is improved, the abdominal organs go back to their proper position and proper eating habits are established so as to eliminate the gases that produce extreme pressure and soften the bowel wall.

Benefits of the Slant Board. One exercise that will help these tissues most is the use of

A good remedy—Lavatory built at the level of the floor and especially good for hemorrhoids.

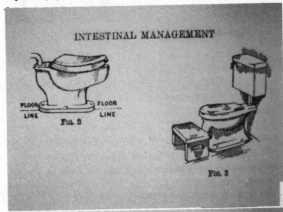

INTESTINAL MANAGEMENT

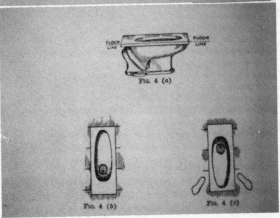

the slant board. The abdominal exercises as described for the slant board are of utmost importance in all rectal conditions.

Adopt a Bland Diet. It may be necessary to adopt a bland diet, eliminating seeds, skins, rough foods, and raw vegetables until the rectal condition is improved. It is advisable to be under a doctor's care. The above suggestions are given only as a home treatment. A specialist in the treatment of your specific condition should be consulted to determine the most effective means of improvement and possible correction.

Foods and Bowel Problems

Learn the foods to Use. There are a number of things we can do to avoid gas in the stomach and the intestinal tract:

1. Too many rough foods can cause a great deal of disturbance in the bowel. You would not run sandpaper over a sore, would you? You would not run lemon juice or citrus fruit over a sore, would you? Whenever there is an accumulation of gas there is a sensitive bowel.

2. However, one of the remedies for gas is putting a little lemon juice in milk.

3. Clabbered milk is a wonderful remedy. If milk is difficult for you to take, then leave it out.

4. Barley gruel and rice gruel are wonderful for those suffering with gas problems. These foods are high in vitamin B, necessary to solve gas problems.

5. Sometimes it is best to avoid too many liquids.

6. Eating drier foods will often help. Dry graham toast or soybean toast will ease a gas condition.

7. Flaxseed tea is wonderful for dissipating gas. If it is difficult to take by mouth, use it as an enema.

8. A warm pack over the abdomen for half an hour or so after eating will help to bring relaxation to the body; relaxation is a wonderful aid in dissipating gas.

Cautions—Food to Avoid. Here are some foods that we should leave alone if we are having bowel problems:

1. Although tops of the vegetables and other greens are good and necessary foods, sometimes they can be very gas-forming. Many are too rough as, for instance, are the strings in turnip greens.

2. Sometimes the sulphur foods, such as cauliflower, broccoli, Brussels sprouts, cabbage, and onions have to be eliminated for a short time, and more bland foods added, such as carrots, beets, string beans, spinach, collards, endive, and watercress.

3. Sometimes salads must be cut down.

4. Even vegetable juices, when drunk alone, can cause gas.

5. Adding a little milk or a little vegetable broth to the juice will reduce the activity in it.

Foods That Digest Easily and Act as Remedies. Here are some foods that will help us:

1. Soaked and peeled dates in milk is a wonderful combination.

2. As a soft food, grapes are wonderful if skin and seeds are eliminated. Acidophilous culture to help change the intestinal flora is a wonderful aid. Whey is also good. If it's powdered, take a tablespoon three times a day. Massaging the abdomen with olive oil will sometimes help until a good balanced system is established.

Exercise is necessary also. You cannot get well without exercise. One of the finest exercises for the bowel is to take an orange or a lemon, or a tennis ball, and work this around the abdomen fifteen to twenty-five times, until a good balance is established in the body. Charcoal tablets can be used for gas troubles. However, if taken continually, use vitamin A long with them.

3. Be sure to always use green leaf lettuce, such as bibb, romaine, or red-tipped. Bread causes a dry, hard stool, because the heat used in baking it dries the oils in the grain. Use cereals instead, and vary these to include brown rice, yellow corn meal, millet, rye, and ground wheat. Ground wheat is a won-

derful food for good bowel activity. Prepare it by placing one-half cup of ground wheat in two cups of hot water. Put this in a thermos bottle, cork it, and leave overnight to soak. In the morning it is ready to eat. Sweeten only with dried fruits, never with sugar.

4. Beets are good for the gall bladder and the liver. They are good for building blood. Shredded beets are one of the best things served. Use an amount the size of a golf ball once a day. If fresh beets are not available, use beet tablets.

5. An element that comes from black horseradish is one of the finest herbs to get the bile to flowing. It clears out the gall bladder and the liver.

6. Dandelion is good for the gall bladder and the liver. The fresh leaves can be used in raw salads in early spring or they can be steamed. Dandelion root coffee is an excellent remedy for the liver.

7. Flaxseed tea contains vitamin E and is one of the finest teas for the mucous membrane of the bowel. The tea is fine boiled, but for the best results, add a quarter cup of flaxseed to one quart of hot water and let it stand overnight. Strain off the seeds before drinking. This method preserves more of the vitamin E. Never reuse the seed after you have boiled or soaked it. In cases of constipation, you can use the whole seed by putting it through a grinding mill.

8. Winter squash is another great food for intestinal disturbances.

9. Flaxseed is one of the best remedies for ordinary constipation. Take one or two heaping teaspoons of ground flaxseed meal twice a day, every day, for several weeks or even months. Be sure to mix it with a liquid so it will not stick to the roof of your mouth.

Flaxseed contains 30 percent vegetable oil by weight. Introduced into the colon, it acts as a laxative by softening the feces and lubricating the canal. Doctors have recognized for years that flaxseed tends to stimulate peristaltic action (bowel action) of the intestines. Flaxseed tea also works well.

Whole flaxseed swells to approximately three times its own size when water, milk, or other liquids are taken. Because of this expansion, whole flaxseed furnishes added bulk, which is so important in cases where there is a lack of bulk in the diet. Flaxseed is not a harsh irritant or purgative.

Here is a smooth laxative combination of flaxseed meal and slippery elm:

1 tablespoon flaxseed meal, 1 teaspoon slippery elm, 1 tablespoon whey. Mix in a glass of apple juice. Take first thing in the morning.

This laxative of slippery elm helps us in mild forms of constipation:
1 teaspoon slippery elm, ¼ cup water. Blend two or three minutes. Take before breakfast.

DEATH BEGINS IN THE COLON. Pocketed conditions in the bowel usually occur as an inherent sickness and it is within these pockets that we have intestinal putrefaction and fermentation developing from this particular part of the colon. Reflex conditions to various organs in the body can develop as the toxic material is picked up from these pockets and carried by the blood to the next weakest organ in the body and usually settles there as a catarrh, phlegm, mucus and to be eliminated by another eliminative organ. (From "Science and Practice of Iridology" by Dr. Bernard Jensen, D.C.)

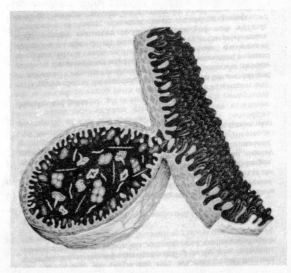

10. Figs are excellent for the bowels if taken when fresh (one to three days old). They contain a high amount of magnesium, potassium, oxygen, and papain. I have obtained excellent results in the treatment of arthritis and rheumatism with fresh figs and raw goat milk. Figs, ripe from the tree, are wonderful energy foods. They are high in a natural sweet, and the seeds have a natural laxative coating which is important when a patient is in distress.

11. Other laxative foods are Agar Agar (Irish moss), used for constipation, containing manganese, nickel, iodine, copper, and vitamin D; Peaches, containing phosphorus, sodium and mangenese; Yellow fruits and vegetables; Alfalfa tablest, whey, mulberries, cherry concentrate; Liquid chlorophyll, mixed 1 teaspoon to a glass of water and then taken 3 times daily; and herb combination for lower bowel system: barberry bark, cascara sagrada, red clover, lobelia, ginger, capsicum.

12. For a laxative, the following formula has been used by a doctor from the famous Mayo Clinic. (It is also an aid in overcoming arthritis).

Dried Natural Fruits
(one week's supply)
21 Prunes
14 teaspoons of Raisins
14 halves of Apricots
7 halves of Pears
7 halves of Peaches
7 Figs

Put in a large pan, pour boiling water over fruit to cover entirely. Cover with loose lid, let stand for four days at room temperature, adding water to keep fruit covered, then store in lower compartment of refrigerator. Each day take: three prunes, two teaspoons raisins, two halves apricots, one half pear, one half peach, one fig. (If desired, grind these dry with senna leaves.)

13. A coffee enema was used a great deal by Dr. Max Gerson, a New Jersey medical doctor in the 1930s. Many of his patients would set alarms to get up in the middle of the night to take enemas. They would take two or three a night to get rid ot toxic waste that the body was breaking down and throwing into the colon. He made sure the toxic waste was eliminated consistently. The formula for making the enema is as follows: Take three tablespoons of ground (drip) coffee (not instant) to one quart of water; let it boil three minutes and then simmer 15 minutes more. Strain and use at body temperature. The daily amount can be prepared at one time. This enema can be used three to four times daily or anytime to relieve pain in any part of the body. It is good for helping the liver eliminate stagnant bile.

14. Retention enema. In blender mix one teaspoon apple cider vinegar and one tablespoon slippery elm powder. Use as an enema with one and one half quarts of warm water

15. It is helpful to know the effectiveness of different enemas. A water enema can irritate the bowel. Flaxseed tea makes a soothing enema. Buttermilk feeds the friendly bacteria when used as an enema. Coffee used as an enema stimulates the bowel and brings the bile down.

Constipation
In dealing with constipation, we must deal with the individual. A highly nervous person can produce constipation from nervous reactions and the tensions he may carry during the day. His workload must be considered, both physically and mentally.

Also, there are some people who are just plain dehydrated. They do not have enough water in their systems because they do not drink enough water. The result is a hard stool. Some people become more constipated living in a high altitude and dry climate. They must learn how to combine their foods properly. They may eat too much starch without the water-carrying vegetables. Without looking into the trouble, they turn to laxatives. This can be dangerous. It is unfair to the intestinal tract and to its health. More harm than good can result from taking laxative.

Correction of Constipation. If the history of an adult patient reveals no apparent reason for the onset of constipation, we would suspect an organic disorder of the colon. There are over 30 million people taking laxatives regularly, but this does not mean that it is the proper procedure for treating constipation. In our practive we discontinue the use fo laxatives. We teach people to have natural bowel movements through eating properly. We restore the defecation through reflex, by teaching people to answer nature's call, not "putting it off." Our main object is to reestablish the peristaltic action to a normal rhythm. This is done through exercise, the use of foods laxative in nature, and giving up those foods that are constipating.

Fibrous Residue Is Essential. We must have a certain amoung of fibrous residue in our diets, otherwise we have a decreased frequency in bowel movements. Insufficient fluid intake can cause many disturbances. A diet low in vitamin B-1 is found to produce a balloon-like bowel. This is a bowel that has lost much of its capacity to react to normal stimulus. Many times the nerve stimulus through the spine must be cared for through physical minipulation to bring the bowel well back to normal reaction. A lack of bile flow may produce contipation.

Diarrhea. Some people have a hypersensitive bowel, and the least little roughage or the least irritation to their nervous system, even through their mental attitude and their environment, will cause a loose bowel movement. There are foods that will balance and control it if we know the proper constipating foods to use for this condition. You can use blackberry juice to flavor a gelatin dessert and add pineapple juice to cut down the strength of it. Consider a variety of juices in your diet. Blackberry and black cherry juice can be used several times over a period of a month.

Blackberry juice and black cherry juice are wonderful mixed with gelatin. Most people can take gelatin very well. Many people complain about the aching joints in their bodies. Gelatin is made from the joints of animals and is a good material to use for aching joints. Gelatin mixed with black cherry juice is sweet enough; you won't have to add any other sweetening. If you are going to use any other sweetening, make sure it is honey.

There are ways of mixing prune juice with blackberry juice so that you have a laxative juice. In cases of diarrhea, we use blackberry juice to control it. The juice has been used for ages for this purpose. We find that a black-berry compound can be purchased in a drugstore today for the control of diarrhea. Another good remedy for diarrhea is a potato, cut in one-inch squares and boiled in a quart of milk for ten minutes. Sip it like tea.

Internal Water Cleansing Treatments. A water treatment can help constipation, eliminating toxemia in the body, cleaning out kidneys:

First Day: 1 glass of water 1 hour before breakfast;
1 glass of water ½ hour before breakfast; and
1 glass of water immediately before breakfast.

Second Day:
2 glasses of water 1 hour before breakfast;
2 glasses of water ½ hour before breakfast; and
2 glasses of water immediately before breakfast.

Third Day:
3 glasses of water 1 hour before breakfast;
3 glasses of water ½ hour before breakfast; and
3 glasses of water immediately before breakfast.

The water should be warm and exercise should be taken each halfhour before drinking water. Stay on your regular health schedule diet. The water is just in addition to regular meals. This water treatment should be taken for one month.

Stomach Washes. In washing out the stomach, tepid water should be used. Drinking water is good for constipation, providing it is used cold and taken upon retiring and arising. Soft water is excellent for concretion and troubles with the urinary organs, kidneys, and stomach. A man who suffers from kidney trouble should drink much pure water, save his strength, change his diet, call his skin into action, and stimulate his bowels. Distilled water can be a solvent in the the body and can penetrate every fiber and cell of the organism, carrying away impurities providing the water is pure and soft. Hard water adversely affects the liver, kidneys, and bones, developing chronic diseases that are difficult to cure. Soft water is the best. Rain water and fruit juices are the best liquids for man, provided the rain water is collected after the atmosphere has been washed by the rain for one hour before the rain water is collected.

Bowel Wall Inflamation. Bile is the fluid that stimulates peristaltic action. Inflammation of the bowel, which occurs when a person has not eaten the right foods to feed the bowel walls properly, may result when harsh, rough foods are taken.

Diverticulitis. Bowel pockets can result in this bowel condition. Metal poisonings from substances such a lead, phosporus, mercury, or arsenic can be responsible for spastic constipation, although nervous tensions are usually more responsible for hypertoxic colon conditions. Never neglect the need to have a bowel movement. Develop a regular time to go to the bathroom each day, to reestablish the defecation reflex. Laxatives should be used on a temporary basis only. Tight girdles and improper fitting trusses are some of the mechanical things that can disturb the normal function of the bowel. Adhesions, foreign bodies, fecal impactions, and prolapsus can also disturb the normal flow of toxic waste in the colon. We have to make sure there are no obstructions. We'll need to see a doctor to be certain. Those who have this ailment may receive from their doctor a temporary special diet to follow.

Abdominal Exercises

All abdominal exercises are recommended when you want to overcome bowel problems. Here are just a few of the best:

Chest-Leg Pull-Up. In the chest-leg pull-up exercise you sit on the edge of a chair with your feet straight out in front, toes pointed upward, and body straight toward the back of the chair. In this position, you are almost in a straight line. Now lift your heels slightly above the floor, just an inch or so. You will find it took all the abdominal muscles to lift those legs when they were straight out. Your abdominal muscles become solid and tense— and stronger. As you keep your body in that straight line, lift the legs slightly. Hold onto the arm of the chair, pull the legs up, with the knees up to the chest; then bring them down to the floor without touching the floor and repeat. Do this two, three, ten times if you can. This develops tone in the bowel. Within three months, you will have developed the tone of the muscles in the bowel to match the better food you have been eating for the past three months. You will also help rejuvenate your abdominal tract.

Exercises to Rejuvenate the Colon

Use the slant board for stretching the abdomen and rejuvenating the colon. While lying flat on your back, stretch your abdomen by putting arms above your head, then raise and lower them to the sides. This stretches the abdominal muscles by pulling them up toward the shoulders. Do this exercise ten to fifteen times daily.

To rejuvenate the colon, lean to the left side and stretch. Pat stretched side of abdomen vigorously with open hand. Change side and lean to right. Stretch and pat vigorously fifteen to twenty-five times each side. Reverse sides three to four times.

The slant board is one of the best remedies I know for getting the dropped transverse colon back into position. It is the finest thing for those people who have falling hair and want to get more blood back into the head and into the eyes. The basic position on the slant board is the finest position for resting to compensate for overwork, especially when you are mentally tired. Exercise is an important part of any health program. Food will not do you any good unless you exercise to get the blood to the place where it is needed.

Twisting. Standing alongside a chair, twist your knees from side to side. Squat, put arms out to side, and twist side to side.

Stretching. Put your left arm high above your head and reach down and touch the right foot with your right hand. Then throw your right hand straight up and go down with the left hand, touching the toes. This stretches one side of your abdomen and then the other.

Rest. The good of all exercise is developed in rest. Exercise can be good for you, but you can't exercise 24 hours a day. A time comes when you need absolute rest. I think everybody should have one day a week of absolute rest. It could be a fast day, or a juice day, but do nothing on that day!

Resting from food while you see how hard you can work physically is not fair to the body. When you cut out food for one day, lay yourself out prone and don't do anything. Let your body recuperate. That is the day when you take the phone off the hook; that is the day you don't gossip; that is the day when the outside world comes to an end. We should learn how to rest. Very few people really know how to rest. Some people would get well if they would just shut their mouth for a whole day. I remember hearing my professor say, "If you want to be a success in life, keep your mouth shut and your bowels open."

ELEVEN

Beauty starts with the skin

THE SKIN — the most diversified organ and the largest organ of the body. The other organs are compact and take up as little space as possible. The skin on the other hand is like "dough." It is rolled out as extensively and as thinly as possible.

The skin weighs twice as much as the liver or the brain. It receives one-third of the circulating blood and its surface extends over ˙3,100 square inches (20,000 square centimeters). Each square centimeter contains 100 sweat glands, 15 sebaceous glands, and hundreds of signal apparatuses.

The skin is sometimes called the third lung or the third kidney. We actually throw off toxic materials through the skin. The skin aids in the elimination of all toxic wastes in the body. It is one of the body's most important organs: it has 120 billion cells, 100 million organs of scent, three million nerve points, two million perspiratory glands, 400,000 points of pressure, 300,000 fat yielding glands, 100,000 minute hairs, 300,000 feet of nerve tissue, and 150,000 feet of veins.

On hot days when the skin eliminates a great deal, the kidneys do not have to eliminate too much, and the urine usually is quite concentrated. The opposite is true in the wintertime. The urine is very heavy and we do not eliminate much through the skin. The skin and kidneys work hand in hand.

Care of the Skin

The skin needs water. Insurance statistics show that an average of five years longer life belongs to those who drink an abundance of water or even the needed amount of water.

A shrivelled appearance of the skin indicates a manganese deficiency. Scaly skin indicates a fluorin deficiency; to correct it increase your intake of fluorin as well as vitamin A. If you skin is sticky, you have a sodium deficiency. Rashes or pus indicate silicon deficiencies. Itching indicates a phosphorous deficiency; and to help soothe this condition rub Aloe Vera juice on skin and take nasturtium juice, which is an antiscorbutic and helps to purify the blood. Scar formations can be smoothed by rubbing Aloe Vera on the skin, and take marigold herb tea. For skin sores, use a flaxseed poultice, use a grape pack, garlic paste, a salve made from garlic and lanolin, and wash with apple cider vinegar solution. Runny sores indicate a calcium deficiency. For skin eruptions, use a chlorophyll supplement.

With any skin problem remember to take care of the kidneys first. Iodine foods are needed.

We must recognize that the skin has to have another remedy, and that is silicon. This element is found in sprouts, particularly alfalfa sprouts, and oat straw tea, as well as in many natural foods. Barley, tomatoes, spinach, figs, and strawberries are all good sources of silicon.

Good herb teas for the skin include horsetail tea (high in silicon), bay herb tea as a stimulant, basil and bay combination, oat straw tea, sweet marjoram, and tarragon.

The Beauty Element—Fluorin. Beauty is not possible without fluorin. The body requires a reserve of this "beauty element" for good health.

Fluorin is one of the most important chemical elements to the human body. It is liberated into air by cooking, heating, steaming. If the system lacks fluorin, trouble arises with the spleen and blood, especially the red corpuscles. When symptoms such as putrid odor of feet, bleeding gums, dark blood, disorderly mind and habits, brain congestion, and chronic catarrh are evident, all relate to fluorin hunger. Other symptoms include pus and toxins in the body, aggravated emotions; awkward movement; swollen, granular, gluey eyelids, unreal emotions, hallucinations, dirty, cold, puffy, scaley, greasy, thick skin; crumbly bones and teeth; decayed taste in mouth, sadness and deafness in morning hours; aching eyeballs; running saliva; puffy face, neck, and forehead; sudden blindness from stooping; puffy lower abdomen and thighs; poor circulation in chest; cold body, hands, and feet.

The chemist terms fluorin the "antiresistant" element of the body. When calcium and fluorin hardness is present in the body, long life and resistance are encouraged. Germ life is combated in the body and disease is unwelcome. Tooth decay is prevented by the proper amount of fluorin. Uncooked foods contain more fluorin, as all heating destroys it. The outside of bones is very hard because it is the fluorin-containing portion of the bone structure, the reserve section of the body for fluorin.

Goat milk is one of the highest fluorin foods. Raw black bass is the highest. Green quinces, rye flour, avocados, raw sea plants, sea cabbage, goat cheese, cream, whey, cottage cheese, and Roquefort cheese are all high in fluorin.

Skin and Complexion. For a clear complexion drink cocktails made of apple juice concentrate with cucumber juice. This is a very good summertime drink: cucumbers are high in sodium, which helps to keep the body cool. Sodium also helps to keep the skin from wrinkling. Another very good treatment for wrinkles is to use a Honey Pat ten times a day for two months; comfrey root poultice is also very effective. For dry skin use lecithin balm.

Apricot kernel oil is one of the finest things for a lovely complexion. This is what the Hunzas use in that extremely cold air they live in. They have lovely complexions. It can be used as a cleansing oil for keeping the skin free from wrinkles. It is also good night oil and can be mixed with Aloe Vera to give it astringent qualities.

Brown Spots. Many people complain about the brown spots on hands and body. In most places it comes from an internal condition involving either the liver or glandular structure. We have used Aloe Vera with some effect.

Skin ulcers. A good remedy for skin ulcers is one green pepper cut into ½ cup oat straw tea to one quart of water; simmer for 40 minutes; strain off and drink one cup of the tea two or three times daily. A mixture of equal amounts of lanolin and garlic oils is the best salve for skin disturbances such as ulcers.

Whiteheads. Whiteheads found on the forehead, around the nose, and on the face are usually caused from a lack of starch digestion. A pancreatic substance added to the diet will help immensely. Using clay packs on the face or using Aloe Vera as a lotion or a salve will help. Start from within, with the pancreas. Cut down on the heavy starches, breads, and heavy cereals for a while. There are a few starches that especially bring whiteheads on: wheat, oats, rye, buckwheat, and potatoes. Eliminate these for a while. Turn to millet and rice.

Suntanning. Ultraviolet light acts on the tyrosine in the skin, transforming it into the brown pigment melanin, which is deposited in the superficial layers of the epidermis and protects the skin against further action of the light rays.

In order to understand the problem of the sunbath, one must remember that sunlight not only acts on the parts of the skin that are directly exposed to it, but it also produces substances in the irradiated skin which pass with the blood into the interior of the body and act on the entire organism. If one's feet are exposed to the sun's rays, substances elevate the blood pressure, excite the heart, and vitamin D passes into the bones. Exposing one's skin to the sun's rays is equivalent to swallowing one teaspoonful of medicine every five minutes — a medicine which is by no means harmless. For this reason one must be careful. For the average person, ten minutes of sunbathing a day is all that is needed. Sunbathing is necessary to keep up the vitamin D and A content of the body. Vitamin D is necessary to control body calcium.

When too much sun is taken, the body develops a suntan, which is a defense pigment that filters out the harmful rays of the sun. The body can absorb only so much vitamin D daily. Too much sun seriously affects the entire nervous system, but a moderate amount of sun improves poor skin conditions and helps to eliminate skin blemishes. Good sunburn remedies are Aloe Vera and sesame seed oil.

Air Bathe Daily. The daily air bath is a definite aid to good health, toning the skin and improving its texture. Body air baths in the privacy of your own room gradually build up your resistance to a cooler temperature; they may then be taken throughout the year.

Perspiration. Under normal conditions an individual loses 500 calories daily, one-eighth of his total heat loss, as a result of perspiration evaporation. The skin contains two million sweat glands. If all the sweat glands were placed end to end, we would obtain a tube six miles in length. Perspiration is acid. It contains salt, potassium, iron, sulphuric acid, phosphoric acid, lactic acid, and above all, urea. The skin excretes as much urea as the kidney, so that it has been correctly described as a third kidney. If one prevents the skin from giving off heat, sweat, and waste products, the body suffers from poisoning and overheating.

Perspiration Methods to Remove Toxic Wastes. Steam bathing and the electric blanket method of perspiring are not harmful unless used immoderately, and are a good means of eliminating toxic wastes from the system. As a means of reducing, they are only a temporary measure. If you use these baths, use them along with a reducing and health diet routine for the best results. This type of bathing is best done under supervision. It is much better to avoid fat to begin with than to melt it off later.

Consider a bath as a worker of good health. The skin brush bath, the sun bath, and the air bath are daily *musts* in your health-building and weight-reducing programs. Any other baths you may choose are an added bonus measure.

Bathing. The body should be bathed and cleansed three or four times per week. The breathing process not only goes on in the lungs, but in the skin cells. Impurities and poisons find their way out through the skin pores. Dirt clogs pores. Many internal eliminations can also cause clogged pores. Over three million pores cover the body. If they were closed a person would die within one hour. This is why many people are half dead today—skin is neglected. Skin brushing is invaluable in caring for the skin.

The temperature of the room, drafts, the temperature of the bather, the time of day, the exhausted condition of the bather, the amount of food in the bather's stomach are all important considerations in bathing. Never take a hot bath in a very cold room or your system will be filled with moisture, which may produce pneumonia. The temperature of the room should never fall below 68 degrees when you're bathing. Neither should the temperature exceed 96 degrees or 97 degrees except in extreme cases. Always let the body accustom itself gradually to extreme measures. Local applications or baths assist the part on which it is applied, but do not affect the general body.

Never bathe within two hours after eating, nor when exhausted, nor when you cool off after perspiration. Never bathe in the open air when chilliness follows the plunge. Bathe when the body is warm, and lose no time in getting into the water — never chill yourself while undressing before a bath. Bathe before retiring and take your cold sponge bath when you arise. Those who are strong may bathe early in the morning on an empty stomach. Those who are young and weak should bathe three hours after a meal, and about three hours after breakfast.

Cold Baths. Cold baths produce greater internal oxidation in the tissues, providing sudden and vigorous friction is taken after the bath. A cold bath increases the absorption of oxygen and the elimination of carbonic acid from the system. A cold bath increases urea.

Sheet baths or compress baths are used in fevers, high body temperatures for stimulation of the skin and pores, for soothing inflamed and irritated nerves, for lowering the temperature of the brain, for reducing abdominal inflammation, etc. This procedure consists of wringing out the water from a large linen sheet that was previously immersed in water of a temperature of 60 degrees to 70 degrees F, then wrapping the sheet around the body while lying on a rubber blanket for bed protection. Cover up well with blankets to rest or sleep for a while, perhaps about 40 minutes to one hour. If chilled, remove the compress and normal body temperatures will return. This sheet bath or compress is variously used: water, milk, milk whey, brine, alfalfa, water, starch water, red clover water, clay water, etc., may be used either warm or cold or lukewarm as the case may require. Such packs, sheets, and compresses fomentations are often highly beneficial either for reducing bodily heat, inflammation, fever, or for increasing body heat, in which case either hot fomentations or hot packs are used.

Russian Baths. The Russian bath is the same as a vapor bath. Water is thrown upon red hot stones, bricks, or metal, filling the room full of vapor for us to breathe. It also heats our body to the point of flowing perspiration. Then follows a cold douche and a vigorous skin friction. If a person feels chilly he should never take a cold bath. If he takes a cold bath he should always have his feet comfortably warm before and after taking the cold bath or it will affect the chest.

Sunbaths. The more delicate a person is, the less vitality he has. The less animal heat he has to spare, the more debilitating a cold bath is to him. It is dangerous for him to even undress in a cold room. Neutral baths, sponge baths, sun baths with massage are the very best for him. In the sun bath greater nerve metabolism and brain nutrition takes place in the nervous system when the body is naked — proving the sun is not too hot, the atmosphere is not cold, and the person is protected. There is nothing better for the nerves than a sun tent in a big luxuriant tree with massage in the sun, sleep among the branches, fresh air solarium, and a brain and nerve building diet.

Herb Tea Baths. These should be taken with savoy, thyme, or pineneedle.

Special Baths with Cold Water

Eye Bath. Take cold water in your cupped hands, place eyes into it, then open and close eyes in the cold water two or three times. Do this twice a day.

Mouth Wash. Take a mouthful of cold water, swish it around in mouth until it is warm, then spit it out. Repeat. Do this twice a day. It is very good for the gums.

Abdominal Disorders. Wet and wring out a small Turkish towel in very cold water and fold into a square large enough to cover abdomen. Wrap and pin a large Turkish towel snugly around back and abdomen, covering the small towel and holding it in place. This top towel is dry and it is vital that it be wrapped so the air does not go in under it. Leave this on for one or two hours daily, or all night, according to doctor's instructions.

Foot Baths. To overcome stagnant circulation, use the hot and cold foot baths. The alternating effect of hot and cold foot soaks with the temperature of the waters not too extreme wakes up a lagging bloodstream and helps the skin.

Daily Bathing. Cleanliness is indeed next to Godliness and starts from within. Unless you have a clean skin with good tone you cannot have the right eliminative activity, and without proper elimination you cannot have "inner cleanliness" or the right mental attitude toward yourself. Think of your bath as an aid to cleanliness and as an aid to good health as well.

A warm, then a cool shower is an invigorating start for the day. The full force of the spray is like a gentle prick of needles on the skin, stimulating the body until it fairly glows with health. After you have turned down the warm water and the cooler water hits your body, there is a moment when your breath will quicken. When you first begin to take the breath in sharply, that is the moment to complete your shower. Your reaction is good then. If you remain longer, the prolonged cold may be detrimental to your health. Avoid a cool or cold bath if your vitality is low.

Warm baths relax aching muscles and tensed nerves and have a soothing effect upon the body, inducing sleep. Take your warm bath before retiring, both as an aid to relaxing sleep and to avoid body chills. Follow all intensive exercises with a warm water bath to relax the overworked muscles, then a few quick dashes of cold water to close the pores.

Too frequent tub baths, soaking in soapy water, is not recommended; this is a poor way to cleanse the body. When the pores are open, the skin absorbs the toxic wastes eliminating through the skin back into the pores again, as well as absorbing the soap in the water. Use less soap for body cleansing, and take care to rinse all soap from the body to avoid clogging the pores. Castile and pure vegetable oil soaps are least drying to the skin.

Skin Brush Daily. Daily dry friction brushing, or skin brushing, creates greater activity for the pores of the skin, is far more cleansing, eliminates more waste material than any soap and water bath, and lets the skin retain its natural oils. Soak a dry Turkish towel in cold water, wring out the excess water, and then rub towel vigorously over the entire body. The friction of rubbing the skin, the skin brush BATH, tones the skin, develops good circulation, and aids in eliminating mild skin conditions.

Sandow, the "Saxon Giant" who performed almost incredible feats of strength, had a skin of velvety softness that any woman might envy. Part of his training to keep fit was the regular use of a hard, coarse, flesh brush for dry skin brushing.

To become accustomed to the dry rub, use a soft flesh brush at first. Then change to a *soft scrub brush*, which you can purchase in most variety stores. The bristles are stiffer and the friction is more satisfactory. Use a soft face brush on the face, since the blood vessels that lie near the surface are easily broken down with too harsh rubbing. Do not use a nylon brush, but rather a long-handled dry bristle vegetable brush.

Use both face and body brushes without water. With your face brush, start at the forehead and work down over the eyes, along the nose, cheeks, chin, ears, and finally the neck, using a firm, brisk, rotary movement. With the body brush, brush the limbs with an upward movement, or towards the heart, brushing the entire body gently at first until the skin becomes conditioned. Avoid brushing the breasts entirely. Devote at least three to five minutes, morning and night, to this type of bathing. Your skin will become stimulated to better function and actually becomes softer; your health improves without question; and you will have lasting returns in both health and charm. Rubbing the body with salt is also a fine health measure; rinse it off as you shower.

I believe skin brushing is one of the finest of all baths. No soap can wash the skin as clean as the new skin you have under the old. You make new skin every 24 hours on the body. That new skin is as clean as the blood is.

Skin brushing removes the old, dead layer. This helps to eliminate uric acid crystals, catarrh, and various other acids in the body. The skin should eliminate two pounds of waste acids daily. Keep the skin active. No one can be well wearing clothes unless they brush their skin. It is the greatest method to remove the scurf-rim (found in the eye) which denotes an underactive poorly eliminating skin. Do your brushing first thing in the morning when you arise, before your bath.

Clothing Can Be Bad. Most people who wear clothes have skin troubles and develop underactive skin. I believe that wearing clothes was the beginning of our diseases, but I do not think that society today is geared to having nude people running around on the streets. As long as we have to wear clothes, we should brush the skin. Take a vegetable bristle brush and rub the skin three to four minutes in any direction. This will keep the skin active. Every squre inch of skin has two hundred pores made up of muscle structure that must be exercised to get rid of toxic wastes.

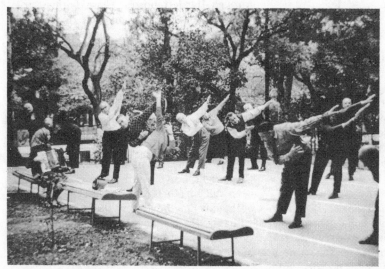

RUSSIA—Exercising in the parks. We found that every morning between 8 and 8:30 the men exercise to music. This is done throughout the regions around the Black Sea.

TWELVE

Get moving with exercise

DUE to the civilized world in which we work today, and due to the abnormal positions under which we work, it is necessary if we choose to stay well to consider some form of compensational exercise.

Physical activity of the body is an absolute necessity. Our bodies were made to move. If they are not kept supple and moveable they will deteriorate, giving poor service. Through actual experience with patients, we have found one objective extremely advisable to work toward in all cases. We must keep the abdomen in good working order and the spine limber. To keep the spine limber muscles must be developed evenly on both sides of the spine, then a perfect lymph supply is able to get into the cartilages between the vertebrae. Lymph is necessary, since we have no blood vessels to keep these tissues alive. With exercises one can do more work without a breakdown. Exercise helps to develop greater room for the nerve liners that pass through the foramen in the spine.

Deep Breathing Exercises

Few of us breathe deeply enough to oxygenate the blood. The deep breathing vibratory exercises explained here are highly concentrated to drive the oxygen into the blood stream, benefiting the nerve, muscular, and glandular system. These exercises benefit all ages. They are especially good for those over forty, when one leads a less active life. Through these exercises you receive the equivalent of two and one half to three hours of the usual form of very active exercises.

A. Benefits the Liver and Spleen. The liver is the detoxifier in the body. The correct posture for this exercise is to sit up straight with no curvatures in the spine. Take a deep, full breath in through both nostrils. Hold your breath. Drop head gently back (don't strain). Then bring head forward, expelling breath through the nostrils strongly. Do this from 10 to 15 times.

B. Benefits the Heart. Close the right nostril. Take a deep breath in through left nostril. Close both nostrils and hold your breath as long as it is comfortable— then let the breath out slowly through one-half of the right nostril. This is highly concentrated and need be done only once.

C. Especially Good for the Thyroid Gland. This exercise normalizes weight through correctly balanced metabolism, it also calms the nerves. All the blood in the body goes through the thyroid every 1½ hours. The thyroid works the oxygenation process. The thyroid produces thoraxin, which burns up toxins, breaks down and builds up tissues, and controls calcium and sex functions.

Start by sitting up straight. Using the thumb of the right hand, close the right side of the nose. Take a deep breath in through the left nostril. Close both nostrils for a few seconds, then open right nostril halfway and let breath out slowly. Now reverse the order. Close the left side of the nose, and take in a deep breath through the right nostril. Close both for a few seconds, then open the left nostril halfway and let breath out slowly. Do this alternately 10 to 15 times.

D. Lung Purifier and Strengthener. This is a way of getting rid of all stale air in lungs. Close right nostril with right thumb, take a deep full breath in through left nostril, close both, expelling breath out through the mouth with a "HA" sound. Alternate this same procedure, first one side, then the other, for approximately 10 to 5 times.

E. Abdominal and Bowel Constipation Breath

Exercise. Exercise of the bowel is very important; even more so than diet. These exercises strengthen the bowel and its entire digestive system. We must have good muscle structure to support the abdomen and keep the intestines in their proper place.

These exercises strengthen the abdomen structure, revitalize internal organs, prevent food from sticking to intestines, stimulate peristaltic action, and lift the ascending colon.

An excellent practice is to hold the abdomen in at all times; discipline yourself to do this and you'll see an improvement in your digestive and bowel action. Also keep the chest up.

1. Stand up, taking in a deep, full breath through both nostrils. Hold the breath while pounding with closed fists the abdomen below the navel, in a circular right to left motion. Do this 30 times and then let the breath out by blowing it out through the mouth slowly and gradually.

2. Sitting down, sit up straight. Pull in lower stomach or the abdomen. Pull it way in, then let it out. Do this ten times; then relax. Now pull in the left side of the abdomen ten times. Relax. Now pull in the right side of the abdomen ten times. Relax. Now roll the entire stomach/abdomen around right to left 25 times, while holding the breath, then blow breath out.

F. **Vagus Nerve Exercise**. This exercise is for the ears, power of hearing, heart, and digestive organs.

Standing, take a deep full breath and while holding the breath circle head from right to left all the way round. Beginners ten times each way—slowly at first. One who is thoroughly accustomed to this exercise can do it 30 times rapidly, with shoulders participating in the same circular movement. Relax. Now do the same exercise the reverse way, left to right. Always let the breath out through the mouth slowly or gradually after holding it. If you get dizzy, bend back and forward from the hips. Any grating in the neck is good: you are breaking up excessive calcium deposits.

G. **Sleep Breath**. This induces right, peaceful sleep and helps to eliminate snoring. This exercise also balances the thyroid gland function. Fear, sorrow, and destructive mental emotions immediately show their effects in the pancreas and thyroid gland and destroy the enzymes. Fear destroys the iodine in the thyroid gland.

Close the right nostril with right thumb, while repeatedly and rapidly opening and closing the left nostril halfway with the index finger of the right hand. Do this 75 times. Repeat, closing the left nostril with left thumb, while opening and closing rapidly the right nostril with index finger of left hand. Do this 75 times. Breathe normally throughout. All these exercises go to develop muscular tone and flexibility in the abdomen.

H. **Circulation Breath**. Sit forward slightly in a straight chair. Place hands on knees, head forward and pant with open mouth in and out 100 times. When just beginning, pant only 50 times, and build up gradually to 100 times. This also stimulates the salivary gland juices.

I. **Pituitary Gland**. The pituitary gland is the master gland that controls all the other glands in the body. This exercise feeds the brain by improving circulation, improves thyroid gland, and acts as a beauty treatment by bringing blood to the neck and face. It produces flexibility in the spine by stretching vertebrae and spinal nerves.

Stand with feet wide apart. Close right nostril, take in a deep, full breath through left nostril, close both, bend knees slightly. Place right hand on head, then bend slowly down, concentrating on each one of the spinal vertebrae all the way, letting the neck drop loosely. Hold the breath in this position as long as you can. Come back up still holding the breath and feeling each one of the vertebrae pull up. When you are straight up, open the right nostril halfway and gradually let the breath out. Do this exercise only twice, since it is highly concentrated. THIS EXERCISE IS NOT FOR PEOPLE WITH HIGH BLOOD PRESSURE.

J. **Vibratory Breath for Pancreas Gland**. The pancreas digests all the body's proteins and starches.

Close right nostril with right thumb, take in a full breath through left nostril, close both nostrils, and moisten lips, letting the breath out gradually through the lips while vibrating them, pulling up the diaphragm at the same time. Relax, then repeat twice.

K. **Vibratory Throat Exercise**. Another excellent vibratory throat exercise is to take breath through both nostrils. Bend head to right and tap up and down the throat while you HUM the breath out through the mouth. Reverse and do other side of neck.

L. Vitality Breath. Sitting up straight, with no sway back or front droop, sniff breath in and out through both nostrils in rapid succession from 75 to 100 times. Beginners who have to can do it 25 times, then stop and relax, then repeat 25 times more, then stop and relax, and so on until you build up your breathing ability and capacity.

M. Vocal Cord Breathing and Exercise. This exercise works out and clears up mucus and energizes the entire abdominal region. Sit up straight, take in a full breath through both nostrils and hold. Put three fingers of the left hand on the right side of the Adam's apple or Eve's apple, pulling the apple to the left. Turn the head full to the right; hold it for a few seconds, then bring the head forward and let breath out gradually, blowing through the mouth. Relax, then repeat this same exercise twice more. Reverse the exercise, taking a full breath through both nostrils, putting the three fingers of the right hand on the left side of the Adam's apple or Eve's apple. Pull the apple to the right as you turn your neck and head full to the left, hold for a few seconds, bring head front, and let breath out slowly, blowing through the mouth. Relax; and repeat two more times.

N. Pancreas Breath. This is for greater confidence, increased energy, and chest expansion. Mental disturbance affects the pancreas instantly. You cannot get well unless you have chest expansion.

Standing up, in one breath, sniff in four times so that the chest is fully expanded. Then let the breath out in one snort through the nose. During the entire exercise, swing the right arm to shoulder length. Raise the left knee and foot to take in the first sniff. Then raise the left arm shoulder high with the right kneee and foot raised on the second sniff. Then raise the right arm and left knee and foot with the third sniff. Then on the fourth arm and leg lift, snort breath out through both nostrils. Rest for three counts. Keep this up for 15 to 25 times. This same sniff breath can be done while walking. These exercises help you to breathe deeply, which promotes good health.

O. Parathyroid Neck Exercise. Keeping spine straight, drop head slightly forward. Then place the three center fingers of both hands at the top of the neck. Take in a full breath and hold as you pull both hands, slowly but hard, around to the front of the throat just above the Adam's apple. Let breath out by slowly blowing.

The second time vary the exercise by beginning the hard pull from the center so that the neck shows red; blow breath out and relax.

The third time begin at the base of the neck and pull the fingers around the collar bone. Release arms, blow out, and relax.

Excessive mucus is the beginning of all disease. All these exercises stimulate the eliminative processes in the entire system and help get rid of excessive mucus.

P. Exercise for Pituitary, Thyroid, and Adrenal Glands. Put feet together and stand erect. Take in full deep breath, with hips forward and no sway back; pull up stomach and abdomen; bow arms by slightly raising out to the sides. Turn head full sideways to right; hold a few seconds; then bring head forward and relax arms down while slowly blowing breath out through the mouth. Relax. Repeat this two more times. Then do it three times turning the neck and face sideways in the opposite direction. Relax.

Remember: The glands must be fed constructive mental enotions, joy, love, beauty, peace, music, etc., which we must consciously practice. The glands must also be fed nourishing food and proper exercise. As soon as you stop destructive thinking you will not have any thyroid trouble.

Four Special Throat and Face Exercises for Circulation and Muscle Tone

1. Sitting down, smile very exaggeratedly, stretching the throat cords and upper chest 15 times. Relax.

2. Alternate each side of the mouth the same way. Tense right side, then relax. Tense left side. Relax. Repeat 15 times.

3. Tilt the chin upward and move it in a chewing motion. Stretch the throat 30 times. Relax.

4. Close the mouth and squeeze the facial muscles, under the skin, up to 30 times. This is good to keep the under-face muscles firm, which keeps the skin from sagging and lifts the mouth muscles.

Special Eye Exercises

1. For eye vision, to develop quick, keen, and alert near and far eyesight: Put the right index finger up directly a foot in front of the eyes. Pick out the smallest object you can— at least a mile away, look at the finger tip, then quickly look at the distant object. Do this 20 to 30 times, looking only at the tip then directly at the distant object.

2. Eye Circulation Exercise. Place the left middle finger over the right eye, lightly tapping the first joint of the middle finger with the index and middle fingers of the right hand, moving the left middle finger joint all around the right eye. Then repeat the same procedure with the left middle finger over the right eye.

3. To Show Your Fusion Is Good. Hold up right index finger about a foot and a half in front of your eyes, look way out in the distance until the finger makes two, then look out between the two fingers.

4. Eye Muscle Exercises.
Put the right index finger up in front of the eyes and, while looking at the finger tip, move it in close to the eyes, feeling the eye muscle pull in, then move the finger out two feet, feeling the muscle relax out as you do this 15 to 20 times. Relax arm down.

Keeping the head straight ahead, throw the eyes way up to the upper right, then down lower left, swing them fully up and down. Then reverse procedure, upper left down to lower right, 15 times. Relax.

Raise the eyes up to the sky, also lifting the lower lids upwards, then lower the eyes to the ground, always keeping the head straight ahead. Do this 15 times. Relax.

Roll the eye balls around in the eye socket from right to left in a full circle, feeling the muscular action, then reverse the eye action. Do each 15 times. Relax.

5. For Full Wide Eye Vision. Put the two index fingers out in front of the eyes about two feet apart, bringing them slowly back toward the ears, until you can no longer see the fingers from the sides of the eyes. Keep the head and the eyes straight ahead. Do this procedure 15 times.

6. To Rid the Eyes of Tension. Look through the sun, blinking the eyes rapidly, while moving the head from left to right for several moments. At the same time rub the palms of the hands together, working up the natural healing warmth of the palms. When they are warm, place the center of the right palm over the right eye. Then place the center of the left palm over the left eye. Open your eyes to see that all the light is shut out, and adjust palms until all light is shut out. Then close the eyes and without any pressure on or around the eyes from the hands— or any tension in the neck, shoulders, or any part of your body— meditate in this position, elbows resting on a high enough support to prevent any awkward strain, for at least eight to 15 minutes. This can be done several times during the day, time permitting.

A meditation I enjoy is based on my profound feeling words: "*I FEEL WONDER-FUL.*" Within this statement is the very basic feeling of having perfectly natural good health. It is based on the original truth that as you feel in your heart and mind so shall you be. This is the profound secret of well-being in all aspects of Life, Spirit, Mind, and Body.

To Circulate Blood through Every Organ

To circulate blood through every organ of the body is the second most important requirement in getting well. This is done through exercise.

Walking and hiking are a stimulant to the flow of blood throughout the body. Swimming is the best form of exercise. It uses the whole body evenly in a prone position and promotes perfect circulation to the head, where the fatigue center exists.

There are many forms of exercise which may be used. I believe that tensing and relaxing the body is very good. Any time we tense a muscle in the body we tend to make the tissue anemic, forcing the blood into more relaxed parts. If we follow this tensing with relaxation, blood automatically fills these relaxed tissues. Many times muscles can be squeezed and contracted without bending the joints. to squeeze and relax muscle structure without involving the joints allows for greater repair of tissue with the least amount of acids forming.

Muscle Tension Exercises

These exercise the entire body, especially the spine from top to bottom. A strengthened spine opens all nerve lines and aids the thyroid gland. It gives poise to body and causes true, right relaxation. Tension and relaxing exercises produce lactic acid in the system. The more tension you produce the better the relaxation after the tension.

1. Raise arms up over head, claw hands, and with great tension draw arms down to chest and hold very tense for a few seconds. Then relax completely. Do this three times.

2. Arms to sides, claw hands, pull up toward chest all the while tensing arms, hold tension for a few seconds, then relax completely. Do this three times.

3. Arms out front. Claw hands and pull in to chest. Hold tension a few seconds. Relax completely. Do this three times.

4. Hands interlaced, right elbow way back on your right side, left pulls right arm down across chest, resisting at the same time. Then do the opposite. Keep body straight as you pull the arms across the chest.

5. Intertwine hands in back, pull apart and move hands up and down the spine.

6. Abdominal exercise: Knees stiff, bend forward, put hands together way out to right side and push one against the other, resisting all the way to the left side, then do it the other way to right side, feeling the pull in the abdomen.

7. Put right leg slightly in front of the left. Tense calf, then thigh. Relax both. Then repeat with the other leg. Do each leg eight times. Excellent for building and strengthening circulation and leg muscles, giving correct contour to the leg.

8. Head way forward, hands entwined on back of head. Push head back slowly as you resist with hands and arms all the way back, then relax. Now start with head back, both hands clasped in back of head. Bring forward, resisting hard with neck. Turn head way to left side; place left hand on side of head and push head to other side. Do other side the same way. Keep shoulders and body straight ahead.

9. Hands together in prayer, push from left to right side, then from right to left, resisting hard each way.

10. Hands together in prayer at stomach, push against each other all the way up over the head while pulling the entire stomach way up; then relax.

11. Put left hand and arm over left shoulder, reaching down back, while the right arm and hand is bent up the spine. Clasp fingers together; pull up with left and down with right; let go and relax. Then do opposite hands and arms.

Tension/Relaxation

We are now beginning to recognize the importance of lactic acid in the body. We definitely know that it neutralizes nerve acids. Lactic acid nerve injections are being used for the mentally ill. Those who are nervous, emotionally upset, and suffer from nerve depletion are the people who have not taken the right foods and have not had the proper kind and amount of exercise. Lactic acid is produced in the body as an end product of muscular metabolism. It gives us the energy to accomplish physical expression. It helps to neutralize many of the fatigue acids in the body.

The ordinary calisthenic exercises are apt to create too many fatigue acids and so we recommend our own relaxation and tension exercise, as explained both above and below, which produce the greatest amount of lactic acid and the least amount of fatigue acids.

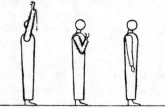

Chinning Exercise. Tense the muscles by clawing the hands, holding them above the head and act as though you are chinning yourself. Tense all the muscles as you bring the hands down toward the shoulders. When you have reached the shoulders with this extreme muscle tension, then relax. It should take three or four seconds to bring the arms down. Do this three times.

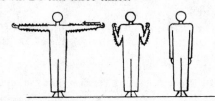

Tension Exercise. The same exercise can be done with the arms directly out at the sides.

Do not close the hands in fist fashion. Keep the fingers half closed so that you can tense the body more, if you desire. Bring the tensed arms in from the sides to the shoulders and when they reach the shoulders, drop them and relax them.

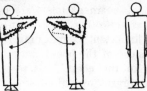

Tension- Relaxation Exercise. Place the fingers of the right hand in the fingers of the left hand. Raise hands in front of you and a little to the left, and about even with the head. Pull down with the fingers of the right hand and resist with the left hand. Both hands should be tensed and should be pulling against each other. As you pull and resist, you are gradually bringing the left hand down with the right hand. Bring it down as far as you can and relax.

Do this same exercise by placing the hands in front of the body and to the right, at an angle. This time pull the right hand down with the left hand, using resistance in the fingers of each hand. Bring down as far as possible and relax. This exercise should be repeated three times on each side.

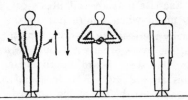

Back Exercise. Place both arms straight down in back of you. Tense the muscles and pull one arm against the other. Then raise the hands up toward the shoulders, all the while keeping your hands locked and tensed. Then slowly bring them down to position and relax. This can be done under tension, three or four times and then rest.

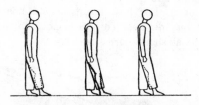

Leg Exercise. Put one leg forward in a relaxed position, then tense its muscles, and relax. Repeat this exercise for the other leg. This exercise may be repeated from three to six times for each leg.

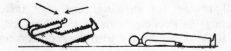

Master Exercise. Lie on the floor or a bed, arms down at the sides and legs and feet straight. Bending at the hips, bring the head and feet up toward ceiling, tensing all the muscles of the body, including the arms, legs, stomach, etc. Hold for three seconds in this position and relax. Do this three times.

Spinal and Nerve Exercise

Standing, place feet apart. Turn toes in pigeon fashion, get a good firm gripping stance, so hips are held absolutely straight, then swing loosely from hips up, from left to right, letting arms, hands, and neck go very free and relaxed. Do this 20 times. This is a wonderful spinal exercise and if done properly will cause the spine to make its own correct adjustment.

Prolapsed Organs

Everyone in ill health has prolapsed organs. Prolapsed organs come from denatured, devitalized foods, occupations that keep us from exercising properly, not enough sleep, too much standing, improper posture, overeating, and too many starches.

To overcome prolapsus, which can cause bladder and kidney irritations, pressure on the sex glands, interfering with proper functions, pressure on the heart, improper breathing, inferiority complex, acidosis, and painful menstruation, it is absolutely necessary that we learn how to live. To live properly is to start a cleansing process, a tearing down of old cell structure material and a rebuilding of new. It requires a real housecleaning, which sometimes is not very pleasant. But years from now you will recognize it as the greatest thing you have ever done for yourself.

It is important with prolapsus to eliminate while squatting. It is also good to take enemas for a good cleansing. By following the Daily Diet Regime, over a period of time your body will absorb the chemical elements that will give your flesh tone and firmness. If you do the exercises and learn the proper posture, the abdominal organs will all go into place and stay there.

In extreme prolapsus, raise the foot end of the bed about two or three inches so that when you are lying down the organs will fall toward the shoulders and stay there during the sleeping hours. A useful exercise is to lie across the bed with the shoulders on the floor, allowing the organs to fall down toward the chest cavity.

Slant Board Exercises

(For Prolapsus and Regenerating the Vital Nerve Centers of the Brain)

When there is a lack of tone in the muscles we can expect prolapsus of the abdominal organs. The heart, lacking tone, cannot circulate blood properly throughout the body. Likewise, arteries and veins cannot contract to help the blood go against gravity up into the brain tissues.

There are some people who apparently have tried everything to get well and their organs are still working under par. Many people do not realize that all the quickening force for every organ of the body comes from the brain. People whose occupations require them to sit or stand continually are unable to get the blood into the brain tissues because the tired organs cannot force the blood uphill. If we continue to deny the brain tissues enough good blood, eventually every organ in our bodies will suffer.

The heart gets its start from the brain and continues its everlasting pumping because of it. No organ can do without the brain. Slant board exercises help the brain become healthier and are absolutely necessary to regaining overall perfect health.

Slant board exercises have done phenomenal things for people with prolapsus and lack of tone in the abdominal walls. A Mr. C. M. Pierce did wonders in rejuvenating his body through the slant board when he was in his seventies. We quote from *Health News* of September 26, 1941: "One night three years ago I saw Dr. Jensen demonstrate the slant board and instantly saw how to make my system much easier, and on the way home I told my neighbor, "I am going to make a board like that." He then went on to make many slant boards, selling them throughout the country.

But there are many cases where the board is contraindicated. It is best in most cases to get professional advice, for some people have had unhappy experiences due to the very fact they started too strenuous a program to begin with. If you haven't done much exercising of the abdominal muscles, it is well to begin slowly and gradually increase them as you get stronger.

Do not use the slant board in cases of high blood pressure, hemorrhages, some tubercular conditions, cancer in the pelvic cavity, appendicitis, ulcers of the stomach or intestines, or pregnancy, unless you are under the care of a physician.

The slant board exercises are practically the same as any other lying down exercises. The most important exercises involve holding onto the sides of the board and bringing the knees up to the chest. This forces all the abdominal organs up toward the shoulders. while in this position, twist the head from side to side and in all directions, thus utilizing the extra force to circulate blood to congested areas of the head, especially bringing the stomach and abdominal organs up toward the chest while holding the breath.

Slant board exercises are especially good in cases of inflammations and congestions above the shoulders, such as sinus trouble, bad eyes, falling hair, head eczema, ear conditions, and similar troubles. Slant board exercises have helped more than any other treatment in cases of heart trouble, fatigue, dizziness, poor memory, and paralysis.

The average person should maintain the foot end of the board at chair height for all exercises, but if it makes him dizzy, he should lower foot end of the board a bit to begin with. Exercise only five minutes a day. More is too much when you're just starting out. Gradually increase the time spent on the slant board; the average patient should be able to lie on the slant board approximately ten minutes around 3:00 P.M. in the afternoon and again just before going to bed. After retiring lift the buttocks up to allow the organs to return to a normal position.

Some General Slant Board Exercises

Use ankle straps while doing the following exercises:

1. Lie full length, allowing gravity to help the abdominal organs into their proper position and letting the blood circulate to the head. For best results lie on board at least ten minutes. This basic position should climax all slant board exercises.

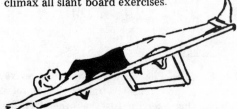

2. While lying flat on the back, stretch the abdomen by putting arms above head. Bring

arms above head 10 to 15 times; this stretches the abdominal muscles and pulls the abdomen down toward the shoulders.

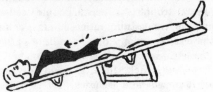

3. Bring abdominal organs toward shoulders while holding your breath. Move the organs back and forth by drawing abdomen upward, then allowing it to go back to a relaxed position. Do 10 to 15 times.

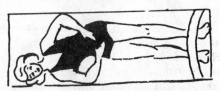

4. Pat abdomen vigorously with open hands. Lean to one side then to the other, patting the stretched side. Pat 10 to 15 times. Reverse sides three or four times.

5. Bring the body to sitting, using the abdominal muscles. Return to lying position. Do three or four times, if possible. *But do only if doctor orders.*

Hold on to the handles, feet out of straps, while doing the following:

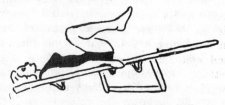

6. Bend knees and legs at hips. While in this position (a) turn head from side to side five or six times; (b) lift the head slightly and rotate in circles three or four times. Reverse. Repeat each set two or three times.

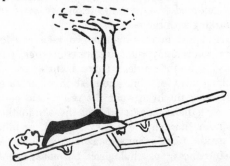

7. Lift legs to vertical position and rotate outward in circles eight or ten times. Then

change direction to inward circles. Increase to 25 times after a week or two of exercising.

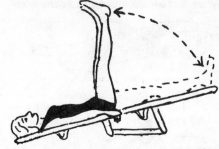

8. Bring legs straight up to a vertical position and lower them to board slowly, first right leg, then left, keeping each straight. Then raise and lower both together. Repeat three

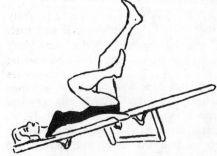

or four times. Bicycle legs in air 15 to 25 times.

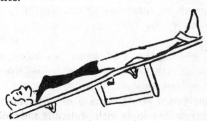

9. Relax and rest, letting the blood circulate in the head for ten minutes.

The side roll. The Side Roll is especially good for conditions of sciatica and lower back pains and for relaxing nerve tension in the lower and middle back and for directing nerve supply to the lower abdominal organs.

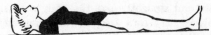

Lie upon a firm bed so that when the leg is extended in this exercise it will be at a lower level than the body. Turn on left side,

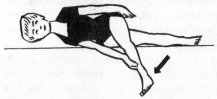

raise the right leg to a 45 degree angle across the body. Grasp ankle with left hand and pull leg up toward the head and at the same

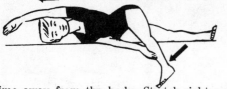

time away from the body. Stretch right arm up and back, pulling the spine in the opposite

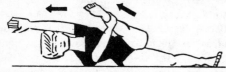

direction. Reverse and repeat on the other side.

This is an extreme spinal stretch with the greatest amount of muscle pull on the lower back.

Standing Mule Kick. One important factor in civilization today that affects the physical organism is the restriction of activity. We do not walk, bend, stretch, and straighten up enough so that the veins and arteries can carry the blood freely between the heart and the lower extremities. When we sit for any length of time, having our legs bent at the hips, we are exerting extra pressure on the heart.

Every time the heart beats the blood is carried through the arteries which lead from it through all parts of the body, alternately expanding and contracting. When the heart beats while the body is in a sitting or bent position, there is an obstruction or a slowing up of the free flow of the blood, and pressure takes place, affecting the heart.

This organ is the strongest one in the body, but if it is constantly subjected to undue pressure, it will ultimately cease to function normally. The result could be a heart attack.

If we have been in a sitting position for any length of time, it is good to get up frequently and straighten out the body so that the blood may flow freely. When traveling in a vehicle, stop at intervals, get out, and walk around a little. Do not sit at a desk or in a seat hour after hour without getting up for a stretch or a walk. To straighten out and activate the arteries and the legs, the Mule Kick is of uppermost importance.

To straighten out the nerves is also important. To get circulation into the lower extremeities so that the joints may be fed properly demands this straightening up

process, especially if you have a sedentary occupation or habits and have indications of trouble in the nerves or joints. In addition to heart trouble, a person could develop lymphatic congestion, varicose veins, cramps in the legs, and many other conditions affecting the legs.

The Mule Kick, then, is good for those with lumbago and sciatica, for sedentary occupational workers, and for those who go through long hours in a sitting position.

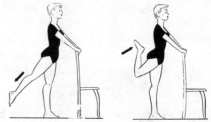

The Mule Kick is done best by standing in back of a chair and grasping the chair with both hands. Raise the right leg backward, bending the knee so that the heel touches the buttocks. Kick back with a fast jerking movement, like a mule would kick. Then extend the same leg straight back as far as possible and parallel with the floor and kick back with a sharp thrust. Alternate the legs, kicking three times each.

Draining the Neck Lymph Glands. This is excellent for enlarged tonsils, neck tension, congestion of the eyes, ears, sinuses, antrum, head, headaches, migraine headaches, head noises, lymph nodes, toxic thyroid function.

Much could be said in regard to taking care of congestions and disturbances that occur in the head area. Many times the cause is remote, involving the extremeities of the body. The head can be the source of many catarrhal congestions when the circulation becomes sluggish, which would cause poor drainage in the neck and poor blood exchange in the head and lymph glands of the neck. To eliminate sinus congestion, we start by working with the neck.

But we must remember to take care of the whole body when we are concerned with any local infirmities. There is little use in taking care of sinus congestion or diseases affecting the head when the rest of the body is even more congested and the elimination is poor through the kidneys, bowel, or skin. Pressure from occupational factors; financial disturbances; psychological mismanagement of situations involving one's children, family, job, or human relations can result in neck tensions. We must remove these pressures as much as possible and as soon as possible, when we experience ill effects in the areas of the head and neck. The condition may often be relieved temporarily through the practice of the following exercise.

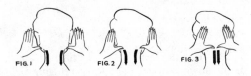

1. Press thumbs behind both the ears at the base of the skull, then push under the skull into neck with firm pressure, slowly going down towards the collar bone.

2. Press thumbs one inch further in on both sides.

3. Press thumbs still further in along side vertebral column.

4. Repeat.

Be sure to press under the skull with the thumbs, then down into the neck to the shoulder level. Do the above exercise once or twice a day to relieve head and neck congestion.

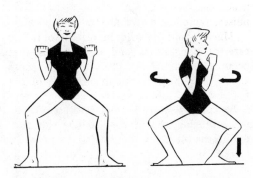

The Wrestler's Stance. This is an old Japanese stance that has been used by the wrestlers whenever they enter the ring. It is excellent for development of the muscular structure in the hips and the calves of the legs and also for developing circulation and muscular strength in the lower abdomen. The Wrestler's Stance is good for lower abdominal muscle development, prostate gland, congestion in any part of the lower abdominal cavity, and for strengthening the upper legs.

Stand with feet apart and knees bent.

Twist from side to side, from the hip up. Bend arms at elbows.

Gradually do a knee bend, going down as close to the heels as possible. Come up slowly, tighten the buttock muscles, and continue the same twist. Do this up and down motion four or five times.

The twisting motion helps develop the muscular structure on each side of the abdomen so that hernias and ruptures will not develop. Tightening the buttocks when rising to a standing position also helps to get a better circulation of blood into the rectal areas and the prostate gland.

Circulation and "Muscle-izing" Exercises

The following exercises are to be performed morning and night. They free encumbrances, give muscles tone, and build better circulation.

You are expected to start slowly and build up to a point of reasonable fatigue, but never to a point of overexertion. Make each muscle work by squeezing hard, concentrate on every movement, and do not jerk the muscles. Do only that which your body is capable of doing.

Generally all these exercises can be used three times each; the easy ones can be done more than three times. Do the same exercise on both sides, so as to develop a well-balanced body.

Sitting Exercises

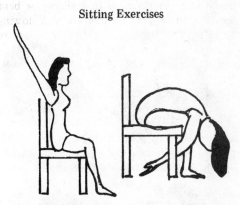

1. Sit upright—feet and knees well apart—and stretch arms straight over head. Bend body forward, swinging arms well under the chair, keeping your chin on chest. Put head as far under chair as possible, stretching back muscles. Return to sitting position with arms still above head and the upward stretch tensing the abdominal muscles.

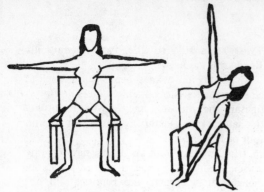

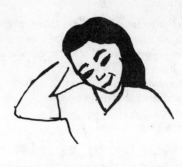

2. Sit upright—knees and feet well apart—arms sideward, shoulder height. Bend over and turn trunk to left while left hand touches right toes and right hand stretches well above the head to produce tension on side of abdomen. Turn trunk in opposite direction and reverse exercise.

7. Stand with feet 12 to 14 inches apart. Look down toward right foot, bringing right arm up and placing palm of right hand at the back of head and drawing steadily toward right foot. Do the same on other side and with left arm.

Standing-Up Exercises

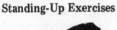

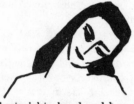

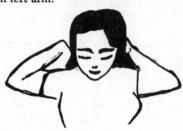

3. Look straight ahead and lean head over on shoulder while keeping eyes straight front. First lean to one side then to the other.

8. Clasp both hands behind head and pull straight down toward feet.

4. Turn head from side to side, stretching as far as possible.

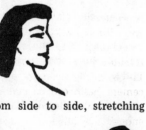

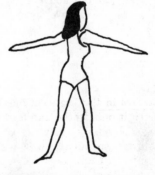

5. Drop head forward. Turn head in circular motion, keeping face and eyes straight ahead. Do this three times in each direction.

9. Feet apart—arms to side—twist body at hips, swinging around first to one side and then to the other.

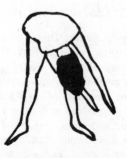

6. Drop head straight backward and forward as far as possible, omitting circular motion.

10. Bend forward allowing hands to drop down to toes, and throw arms together, first up to one side and then to the other.

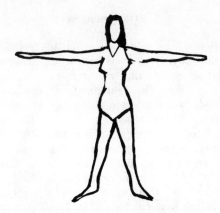

11. Raise arms sideward, level with shoulders, and make circles with hands (backwards) about 15 to 16 inches in diameter.

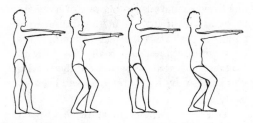

The Calf Stretcher
1. Stand up straight, putting one leg directly behind the other, toe touching heel.
2. Keeping erect, bend slowly at the knees. Do this ten times. This pulls on the long muscles of the leg.
3. Change over so the other leg is in front and repeat another ten times.
4. Repeat.

Muscle Cramps in the Legs. Put one leg on a chair, stretch it out tightly, and lean towards the foot that is on the chair. Reach for the toe with the corresponding arm. This stretches all the leg muscles from the hip down through the heel and allows for better circulation, break-up of congestion, and removal of blood stagnation.

Exercise, Breathing, Water Treatments, and Baths

Breathing exercises, such as were taught by Dr. Hanish, are very helpful. Quick inhalations with slow exhalations help the body tremendously. While we are inhaling slowly, we should try to tense the body.

Forcing against your own body, or another's body, in a pulling-pushing fashion, is a form of mild wrestling which is good. Aesthetic dancing is very good. To really stimulate the bloodstream investigate square dancing.

A mild form of exercise that can be prac-

ticed by most people is jumping up and down in one spot, just as though you were running.

Water treatments are probably the most important of all to think of. This is a method of getting blood into the various organs of the body without exercise. Cold water forces the blood away from the tissues, wherever the cold pack is used. Warm water relaxes the tissues, allowing blood to be brought to the tissue wherever the hot pack is used.

By using alternate hot and cold packs, we are then able to drive the blood into and draw it out of the various organs of the body. Using hot and cold packs on the shoulders, knees, feet, and abdomen is very beneficial. It moves along the stagnant blood. In using the alternate packs, consider one-half minute cold and one minute hot, with eight changes. Of all the baths that we use, I believe the sitz bath to be the best. This may be used alternately hot and cold also.

There is a very wonderful bath called the cosmo-vital bath. The method is to lie on the back in four inches of cold water from one-half to one minute, while the exposed part of the body is in the hot sunshine. The blood will thus be drawn to the upper parts. Then turn over, so that you are face down in the water, back exposed to the sun, and the blood will quickly be drawn to your exposed back, while the front parts are now being cooled in the water.

Stay in this position one-half to one minute. This is the most natural of all baths. Lie with the head to the north. A shallow cement basin can be made just for this purpose, with walls four inches high and large enough to allow the human form to lie stretched out in it.

Tai Chi
Tai Chi—short for Tai Chi Chuan—is an exercise that is used in Taiwan and the internal parts of mainland China. It is used in the morning before going to work as an exerciser and a conditioner for the body. Tai Chi does not give you any heavy breathing or exhausting gyrations such as we have in our typical calisthenics. It is a nonstrenuous, pleasant conditioner. It is one of the old martial arts that has been slowed down to an activity that the average person can use; it helps to develop small muscles of the body which we use so much in our daily activity and helps to take care of the internal arterial system and venous blood system. Many people just don't do enough from a physical exercise standpoint. People in America have sedentary

jobs, exhausting mental activity; they need a hobby or exercises to balance this out. Tai Chi could be used every day by everyone. The Chinese use it in all ages, from when a child is young right on through to 70 and 80 years of age.

You will find that Tai Chi is a well organized program and takes in the development of the whole body. I personally believe that Tai Chi is the greatest emotional balancer that we have for the body. It is a wonderful exercise in developing the longevity pattern in a person and for producing the best of health.

Tai Chi gets in and develops all of the joints of the body, takes in all of the small muscles, and helps to keep the circulation going in all parts of the body. It is a very wonderful exercise because when we are finished we have rounded out or have given round circulation exercises to all the joints of the body. This is important because many exercises just go forward and backward, side to side, and do not give the circle exercises to the joints.

Tai Chi Exercises. These are practiced in the parks in Hong Kong, Taiwan and the internal parts of mainland China. This is an ancient art that we could take a good lesson from and use well in this country. It is now being taught in many centers throughout the United States. These pictures were taken in the park in China.

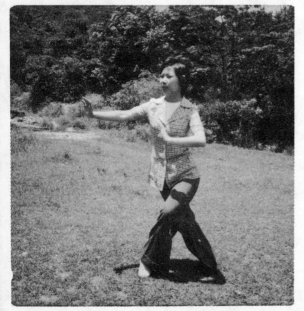

Overcoming Tension

Renew the Mind. Relaxing and revitalizing the body has to come from within. The source of all change and improvement is within us. If we learn the right principles, the physical body will respond in well-being. The physical body is the temple we live in. The stones are set according to our relationship to life. That is going to determine the condition of every cell in our bodies. Every thought will finally find an expression in the physical body. By thinking the very best thoughts, we can have the kind of body we truly want.

In other words, physical perfection is accomplished by the renewing of the mind. This has been a largely neglected factor in our lives. We have been unaware of its relation to our state of health. In the future, we are going to call this neglected factor "life." It is more important than just "health." You are the richest person in the world if you can live by right principles and keep your body well.

You must advance in knowledge, beyond the belief that whatever you eat makes no difference to your health. You have got to know there are such things as good food, good health, and a good mind. Without all these, you are not going to get anywhere. Let us be inspired to live a better life. "When good men do nothing, evil comes in." There are a lot of people who talk about things but do nothing about them.

How to Relax? In experiments with animals it has been found that simply sleep and relaxing bring such rejuvenation that the body has been able to repair itself. If a person could rest and completely relax through sleep for only one-half hour a day, he could recuperate enough to go on for the remainder of the day.

Most of us don't know how to relax and let go. It is something we have to learn. In Germany there is a place where people come just to sleep and rest — they have a three-year waiting list. People are placed in a dark room and are not allowed to see anything or do anything. Then the sound of "rain on the roof" is reproduced. People rest and relax under the sound of rain. This is what we should do with life— let it go.

Cyd Charisse, a famous Hollywood film star, brings on relaxation by stretching out in a chair she had designed to follow her body's contour and release tension. In a newspaper article on relaxation, she says of this chair,

"I use it whenever I feel keyed up. A big mistake is to go to bed when you are excited from work or a party. No matter how late it is, I lie in my chair with my favorite eye pads on until I feel drowsy. Then I can drop off to sleep as soon as my head hits the pillow. I never thought sleeping pills were the answer. The kind of sleep you get from drugs is not refreshing.

"If I am away from my home and don't have my chair, I lie down and put my feet higher than my head. It is good to let the blood flow away from my feet and to reverse the pull of gravity."

This is exactly what the slant board can accomplish for you. It is a great aid to complete relaxation. Anytime you are tired, especially at the rather depressing hour of around 3:00 P.M., a quick way to restore depleted energies is to get on the slant board for 15 to 30 minutes. Just lie there and relax. Exercises followed by rest bring added value. In these days of strenuous living, the slant board is indispensable. Use it as Cyd Charisse uses her chair. Just before bed, relax on your slant board to free tensions and bring on a pleasant desire for sleep.

Cyd Charisse has another favorite relaxation hint we agree with: "After tennis I love to take a whirlpool bath. You can stimulate the circulation and feel the soreness go away, if you stay in it long enough. I think if you can afford it, this type of water massage is an investment in health." We have one of these baths in our clinic and achieve pleasing results with this form of water therapy.

Activity Releases Tension. Taking care of small muscles is most important. The secret in getting relaxation of these muscles is action. Take another leaf out of Cyd Charisse's book. "I am a great believer in exercise — in anything that will stimulate the circulation. Most people don't use their bodies enough, and they get stiff and out of shape. It is what you do every day that means the most. Knocking yourself out on the golf course or tennis court over the weekend may be an exertion and do more harm that good. I have tremendous energy. I think it comes from not letting myself get overly tired and from exercising and deep breathing."

We produce plenty of lactic acid when we use our muscles. Use your physical powers to make happen that which you desire. You must have a hobby or recreative activity. You cannot maintain health and happiness with no greater release of your creative energy than that provided through your work, unless it be something to which you are utterly devoted. Even then, it will benefit you to do other things. There are few people so strong that they can use only the mind and not the body. Without physical activity, you are on you way to a nervous breakdown. Tensions come when we don't relax our bodies. Every time you move a joint you produce a fatigue acid. Fatigue acids are produced in the joints. These affect the lactic acids in your body, reducing their good. We should try to reach the state where we produce a good balance.

The Need for Minerals. Last year there were three billion pills taken as a means to get people to relax. Normal relaxation is impossible if the body is starving for mineral elements. Magnesium, a mineral found in yellow corn meal, is essential. Obtain it from this source at least once a week. "Milk of Magnesia" is used for your bowels as a medicine. Why not get your own biochemical magnesium from your pantry? Phosphorous, a required nerve food, is also found in the yellow corn meal. Concord grape juice is also high in magnesium. Your body can absorb grape juice more quickly than any other sugar. I believe strongly in grape and apple juice.

Silicon is one of the magnetic elements in the body, along with magnesium. Silicon is necessary for the nerves and is found high in oat straw tea, rice bran, rice polishings, and rice bran syrup, which is also very high in vitamin B. Vitamin B is a wonderful food supplement for those who have nervous disturbances. With your intake of vitamin B supplement, you must also get its mineral partner. Natural foods have these. Vitamin B is found in whole grains, wheat germ, and rice polishings — along with other mineral elements. If you want to overcome mental and nervous disorders, lecithin is a wonderful food. Vitamin B will not stay in the body without it. Vitamins alone will not do any good. Don't buy vitamins without minerals. Get all the minerals possible. Vitamin and mineral supplements must be natural. However, if you can keep the body relaxed, your vitamin consumption won't have to be nearly as high. We burn up vitamins through tension.

The richest source of calcuim in the vegetable kingdom is green kale. Calcium gives tone and steadiness. Good sources of calcium are the green tops of all vegetables. The next best are from grain; the highest and most easily absorbed source is barley. You should not use this grain in the summer, as it is heating in certain liver conditions. However, in the winter, often use barley/green kale soup for its high calcium.

Our Attitudes Are Killing Us. I hardly have a patient who comes into my office relaxed. If only the mind could be straightened out, we would be all right. I am convinced that people's attitudes are killing them faster than anything else. We should control our thoughts and keep them positive. Control our speech; there is great power in the spoken word! Keep well by seeing the good. If you need to get well, be spiritually minded about your disease. Dedicate yourself to finding a deeper realization of oneness with all life. This will bring relaxation and then harmony will express itself in your life and affairs.

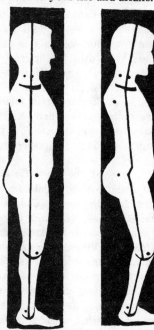

Posture Wise. The Chiropractic Research Foundation has noted that 35 percent of all adults have spinal defects likely to lead to organic disease unless corrected. Standing tall, sitting tall, and walking tall should be our uppermost thought for good posture. Posture habits are formed early in life and these three points should be considered in training and raising our children. The following rules will help in this training:

1. Learn to stand tall, sit tall, and walk tall.

2. Follow a few simple daily exercises to preserve strength and tone of the ligaments and muscles which support the spinal column.

3. Learn to relax completely.

Good posture is the foundation of good health. With correct posture we allow the different organs of the body to have free movement with one another, and no pressure symptoms are produced on one organ more than another. The knees do not become buckled, prolapsus does not set in, shoulders will not droop, and the Adam's apple will not be pressed forward to put pressure on the thyroid gland. Our breathing becomes deeper with good posture. Our chest is carried higher. Good posture does away with lower back curve and the consequent curves that develop in the upper spine. With good posture we walk with our feet straight ahead; the muscles of the legs are strong; the veins and arteries carry the blood more freely; and the nerves in our body carry the messages from our brain to the different organs without any inhibitions or stimulation. Digestion and elemination are improved through good posture.

Another remedy for that big swayback is to walk pigeon-toed every day. If you take care of the swayback, you get rid of the curves in the upper back.

Poor Arches. A remedy for poor arches is to roll the sole of your foot over a golf ball while barefoot. This will help lift fallen arches.

Constipation. It is good to use exercise throughout the bowel. Use soaked prunes, figs, dried fruits with fresh cream in the morning with bran, sometimes a whole grain cereal. Bending, twisting exercises, slant board exercises before breakfast will help.

Gas Pains. Try the knee-chest position several times a day for a few minutes. Sometimes using a rectal (glycerine) suppository will remove hardened feces and help relieve the gas. The knee-chest position will move the gas, which is lighter than air, to pass towards the rectum and be passed off easily.

THIRTEEN

The catarrhal run-off

WHAT Is Catarrh? A catarrhal condition is nature's method of ridding the body of waste materials not handled in the normal elimination process. (The word *catarrh* means "I flow.") When these elimination processes reach the "running" stage that means the body is waging an all-out fight against these centers of infection.

The elimination process should never be stopped, since. any discharge is the natural healing effort of the body to get rid of that which does not belong to it — excess waste material, fatigue acids, etc. Discharge cleanses the body of toxic materials before they harden and become even more difficult to remove from the system. In other words, if we use unnatural methods to stop these acute processes of elimination they will manifest themselves in subacute ways. If the policemen of the body are thwarted in their efforts to oust the petty criminals, the detective may have to be called in later to find the hardened criminal. When we stop a catarrhal discharge we have not effected a cure or conquered a disease; we have merely prolonged the day of reckoning.

Why and How Do Catarrhal Conditions Develop in the Body?

Why do we develop catarrhal conditions? There are hundreds of "little reasons," but basically it all goes back to several major causes, such as inherent weaknesses or constitutional taints in certain areas of our individual bodies. When we know we have an inherently weak colonic system or that our bronchial system is inclined to be affected by adverse weather, etc., we should as a matter of common sense guard against unnecessary attacks — just as we would put a fence around our yard to keep out stray dogs. One reason for the existence of catarrh in any part of the system may be fatigue, because a tired body develops acids which irritate tissues and mucus membranes. This fatigue may be due to habits of work that place undue strain on certain portions of the body. It may be due to overeating or indulging in wrong combinations of food over long periods of time, or the use of narcotics, drugs, or any factor that depletes our normal energy beyond the natural power of the body to resist and throw off such attacks. In short, fatigue may be due to repeatedly breaking the laws of equilibrium or balance which maintain a healthy body.

When we break a public law once, we get off with a small fine or a light sentence. So it is with the body. We may be able to get away with one cold, but if we continue to break the law which resulted in that penalty we will develop a chronic condition and pay for our negligence just as the habitual criminal pays for his law-breaking. If we have already become habitual offenders against the laws of nature, then it is up to us to correct our habits and try to establish law and order again. We need to rehabilitate ourselves! By so doing we can avert serious stages of catarrh as manifested in chronic diseases such as asthma, arthritis, bronchiectasis, diabetes, heart trouble, hardening of the arteries, and cancer.

Getting the Right Start. Much of the ill health in adults has its beginning in childhood. Colds and children's diseases such as mumps, measles, discharges of the ears and nose, etc., should be taken care of by natural methods. We should remember that body cleanliness, correct foods, normal activities, and a happy environment, with plenty of *love*, will prevent most of the ill health found in children. Even those with inherent weaknesses will, if properly cared for, become healthy adults and escape most of the ills of childhood. Are you giving your children the care that is their birthright?

Symptoms of a Catarrhal Condition. There is such a thing as innocently breaking laws that we are unaware of until we are caught, but the body has its policemen who write tickets to enlighten or warn us. These are known as "symptoms." They are in the form of discharges, irritations, pains, and inflammations that occur when we have an accumulation of morbid matter or poisons in any part of the body. These symptoms usually appear first in the mucous membranes. The sign posts grow as we progress down the road to a complete breakdown of the body. From the common cold, which we suppress, we go on to hay fever, which, when dried up, becomes asthma or even arthritis or some other chronic disease.

A weakened body and a sluggish bloodstream and lymph system react to every change in temperature. Every little breeze that blows becomes an ill wind for us. What should be normal adjustments to changing weather conditions such as temperature, humidity, or atmospheric pressures become violent reactions. We can't take them in our stride. We get summer colds, winter colds, attacks of asthma, hay fever, sinusitis, bronchitis, and our joints, which have become corroded with arthritic accumulations, are painful. Accumulations in the arteries cause a strain on the heart and slow the circulation, causing coldness in the extremities. These are symptoms of subacute and acute conditions; they are the result of neglect of small symptoms or the suppression of catarrhal conditions. We are only storing up misery for ourselves and our children when we suppress these small ailments, first discharges, first colds. When we understand that we shall have gone a long way toward maintaining good health.

Nervousness and depression often accompany catarrhal conditions. Many people today have nervous breakdowns, which affect the mental capacity as well as injure the physical body beyond its power to recuperate. This may be due to the strain of living, but disease usually follows tension, and vice-versa.

Fatigue can be a symptom of catarrh, as well as a cause. We feel tired all the time. We can't quite "cut the mustard" at work and we just don't feel like playing. We haven't the energy to carry on our normal activities,

much less the extra vitality needed at times for special occasions. Life becomes dull and burdensome.

Catarrh manifests itself in many other ways. Some of the most common are bronchitis, sinusitis, and tonsillitis.

The symptoms of *bronchitis* are a raw, stuffed feeling in the membranes of the bronchial tubes; poor circulation of the blood, which appears blue in color; sluggish venous circulation; slight or mouthlike inhalation of the breath; weak voice; suffocation; soreness in the chest, developing into a rattle; one red cheek and the other pale; a contraction and tightness in the chest that becomes a hollow cough.

The symptoms of *sinusitis* are similar to those of bronchitis except that they develop in the sinus areas, causing pressure pains in the ears, eyes, and head, with a raw feeling in the sinuses.

Sinusitis affects the various cavities of the head, but we do not treat it as a local condition but as a general thing. When we want to treat the face or the nasal membranes for a local condition, we can use the nasal chlorphyll douche, the salt water nasal douche, or the chamomile tea douche. We could also use hot and cold packs or hot epsom salt packs on the face, along with our catarrh treatment.

We treat *tonsillitis* the same as we do all catarrhal conditions of the body. We do not consider tonsillitis a local condition to be taken care of without considering the whole body. We must build good health. It is part of our work to recognize that what cures disease is found in the prevention of disease, and whatever works to prevent disease can also be used in the eradication of a disease.

When we reach these extreme conditions we know we are old offenders against the laws of nature. We know we have created an abnormal composition of the blood and lymph systems through improper foods or the addition of drugs. Or perhaps we have blocked the normal flow of the blood or lymph by some occupational or recreational habit that puts abnormal pressure on the colon and those portions of the body that act as waste disposal areas. When we block their normal flow, these wastes may eventually get into other areas of the body and cause mastitis, appendicitis, colitis, or any of the many forms of "itis" with which we mortals are commonly afflicted.

What to do. When we get that kind of back

up the first thing we must do is give the body as much rest as possible, because a tired body cannot eliminate, nor can it function. It requires all the energy it is producing to throw off its excess accumulations. Just as it took an abnormal amount of strain to break down the body, so will it take more than an abnormal amount of rest or relief from stress to rebuild it to a normalcy. Any undue stress or strain must be compensated for by extra relief and rest for that portion of the body that is affected. Any accumulations must be taken care of by giving the body the right combination of foods, water, air, sunshine, a normal amount of work, and a plentiful supply of joy. Why joy? Because the body is physical, mental, and spiritual, and the well-being of one is dependent upon the well-being of all the others.

Watch Your Breath. Too many of us do not understand the importance of correct breathing, possibly because we do not know much about this vital function of the entire body. The medulla of the brain is the nerve center that controls the respiration of the lung structure. When we wear down the nervous system this particular center of the brain cannot control the breathing well. There are many people who cannot breathe as they should and who actually lose their lives from nervous breakdowns.

Our breathing capacity has a direct connection with the spinal cord, the muscles and nerves in the neck, and the medulla of the brain. An arthritic spine or tight neck muscles will impair breathing capacity and eventually weaken the brain control over our breathing. Some people with depleted nervous systems and weakened medullas will breathe way down low as little as six times a minute. This is scarcely enough to sustain life, much less enable them to work, play, and enjoy living. Those who are subject to fears will develop a very fast breath. Under emotional stress such as fear, anger, and hatred, the breathing will become staccato, short and quick, as high as thirty times a minute. Watch your breath!

Air that is laden with dust, industrial chemicals, car fumes, carbon monoxide, and other offending materials cannot feed the lungs or the bloodstream with a healthful supply of oxygen, nitrogen, and other essential elements. The body is fighting a losing battle when it tries to extract from such poisoned materials the small amount of good that remains in them, and it cannot help

but develop acute, then subacute catarrhal conditions, then finally chronic ailments.

Keep Clean. In order to have true freedom from any disease, it is essential to have a clean body Keeping the body clean is a must in maintaining good health. Whenever we have debris or an excessive amount of cararrhal congestion in the body germ life is attracted. It has been said that nearly everyone has tubercular germs in the throat area. This doesn't mean that nearly everyone has tuberculosis, but it does mean that if the body is allowed to become nutritionally unbalanced and filled with catarrhal settlements this germ life can become more active and may develop into a serious condition.

I have never felt we should treat this germ life. I believe we should treat the cause. I believe we should cleanse the liver, the gall bladder, and the intestinal tract and thereby increase the resistance of the body to germs. The eliminative organs will throw off the catarrh and with it the germs, because they have no breeding grounds. We do not consider germ life the primary negative condition in the body or the primary cause of disease; rather, it is the secondary effect — it is the effect of a catarrhal build up in the body.

The enema can be very helpful in preventing a catarrh build up, but it should be used principally in an eliminating and fasting regime. It should be used for cleansing the lower bowel only, serving as a slight stimulant to peristaltic action. One pint of plain, lukewarm water is sufficient for the enema. If there is an extreme colitis condition, flaxseed may be boiled in the water; flaxseed is both soothing and healing. A warm milk enema will relieve internal hemorrhoids. For severe constipation, a thorough cleansing of the lower bowel may be accomplished by using a coffee enema four times daily, every four hours. Coffee stimulates a sluggish bowel. Use three tablespoonsful of ground coffee to one quart of water; boil two or three minutes; then simmer 10 to 20 minutes. Strain and use at body temperature.

To develop a clean intestinal tract we must have what we call the proper acid-alkaline balance. If it is in balance we have an 80 percent germ life made up of friendly bacteria, called acidophilous bacteria. The ratio of the germ life within us determines our health. One mix produces a lot of gas in the bowel and until we get the proper balance we are going to have the gas problem. There are very few people who have perfect balance. In nearly every case we have tested, we have found that the sick person has about 20 percent friendly and 80 percent unfriendly bacteria in the bowel. It should be just the opposite.

If we combine our food properly it will build up the friendly bacteria in the bowel. Whey is one of the finest foods we have to create these friendly bacteria. Soybean milk is also good for feeding the acidophilous bacteria. We can also use acidophilous milk, but this does not have the same potency as does the culture. It takes about 365 glasses of acidophilous milk to equal one bottle of culture. Using both regularly is one way to break up the prolonged nutritional deficiency that exists in our bodies.

Acidophilous milk is made in many different ways. We have a culture that can be put in the milk and as it grows we can add another glass of milk, skimmed or whole. The culture can be kept growing for many years.

John Harvey Kellogg brought out a system of caring for the bowel by implanting friendly bacteria in the bowel by means of an acidophilous culture. We use this method at our Hidden Valley Health Center the first thing in the morning and the last thing at night.

Bathing, of course, is of utmost importance in keeping the body clean, both inside and outside. We eliminate pounds of toxic material through the skin every day. This is a form of catarrhal discharge.

Don't forget that friction baths and air baths are very beneficial. Skin brushing, particularly, aids us in getting rid of the catarrh in our bodies. We must use a good skin brush, otherwise we cannot have clean, healthy bodies. Wearing clothing, which is a necessity for many reasons, makes skin elimination difficult, so we must aid it by brushing. Sunshine and exercise also help to bring out perspiration and eliminate toxic material. Exercise and skin brushing develop tone in the little tubules that bring toxic waste to the surface of the skin and make it clean and glowing.

Another way to help skin discharge is through the use of hot and cold baths. When we take a warm shower or bath we should always conclude by taking a cold shower or bath. This closes the pores and drives the blood inward. Then, with a little exercise, the blood is brought back to the surface and is ready to eliminate a full load of toxic waste. Do not use soap in hot water when taking a bath as the body will absorb most of the dirt again as well as the fat and alkali of the soap.

Take a daily sun bath if possible. We should be careful not to overexpose our bodies to the sun's rays, however, since this can be harmful. To begin with ten minutes at a time, is sufficient. The best time for sunbathing is between nine and eleven o'clock in the morning. One should never bathe right after eating. Always wait at least one hour. Bathing is to be used as regular medicine while we are feeling well so that whenever we need a good bath to withstand a cold or a chill, we have a body to meet it. We must have a warm body.

Let us remember, "Cleanliness is next to Godliness." We cannot hope to attain perfection, either physically, mentally or spiritually, unless we keep our "temples" clean.

Remedies for Catarrh Build-up. Coffee, as a stimulant, assists the bronchial tubes in the healing process.

Black horseradish contains a chemical called raphanon, which is a wonderful eliminant for catarrh that has settled in the gall duct and in the gall bladder. Mix it with a little lemon juice and put some on the tongue, then breathe the fumes through the nasal passages. It may lift the top of your head off, but it will open up those passages beautifully. This is one of the many remedies the doctors today are using for gall bladder disturbances. Powdered horseradish in its natural form may also be used in the way I have mentioned.

Another good "catarrh chaser" is a pinch of cayenne pepper in one cup of water. Sip a little every once in awhile for coughs.

A "cough syrup" that is harmless but effective is made by placing six cut white onions in a double boiler. Do not add water. Add a half cup of pure strained honey. Cook slowly over a low fire for two hours and strain. This mixture will stop a cough if taken at regular intervals. The onions act as a bowel cleanser and the honey aids in building the bloodstream. Keep the mixture warm. It is more effective if slightly heated and it will relieve the irritation that induces coughing.

In our morning walk at the Hidden Valley Health Center we take people through the hills and as we pass through the sagebrush we take some of the sage leaves and rub them with our hands and breathe the aroma. This loosens the nasal passages, the antrums, and the sinuses. We can do the same with bay leaves.

Food and Catarrh

Catarrh–Producing Foods
Heavy starches: cereals, bread, potatoes
Dairy products
    Any product from a cow
Eggs (eggs occasionally cause catarrh)

Non-Catarrh Producing Foods
All vegetables
All fruits
Meat — fish
Nut butters
Seeds
Milk substitutes (soy, sesame, almond, sunflower)
Teas

Asthma

Asthma is considered a catarrhal disease. It is a heavy catarrhal condition of the bronchial tubes, the lung structures, etc. Asthma can develop from various causes. We can have a bronchial asthma which invariably can be treated by using some of the instructions given in this book. On the other hand there is the asthma that is caused by the heart, called cardiac asthma. There is also a renal asthma produced whenever we have Bright's disease or a kidney disease in the body.

Bronchial asthma is not usually connected with either kidney or heart disease, but is usually associated with hay fever, a catarrhal condition of the mucus lining the membranes of the bronchial tubes. It is characterized by sudden attacks where the person has great difficulty breathing, has a terrible sense of constriction of the chest and a feeling of choking, wheezes, coughs a great deal, and, as a rule, expectorates a thin, viscid substance that later on in the attack becomes purulent in character. In this bronchial asthma, there is very little or no expectoration except during the end of the attack, when, as a rule, considerable mucus or muco-purulent material is coughed up.

Bronchial asthma can almost always be helped, no matter how old the patient may be and in whom it occurs. The cardiac renal varieties, however, may accompany advanced cases of heart trouble and kidney diseases and will only improve as we treat the heart and the kidneys. There are indeed few efforts that a man is called upon to make that are more wearisome than the toil of almost impossible breathing found in the case of bronchial asthma. In almost every other illness, relief is obtained when lying down in a recumbent position. In bronchial asthma the recumbent position is utterly impossible and the patient is compelled to sit up constantly day and night, until either relief is given or the attack subsides. In most cases he cannot even have his feet placed horizontally on a chair or some other support, but they must hang down or be placed on a low stool or on the floor to make him comfortable. Even the head of the patient cannot be laid backward on his chair nor can it be kept erect. It must be bent forward so it will rest on the arms in front of him or on something that will support his head. The patient's arms must be in a position where it will take the least possible effort to hold them.

Some patients have a diathesis or an inherently weak set-up in some of their organs that brings on a catarrhal condition in the body. When these membranes become inflamed it brings on colds, hay fever, and bronchial or catarrhal asthma. These people are the ones who have to be careful of certain foods. They are the ones whom allergy specialists spend most of their time with, trying to find what protein or what foods bring on such a hypersensitive condition in the body.

Most allergies develop from these catarrhal conditions. Wheat and milk substances usually cause the greatest number of allergies in heavy catarrhal-producing people. Cut out dairy products and substitute soymilk or goat milk products. If we have a tendency toward these conditions, we should look to the cleaning up of the body, making sure that we develop a hearty one, a healthy one, eliminating all catarrhal forming foods, watching our climate and altitude. We need mountain air and the ozone given off by pine trees.

We must get in and obey the laws of life! We cannot follow uncontrolled impulses or emotions. We must not let business or domestic worries disturb us. *We must have poise and control* and eliminate anxiety and fear from our environment.

We cannot sleep without ventilation. We cannot have sexual drain, overeating, improper eating, constipation. We cannot have a body that favors gastrointestinal decomposition and develops a state of enervation that always cuts down on the secretions and excretions of the body.

When we are tired, elimination becomes poor which in turn produces toxemia. Instead of toxemias being eliminated properly through our expiratory organs, such as the bowels, skin, kidneys, and bronchial tubes, they become reabsorbed and are passed on and settle in the weakest organs. In bronchial asthma this would be the lung structure and bronchial tubes. When our blood becomes so overwhelmed with toxemia we are not able to get sufficient oxygen, and purification cannot take place in the air cells of the lungs and bronchial tubes. Our greatest hypersensitive conditions are aggravated by starches and proteins. For this reason we make a good start in our treatment if we eliminate these two items.

We can divide the treatment of bronchial asthma into two sections: the treatment of the paroxysm or the attack, and the treatment of the general catarrhal condition. In the acute attack we should abstain from food and water. When the attack is less severe, a half teaspoon of hot water, if given every five or ten minutes, will many times give great relief. We may also rub along the spine with the hand, especially between the shoulder blades. Wet the hand with cold water. This brings ease many times, providing the rubbing is not carried to the point of irritation. Heat is almost always indicated, usually moist heat on the lower extremities; rub the feet and legs so that we bring on a healthy glow. When the nerve energy is low the feet are always cold and swell badly. If artificial heat is not applied, serious and grave consequences can follow. When we help the circulation in the lower extremities we help the circulation throughout the body. This helps throw off excess waste matter in all the organs of the body instead of bringing it all to the bronchial tubes and the lungs.

Brushing the skin- making the skin more active- is always indicated. After the patient has gotten some relief he can be put to bed, and he should go with as little food as possible for a short time. The length of the fast will vary depending upon the condition of the patient and the degree of enervation and the extent of the toxemia. When eating is resumed, do not start in with a heavy amount of food. That will overwork and use up the energies of the body.

A doctor with whom I studied at one time used the following diet whenever a person had catarrhal conditions, especially asthma: Eat lean meat (no fat, no pork), fish that has scales and fins, vegetables of all kinds and prepared in any way, canned tomatoes, tomato juice, and fresh grapefruit. Always have the canned tomatoes or tomato juice or grapefruit when you have the meat or fish. Otherwise, combine the foods in any way you wish: one at a time, two at a time, or all three to-gether. Make all of your meals on just these foods. Nothing else is allowed except water. No salt or vinegar must be used. You cannot produce any catarrhal condition with this diet.

Another good diet requires omitting all dairy products, anything from a cow. Omit anything from wheat, especially bread. Use soymilk and soy powder instead. Coconut milk is also good. Use vegetables and fruits along with the soymilk, or even follow a cut-up vegetable leaves diet.

Onion packs on the head and throat are also good for asthma, used with garlic oil capsules. This, along with our regular diets and no dairy products, will help to remove the catarrh in the body. Also find a dry climate, high altitude, warm air, and consider everything to build a high blood count.

Some herbs will help with asthma. A good combination for the respiratory tract is comfrey root, mullein, marshmallow, slippery elm, and lobelia. Another good combination is blessed thistle, black cohosh, scullcap, and pleurisy root. Or try ½ ounce of stem of balsam of Peru in hot water and inhale.

Good herb teas are comfrey leaves and roots, hissop, fenugreek, horehound leaf, aniseed, mint, sassafras.

Those with severe asthma must continue to live with the greatest care, avoiding large quantities of food and limiting themselves to such amounts as they can both digest and assimilate. We must take care of the constitutional derangement or the inherent weaknesses in the body and work for as clean a body as we possibly can.

Overeating Creates Chronic Catarrhal Conditions. The habit of overeating develops a state of chronic gastric fermentation. This fermentation is normally thrown off directly by way of the mouth, but it can, through absorption in a body that is not working properly, be thrown out through the elimination of the lung structure. In people who are troubled with a chronic catarrhal condition it many times goes through the nose, attacking the schneiderian membrane. This is an expiratory organ and can become very sensitive in those conditions. When particles of inert dust, lint from clothing, pollen of flowers, odors of all kinds (in fact, anything capable of having an irritating effect on the mucous membranes) are inhaled, they will bring about a highly sensitive, irritated, and inflamed state of the nose, eyes, and throat. if this irritation continues hay fever results. For example, in dry, dusty weather, or in the season of the year when the pollen of flowers is filling the air, these persons are made very uncomfortalbe; but dust or invisible particles are not the cause. Those who have taken care of the cause of catarrh in most cases do not have these seasonal problems. What hay fever really means is that in the haying season when the atmosphere is full of odors and pollen, those with established catarrhal inflammation of the mucus membranes of the nose react to the pollen as a symptom of their catarrhal buildup. The problem is not the pollen or dust, the problem is their health. Often the health problem with hay fever is a deficiency in iron and chloride foods.

Diet can help us with catarrhal problems then. Two salads a day, as the major part of the meal, would be good. We do this because it takes some time to overcome a catarrhal condition– we may spend a solid year getting the body cleaned up. Those who feel they cannot miss any of the good things in life and must indulge in all kinds of food will find it difficult getting well. While trying to cleanse the body, many times we have to lose weight, which may be a little disturbing to some people. But as soon as we have gone through the transition and building stages, we are on our way up. Each case is unique and we should find out as much as we can about ourselves to learn about and deal with any constitutional or inherent weaknesses we may have. It has been said that catarrh is the beginning of all diseases, and to get rid of the root of all of our physical troubles is not any easy job.

In our routine at the Hidden Valley Health Center we handle catarrh by starting with a little fast. Sometimes we use vegetable juices, sometimes fruit juices. We may go only for a day or two at a time and then get back to the lighter foods, cleansing foods, and salad foods. Then we break into a two-day fast again. These diets are best taken during the summer.

The Common Cold

A cold is not a disease in itself but is the beginning of catarrhal elimination. It is a sign that the body is endeavoring to liquefy hard catarrhal settlements in the body and trying to eliminate them. Contrary to the usual attitude of regret — "I have caught another blasted cold!" — the waste thus unloaded is a blessed riddance of toxins.

The common cold is usually the first disorder of any human body trying to eliminate catarrh. If the condition is suppressed by drugs or treatments, the patient is definitely on his way to future chronic disease. Most of the cold remedies have been found by the government to be ineffective anyway.

When we have a cold, we should get plenty of bed rest, take warm baths, and take the proper teas as indicated in this book or as prescribed by the doctor.

Taking a warm bath and sponging off with a little cool towel afterwards is always the way to bring up the energies and to help the circulation. Bowel exercises should be used two or three times a day.

Our emotional makeup must be controlled and a good philosophy developed. Retoning of the skin should be started immediately, according to the methods explained in this book.

At the first sign of a cold, make sure the colon is clean by taking an enema. Take plenty of fresh fruit or juice but reduce the amount of solid food you eat. You may want to fast a day or two. If so, you should break your fast with fruit juices. Vitamin C may be taken frequently, as many as ten 250 mg. tablets a day, but antihistaminic drugs should be avoided, since many have produced bad side-effects. Also, take from 100,000 to 200,000 units of vitamin A for several days. This must be an oil vitamin A as opposed to an acetate or a drug. Within a few days you can reduce the amount to 25,000 per day.

I learned from my Professor Charles H. Gesser (a doctor of homeopathy in Chicago) of a cold remedy that is quite effective; it helps in coughs and helps get rid of mucus and phlegm or catarrh from the body. Use two tablespoons each of the following herbs: Mullein flowers, coltsfoot, slippery elm, and finely chopped licorice root, and mix together. Put in three pints of cold water. Slowly bring to a boil. Simmer for five minutes and strain. Drink ½ cup to a cupful of this concoction every few hours during the day. Use until the cough has ceased. This remedy should be made fresh every day.

Use vegetable broth every two hours. Whey drinks are very good.

Bake a lemon 20 minutes. Put ½ baked lemon in hot oat straw tea or boneset tea. Go to bed, since this will make you perspire.

Use onion and garlic pack on chest.

Deep Breathing. Deep breathing should be developed whenever we have colds. The head cold, or catarrhal condition we call "a cold," generally develops when we have been exposed to chill, dampness, or something of that nature. We say that we contract a cold when our body cannot maintain good balance in face of the elements. When a fluid or moisture evaporates, a chill is produced. For example, if you moisten your finger and blow against it you will see that the side you blow against will feel cold. The skin throws off a certain temperature. The average natural, normal skin should be moist, but if a cold wind comes along, dryer than the humidity of the skin area, the skin will be chilled. When our skin is in good working order we have less likelihood of catching a cold than at any other time.

For That Flu

During the epidemic of influenza stay out of inclement weather and try to avoid atmospheric changes. If you should fall victim to the flu the first thing you should do is go to bed and rest. Keep well covered and perspire, if possible. To encourage perspiration and help drive the virus and congestion from the chest drink boneset tea, to which has been added the juice of a lemon which has baked for twenty minutes.

Do not try to act as your own physician in any serious condition, however. If your condition become serious you should immediately consult a physician and rely upon his advice. It is good, also, to have a doctor prescribe home treatments for you. Be sure to straighten out your kitchen at home to be certain there is nothing on the shelf that will produce the trouble you are asking the doctor to correct.

Skin Care for Catarrhal Conditions. To be healthy skin must be kept clean. I believe skin brushing is one of the finest of all baths. No soap can wash the skin as clean as the new skin you have under the old. You make new skin every 24 hours. The skin will be as clean as the blood is. Skin brushing removes this top layer and helps to eliminate uric acid crystals, catarrh, and various other acids in the body.

The heating and ventilating system of our bodies must be working properly. High humidity combined with high temperature is extremely depressing. However, if the temperature is kept below 70 degrees the humidity may be up as high as 70 and 80 percent without causing discomfort.

Excessive dryness always irritates the nasal membrane. When the membranes of the breathing tract are exposed to extremely dry air they open up; when they are exposed to cold, moist air, they contract abnormally and become congested, which usually leads to a cold. The skin needs an opportunity to breathe. It should throw off moisture and should come in contact with air so that the moisture can be evaporated within a short time. We should not wear air-tight clothing except for a short period of time, as when we wear a rubber coat during a storm. A good rule is to wear just enough clothing to keep us comfortably warm.

In case you become chilled when resting, exercise immediately to stir up the blood circulation. If you cannot practice exercise at that time try some forced breathing. When symptoms of repeated sneezing and especially when exposure chills the body, take a hot bath before retiring. Even a hot water bottle used at the feet and a hot drink will help.

Nerve exhaustion is probably the beginning of many contracted colds. We find there are very few people with 100 percent mental and physical efficiency. Every action in our body is dependent upon an abundant supply of nerve force. When the vital organs of the body are not stimulated by impulses of the nerve force the blood becomes impoverished and the system clogs with poisonous matter. These two factors are the main cause of most ailments. This is the reason we consider taking care of the mind and emotions, one of the most important things in taking care of the body.

Consider Your Nerves in Catarrhal Conditions. Always consider your nerves! Be good to your nerves! There has never before been a time in history when we have had as many nervous breakdowns as we have today. With the black soot, the roaring of the radio, the overworking of television eyes, we are using more of the nervous system today than ever before. It has been said that a man living today sees more in five years than a king saw in a hundred years before.

If there ever was a need for philosophy, for emotional control, it is today. Never were there such rumors of war, such noise conditions to overcome both of which use up the nerve force. Never have there been such atomic blasts or ranting and raving of countries trying to be out in front. Never has there been so much delinquency or problems for parents to handle. City life has made the no-care person of today; but he goes on from no-care to nervous breakdown.

Of course, one reason for the increase in nervous breakdowns may be the type of food we are eating today; it does not feed the nervous system properly. It is possible we will have a nerve plague in the future just as we have had the white plague of the past, tuberculosis, pneumonias, and the flu of 1914. Take care of your nerves, do get plenty of sleep, have good companions, go the uplifted way, let the unimportant things go.

Catarrh is one of the national maladies taken care of with nostrums. It is well to learn how to prevent this condition. Get on a noncatarrh diet, learn to balance your day, place yourself in the proper climate and follow the many suggestions given. Catarrh will automatically leave as the body becomes cleansed and purified. Live a better life and the body will change automatically to one free of all catarrh.

Catarrhal Helpers. When a person has a catarrhal condition how much milk should he use?

First, I don't think that milk is the only thing that produces catarrh. Don't run away with the idea that dairy products are the only things that produce it. I believe starches can produce catarrh; I believe wrong combinations of foods can also bring about catarrh. I also believe that an enervated body can produce catarrh from the best foods in the world. Catarrh and acids are the beginning of every disease. Now, how much milk should we eliminate? I would say the elimination of dairy products can quite often help the person with catarrh. Many times our bodies have been so leaded with dairy products in the past that the simple elimination of improper foods from our diet can easily change the chemical balance.

Chronic Nasal Catarrh. Chronic nasal catarrh can be very uncomfortable and hard to rid oneself of. But there are a few remedies. Put one or two drops of eucalyptus oil in water. Dip a cloth into the water and drape it over your head. Breathe the smell into your nasal passages.

A nasal douche can be made with two drops of Eucalyptus oil in four drops of olive oil. Take this into the nose by sniffing.

Herb teas can be used, such as those made from the following herbs: boneset, ragwort, burdock, cascara, clivers, and goldenrod. Simmer in three pints of water for one hour. Strain after cooling. Use about a wineglassful after each meal.

For nasal catarrh with colds: A tea made with dried elder flowers and peppermint, before going to bed will often nip a cold in the bud. If you develop a heavy cold, this mixture can help: Mix one ounce each of ground ivy, horehound, hyssop, honey. Place

in one pint of water and simmer for an hour. Strain and cool. Take one tablespoon frequently until the cold has subsided.

The Turnip Diet. The turnip diet is excellent for asthma, bronchial trouble, and all other catarrhal conditions. White turnips are higher in vitamin A than carrots and have a most wonderful cutting and cleansing effect.

In the turnip diet use the juice, the greeens, or the turnip itself– raw, cooked, or in soup form. Vary the diet by eating the turnips in various ways along with the regular health diet, or by having turnip combinations alone. The juice can be made very palatable by mixing it with pineapple or apple juice. The raw turnip can be used in salads with cut dates or steamed raisin.

The turnip diet can be taken for a period of from three days to two months. For a long period of time you should seek the direction of your doctor, but three days on a diet of turnips, on your own volition, is a good diet to begin with.

Some years ago it was found that many people who were confined in concentration camps had nothing to live on except turnips. What was the result? Their catarrhal problems, sinus problems, and asthma conditions were cleared up. I have used the turnip diet in my private practice with a great deal of success. Using turnip juice and pineapple juice together helps asthma tremendously. In fact, it helps all hay fever and catarrhal problems.

One of my patients at the center suffered from asthma, catarrhal trouble, and a 240 systolic blood pressure. We put him on a thirty-day diet of nothing but turnips. We give him turnip greens, turnip juice, raw turnips, and cooked turnips. Yes, nothing but turnips for one whole month. When taken off the diet, he no longer had asthma or catarrhal trouble; his blood pressure was normal (140 systolic), and he was down to his normal weight by losing forty pounds. He was a picture of health. Compare this with the pills and potions he had been taking for years. You see, nature has a remedy!

Bronchial troubles need calcium foods, iodine-containing foods (excepting in cases of tuberculosis), onion syrup, onion tea, cream toast, honey, hot drinks, blackberry tea, hot foot baths, dry feet, flannel and warm moisture next to the body, hot applications to the throat, and a warm moist climate.

There is a wonderful liquid chlorophyll put out under the "Garden of Life" brand. Use this as a nasal douche (¼ teaspoonful to ½ cup of water). Sniff it into the nostrils. Drinking one teaspoonful of chlorophyll in a glass of water three times a day (the first time before breakfast) is a very effective treatment for sinus disturbances as well as inflamed nasal membranes.

For a Catarrhal Throat. A fine cough syrup can be made from chopped onions and honey. It is a splendid remedy. Put one or two tablespoons of honey in a dish of chopped onions; let it stand for three or four hours, then drain. Sip a teaspoonful every hour, or, if necessary, every half hour.

It may not sound like it, but this is a very soothing syrup and children will not object to it.

Eucalyptus Honey. Eucalyptus honey is a powerful honey for catarrhal problems, tuberculosis, or swollen tonsils if used with a combination of onions, as in the cough syrup above. This combination goes deep into cells to release harsh toxic materials that settle in the body. Failure to release this harsh material is the reason the skin breaks out so often during the healing process. That is why catarrh runs when we are cleansing the body. Remember that we are striving for a clean body in recommending all these foods.

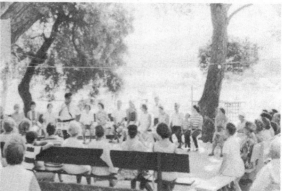

People from all over the world come to Hidden Valley Health Ranch to get the information and material on preventing disease, correcting problems and learning a new pathway to right living.

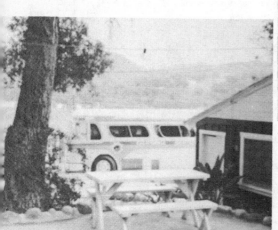

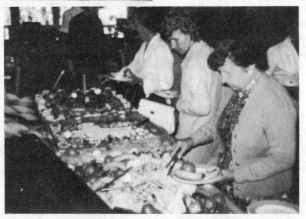

Living it up with natural foods at the Ranch. A fruit night—of fruit, cheese, milk, nut butters, and a simple meal, but all natural.

FOURTEEN

Building a body

I FULLY believe that there was an all-intelligent, all-powerful force that put together a whole wheatberry, whole rice, whole sugar, whole milk that no laboratory could ever duplicate or science could ever construct, reconstruct, breakdown, or put together. God gave us foods to build, repair, and maintain our bodies. I believe the Garden of Eden is still here, but man has made a mess of it.

Man has mistreated God's natural foods through his commercial enterprise, his refining and pickling. He puts artificial chemicals in the soil in which his food is grown. We are having only half loaves of bread. We cook our food too much, cooking out half the vitamins we need for our body.

So we come to feel we need supplements. But most vitamins and minerals are man-made products; they are a fad of the day. They are part of this civilized life we are living and are not part of the whole life we need. They are just to get by. But they can never be the answer to the shortage that develops from unnatural living. There are no substitutes for right living. There is no right way to do the wrong thing. However, if you are going to live the unnatural life, vitamins will get you by until you can get straightened out.

But if you have learned the way to live, the supplements to add to your diet to make up for the shortages in the past, especially for the white rice and white flour, are vitamin B and vitamin E. There is a natural vitamin B from rice polishings; there is a natural vitamin E from wheat germ flakes.

Always try to get the most natural products. Remember, taking vitamins does not build the body. It takes minerals to build the body. Minerals are more important than vitamins. I try to get the vitamins and minerals from the most natural sources possible, with the least man-handling. This is why I say, "Get your iron from black cherry juice, blackstrap molasses, greens, and chlorophyll." These are food supplements that can be taken in between meals or with meals.

In case of emergencies, when vitamin and mineral deficiencies show up as ailments in the body, we can turn to health store vitamins and minerals for the most natural supplements possible to help overcome that emergency moment.

Vitamin A. Vitamin A is good for all infections in the body, such as skin trouble, discharges, leucorrhea, mastoids, and colds. Antibiotics often affect the pituitary gland causing headaches and blurring of vision; this is often helped by vitamin A foods. But there are different kinds of vitamin A. There is a vitamin A acetate; that is a drug. Keep away from it. The effects of a synthetic are not of a healthful nature. Use a natural form of vitamin A, as in oil.

Vitamin B. Vitamin B is for the nervous system. It can come in a yeast form, in an egg yolk, and in fish, meat, and milk.

Vitamin C. Vitamin C is found in all salads, all green vegetables, all sunshine fruits, all citrus fruits– nearly all foods. Green pepper is just as high in vitamin C as citrus fruits. Even potatoes have vitamin C. If you take the foods prescribed in my " Balanced Daily Eating Regimen" (see chapter "There's Much to Learn about Foods"), you will be getting enough vitamin C without taking any citrus fruits. You will get plenty of vitamin C for the various infections we get, unless it is an extreme infection, in which case a doctor should prescribe something for you. Vitamin C is one vitamin you can take in varying amounts without worrying, in most cases. We have given 5,000 and 10,000 milligrams a day without any trouble. The average person can take 1,500 milligrams a day without any side effects. You may simply have to take more water because it will color the urine. Vitamin

C takes a lot of toxic wastes from the body and throws them out through the kidneys.

Vitamin D. Vitamin D controls the calcium in the body. In Sweden, they have a lot of arthritis; the dampness there continues over a period of six months. But when they go to the Sahara Desert, or other places in Africa where they have a lot of sunshine, they get a lot of relief. Why? Because sunshine gives you the vitamin D to control the calcium. And it's an imbalance of calcium that leads to arthritis.

A ten-minute sunbath will last for a period of three days. Especially try to get sunshine on your arms, your legs, and your spine.

If you are wearing eye glasses made of glass, you cut out 85 percent of the sun's ultraviolet rays, and thus cannot control the calcium well in your body. If you are subject to joint trouble, I advise you to get plastic glasses. A lot of people can have joint trouble just from wearing glasses. The plastic glasses may cost a little bit more, but they cut out only 15 percent of the ultraviolet light.

If you live indoors, especially in buildings that have no natural light coming in, or if it is winter, and there is not a lot of sunshine, it is good to take a little extra cod liver oil.

Vitamin E. Vitamin E is a remedy for many things. It is good for people with flabby tissue, varicose veins, or lack of oxygen in the brain. It is a good heart support. Vitamin E is the procreative germ life of such grains as wheat, rice, and corn. But it is removed when they are processed. You have been cheated out of this material for years. That is why in most cases we find people lacking in vitamin E. Vitamin E makes a wonderful remedy for all the glands and for the whole body.

Vitamin F. Vitamin F is a splendid vitamin for healing the tissues that line the intestinal tract and other mucous membranes. Flaxseed tea is high in vitamin F, especially when the seeds are soaked in warm water overnight rather than boiled.

Vitamin K. Vitamin K is the antihemorrhagic vitamin found highest in alfalfa juice. It has saved the life of many women who have hemorrhaged at childbirth. All chlorophyll has a lot of vitamin K. Chlorophyll is a fine blood builder because it is also unusually high in iron and potassium.

Supplementary Foods. We should never con-

sider a remedy or a supplement as a complete correction for any ailment in the body. We should first learn to live correctly and seek good guidance for nutrition. Seek out professional care as to what nutritional shortages exist. I have never found anyone who would not benefit from the daily addition of the following supplementary foods. Keep them by your table.

The first four supplements, in particular, should always be served on the dining table to overcome the fact that most of us have shortages from the past to make up. They can, of course, also be added to any liquefied drink, morning cereal, salad, dessert, and so forth.

Nova Scotia Dulse. Take ¼ teaspoon a day (or one tablet). Only minute quantities of iodine are required by the body, and dulse, being a high iodine food, supplies this need. Iodine keeps us from getting goiter. It prevents wrinkles. Lack of it causes mood swings, tiredness, and dry and brittle hair and skin. Dulse is the highest source of iodine for the thyroid gland.

Here's how you can prepare the dulse: Take possibly two or three big leaves of seaweed and cut it up fine enough to put in a liquefier. Grind it up in hot water. Let it stand for ½ hour, then strain it off and use just the liquid. Use about two ounces of this Nova Scotia dulse in about two quarts of water. This can be flavored with a little cream if desired, or perhaps a little honey. This water can be used in broths, soups, or vegetable juices. Just take a little bit every day — one cup daily is plenty — and you will get the benefit you need.

Rice Polishings. Use a teaspoonful a day. This is high in vitamin B- a vitamin for nerves, appetite, and muscle coordination- and the mineral element silicon, which is the youth element. Silicon is the "cutter" in the body, cleaning out all pus and debris. It is necessary for beautiful hair, nails, and skin. For cold feet and skin disease, take extra silicon.

Sunflower Seed Meal. Use one teaspoonful three times a day. This is one of the finest vegetarian proteins you can use. If the body is protein-starved, perhaps due to overuse of mind in your studies or job, use this to feed the brain and nervous system. All seeds are for the glands, too. Sunflower seeds are high also in silicon.

Wheat Germ. Use one tablespoonful daily.

This is high in vitamin E, the specific vitamin for the heart. It gives tone to the muscle structure, strengthening the veins (varicose veins) and helping circulation. Wheat germ also feeds the glands and nerves and is a good source of vitamin B.

Whey. This is one of the finest of foods. Be sure you always have a bottle of the powder on hand. A very good habit to develop is to take a glass of whey at each meal. It is our highest sodium source. Sodium is known as the "youth maintainer," allowing our joints to remain supple. It also aids digestion and builds the blood. Whey is friendly to the acidophilous baccilli in the intestinal tract, which are important to good intestinal management. It also has calcium, the tone-builder and strengthener, and chlorine, the cleanser. People on slimming diets need not be afraid of whey. Taken before meals, it partially appeases hunger.

Blackstrap Molasses. This is an excellent iron supplement.

Brewer's Yeast. Brewer's Yeast is a good source of vitamin B.

Desiccated Liver. This helps to build the bloodstream.

Supplements and Fortifiers

Tablets, powders, protein and amino acid preparations, mineral and vitamin supplements, oils such as wheat germ oil, capsules (discard the "shell"), medicinal herbs, and other necessary supplementary preparations can be added to liquefied drinks so that you can't tell they are there. Their taste can be camouflaged with a counteracting flavor.

Here are some of the tablets and powders that can be used for health enhancement by including them in liquefied drinks:

Alfalfa Tablets.	For alkalinizing.
Bone Meal Tablets (or Powder)	For extra calcium needed in the body. in the body.
Green Kale Tablets (or Powder).	For extra calcium needed *in the body.*
Lecithin	Good in all high cholesterol cases.
Parsley Tablets.	For the kidneys.
Okra, Celery Tablets.	High sodium content.
Papaya Tablets (or Powder).	For digestion.
Prune, Apricot Powder.	Good for its laxative effect.
Peach Powder.	Good for its laxative effect.
Watercress Tablets.	For reducing (high in potassium).
Whey Powder.	High sodium content.

I do not believe in vitamins made from coal tar; those that always carry the highest potency; those that are made from abnormal or inorganic substances. These prostituted vitamins will cause another disease in the body and one of these days you'll have to be treated for something new again.

To make up for deficiencies in the body, remember these points:

1. Find out what a healthy daily eating regimen is and follow it.

2. Consult with a doctor who knows how to determine chemical deficiencies in the body, or learn how yourself.

3. Find out the natural foods that are high in the minerals and vitamins that you are deficient in.

4. Make sure that everything you eat is close to what God created and meant for you to have.

Summary of Vitamins. Vitamins are more or less on the tongue of every dietician, housewife, doctor, and groceryman today. They commanded attention first, probably, back in 1774, when oranges and lemons were found to prevent scurvy. To date science has found some seven vitamins and will probably find many more in years to come.

Vitamins seem to offer the "kick" to the minerals that enter our bodies. They are little invisible helpers ready to right every wrong that may come about in the complicated processes of building and maintaining a perfect body.

Natural foods contain all the vitamins that have been discovered and will be discovered. Scurvy, pellagra, beriberi, and most all diseases are the result, partially at least, of vitamin deficiencies. Cheat the body of vitamin-rich food and you are on a disease-producing diet. *Quality* foods count, *not* quantity. And remember, vitamins essential to our bodies are best found in natural foods.

What are the best natural vitamin foods?

Vitamin A.	Carrot juice or lemon grass
Vitamin B.	Rice polishings or flaked yeast
Vitamin C	Rose hips tea and persimmon leaf tea
Vitamin D.	Cod liver oil
Vitamin E.	Wheat germ oil
Vitamin F.	Peanut oil
Vitamin G.	(B2)—Yeast extracts
Vitamin K.	Alfalfa juice (chlorophyll)

VITAMIN A

Antiophthalmic — (fat soluble) — Injured by by high temperature

Conditions caused by lack of vitamin A:
Loss of weight and vigor; loss of vitality and growth; loss of strength and glandular balance. Eye infections. Emaciation, acne, poor vision, poor digestion, diarrhea, nephritis, rough dry skin. (Children require this vitamin more than adults.)

Conditions controlled by vitamin A:
Makes tissues more resistant, especially to colds and catarrhal infections in respiratory organs, sinuses, ears, bladder, skin, and digestive tract. Increases blood platelets. Promotes growth and feeling of well-being.

Stability:
Cooking temperatures do not affect this vitamin much, but it is destroyed by heat in the presence of oxygen.

Storage:
This vitamin is stored in the body for future needs. A surplus is depleted quickly under strain and stress.

Foods rich in vitamin A:
Green leafy vegetables and yellow vegetables, spinach, parsley, Swiss chard, green lettuce, cabbage, tomatoes, carrots, green peas, sweet potatoes, endive, beet leaves, mustard greens, Brussel sprouts, green celery, yellow squash. Milk, butterfat, egg yolk, whole milk, cheese, bananas, apricots, peaches, melon, cherries, papaya, avocado, mango, prunes, pineapple

VITAMIN B

Antineuritic - (water soluble) - Injured by high temperature

Conditions caused by lack of vitamin B:
Nervous exhaustion, loss of growth, loss of reproduction function, loss of appetite, beri-beri, polyneuritis, intestinal gas, fermentation, faulty nutrition and assimilation, indigestion, convulsions, soreness, pain, lack of digestive juices, slow heartbeat, impaired insulin secretions, loss of will power.

Conditions controlled by vitamin B:
Makes for better absorption of food and normalizes the brain and nervous system by increasing metabolic processes.

Stability:
Ordinary cooking does not affect vitamin B, although heat might affect it. Soda added to keep vegetables green destroys vitamin B.

Storage:
Limited quantities of vitamin B are stored in the body.

Foods rich in vitamin B:
Yeast, egg yolk, whole milk, lean beef, liver, kidney, asparagus, spinach, tomatoes, peas, turnip greens, mustard greens, chard, celery, potatoes, carrots, cabbage, beet leaves, cauliflower, lettuce, broccoli, onions, peppers, grapefruit, lemons, oranges, bananas, pineapple, apples, melon, peaches, avocados, grapes, prunes, dates, cherries, pears, almonds, walnuts, chestnuts, brazil, pecans, and all legumes. Also whole grains: wheat, rye, corn, rice, barley, oats.

Vitamin B. combines well with Silicone.
Vitamin B_1 (Niamine). Deficiency (as in polished rice) causes beri-beri, nervousness, weakness.
Vitamin B_2. breaks down starches and sugars to give energy.
Vitamin B_{12}. needs cobalt, as found in almond skin.

VITAMIN C

Antiscorbutic - (water soluble) - Destroyed by high temperatures

Conditions caused by lack of vitamin C:
Tender painful swelling of joints, poor health, faulty nutrition, scurvy, loss of appetite, loss of weight, irritable temper, poor complexion, loss of energy, irregular heart action, rapid respiration, reduced hemoglobin, reduced secretion of adrenals, cataract, hemorrhage.

Conditions controlled by vitamin C:
A marvelous health promoter as it wards off acidosis.

Stability:
Destroyed by heat, cooking, low temperature, and oxidation.

Storage:
Vitamin C is not stored in the body- we must get a fresh supply every day in our life.

Foods rich in vitamin C:
Oranges, lemons, grapefruit, limes, melons, berries, apples, pineapple, cabbage, tomatoes, spinach, peas, broccoli, rutabagas, collards, Brussels sprouts, celery, parsley, endive, watercress, turnips, cucumbers, cauliflower, radishes, persimmon leaf tea.

VITAMIN D
Antirachitic - (fat soluble) - Injured by high temperatures
Conditions caused by lack of vitamin D.
Rickets, soft bones, lack of body tone, fatigue, respiratory infections, irritability, restlessness, constipations, ptosis, prolapsus, dental cavities, retards growth, causes instability of nervous system.

Conditions controlled by vitamin D.
Facilitates absorption of calcium and phosphorus from foods, and is consequently a great bone builder. Guards against tuberculosis. Regulates mineral metabolism.

Stability:
Heat or oxidation does not affect vitamin D.

Storage:
Nature expects us to get this vitamin from the sun. We tap our greatest source by exposing the skin to sunlight. This sunlight contains ultraviolet rays, which change the ergosterol in the skin into limited amounts of vitamin D. A limited amount of vitamin D is stored in the body.

Foods rich in vitamin D:
Fish oils, cod liver oil, halibut liver oils, egg yolk, butter, and milk. Green leafy vegetables grown in the sunshine.

VITAMIN E
Antisterility — (fat soluble) — Quite Stable

Conditions caused by lack of vitamin E.
Sterility, loss of adult vitality.

Conditions controlled by vitamin E.
Essential in reproduction, poor lactation, menstrual disorders, miscarriage, dull mentality, pessimism, despondency, and loss of courage.

Stability:
Heat or oxidation do not affect vitamin E.

Storage:
Limited supply is stored in body.

Foods rich in vitamin E:
Milk, cottage cheese, and wheat germ. Vegetable oils, such as olive oil and soybean oil. Green and leafy vegetables, yellow corn, and raw fruits.

VITAMIN F
Growth Promoting - (water soluble) - Injured by high temperature and long cooking

Conditions caused by lack of vitamin F.
stunted growth, sexual immaturity, falling hair, baldness, loss of appetite, skin disorders, nervousness, and eczema.

Conditions controlled by vitamin F.
Vitamin F is necessary for all around development.

Stability:
Long cooking destroys vitamin F.

Storage:
More vitamin F is necessary as the metabolic note increases in the body.

Foods rich in vitamin F.
Yeast, whole grains, and eggs. Root vegetables and fresh spinach. Fruits, particularly orange juice, and nuts.

VITAMIN G (B2)
Antipellagric - (water soluble) - Injured by high temperatures

Conditions caused by lack of vitmain G:
Nerve disorders, irritability, pellagra, skin eruptions, loss of hair, stomach disorders, cataracts, old age, lack of growth, poor appetite, digestive disturbances.

Conditions controlled by vitamin G:
Prolongs life span, increases adult vitality.

Stability:
Heat does not affect vitamin G.

Storage:
A limited amount is stored in the body, it must be added daily.

Foods rich in vitamin G:
Whole milk, buttermilk, cheese, cream, eggs, meats, wheat germ, yeast extracts, green leafy vegetables.

VITAMIN K
Antihemorrhagic – (water soluble) – Injured by high temperature

Conditions caused by lack of vitamin K:
Lack of blood coagulation.

Conditions controlled by vitamin K:
Hemorrhaging at childbirth, bleeding gums, nosebleed.

Stability:
Water soluble.

Storage:
When concentrated will not ferment or spoil.

Foods rich in vitamin K:
Alafalfa, comfrey, greens.

MINERALS IN SUMMARY
Body Content
(Total weight 160 pounds)
Calcium: . . . . 4 lbs.
Carbon: . . . . 45 lbs.
Phosphorus: . . . . 2 lbs.
Potassium: .3½oz.
Magnesium: . . . . 2½ oz.
Silicon: . . . . 1¼ oz.
Iodine: . . . . Trace – 1/14,000 gr.
Oxygen: . . . . 89 lbs.
Hydrogen: . . . . 15 lbs.
Chlorine: . . . . .1-1/3 oz.
Sodium: . . . . 3 oz.
Iron: . . . . 2 oz.

Body chemical deficiencies are usually calcium, silicon, sodium, iodine.

Body Organs
(Mineral Needs)
Thyroid: . . . . Iodine
Bowel: . . . . Magnesium
Brain and nervous
system: . . . . Phosphorus, manganese
Skin and circulation: . . . . Sulphur
Nails and Hair: . . . . Silicon
Spleen: . . . . Flourin, copper
Teeth and bones: . . . . .Flourin, calcium
Adrenals: . . . . Tin
Liver: . . . . .Sulphur, iron

Pituitary gland: . . . . .Bromine
Tissues and secretions: . . . . .Potassium

CHEMICAL ELEMENT ANALYSIS
Abbreviations used:
D – Destroyed or injured by high temperature
W – Dissolves in water
O – Oxidizes rapidly

CALCIUM
Essential Mineral Salt
Calcium: Found and needed mostly in structual system. Tooth and bone mineral. (W;D;O)

Mineral Salt Activity in Body
Tone-building in the body. Builds in the body. Builds and maintains bone structure. Gives vitality, endurance. Heals wounds. Counteracts acid.

Principal Sources
Bran and cheese (very high), raw goat cheese, cottage, Swiss, Dutch edam, or gouda, milk, raw egg yolk, figs, prunes, dates, apricots, cranberries, gooseberries, cabbage, spinach, parsnips, lettuce, onions, tops of vegetables, kale, cauliflower, bone meal, collards, broccoli, turnip greens, kidney beans, soybeans, lentils.

Special Points about Calcium

Calcium is the knitting element.
Blood–clotting problems indicate calcium deficiency.
Metabolism needs vitamin F.
Never use cheese from pasteurized or homogenized milk.
Never use cheese matured with salt.

Calcium Tonic: Put one tablespoon of powdered bone meal in a glass of raw milk once a day. This makes a wonderful calcium cocktail
A good way to control the calcium in the body is to cut up a large leaf of comfrey and put it in any broth or soup or run it through the vegetable juicer. This is one of the greatest ways to build the bone structure of the body.

CHLORINE
Essential Mineral Salt
Chlorine: Found and needed mostly in degestive system and secretions. (D)

Mineral Salt Activity in Body

Cleanser in the Body. Expels waste. Freshens, purfies, disinfects.

Principal Sources

Goat's milk, cow milk, salt, fish, cheese, coconut, beets, radishes, common salt, dry figs, endive, watercress, cucumber, carrots, leeks, Roquefort cheese, Danish blue cheese, Swiss cheese, Italian cheese, and all green vegetables.

Special Points about Chlorine

Deficiency contributes to sluggish liver and glandular swellings.

Goat's milk provides chlorine that is effective in kidney problems because of its germicidal effect.

FLUORIN

Essential Mineral Salt

Fluorin: Found and needed mostly in the structural system, tooth enamel; preserves bones. (D)

Mineral Salt Activity in Body

Disease resister and beautifier in body. Strengthens tendons. Knits bones.

Principal Sources

Cauliflower, cabbage, cheese. raw goat milk, cow milk, raw egg yolk, cod liver oil, Brussels sprouts, spinach, tomatoes, watercress, salad vegetables, black bass (fish), quinces.

Special Points about fluorin:

Combines with calcium.

Stored in spleen, eye structure, elastic tissues. Released from foods when heated, but destroyed by too high temperature.

Spleen stores and uses large amounts of fluorin.

Fluorin, a "beauty element," gives teeth their hard coating and keeps the teeth from decaying. Raw goat milk contains highest content of fluorin foods.

IODINE

Essential Mineral Salt

Iodine: Found and needed mostly in nervous system. Gland and brain mineral (O - D)

Mineral Salt Acitvity in Body

Metabolism normalizer in body. Prevents goiter. Normalizes gland and cell action. Ejects and counteracts poisons.

Principal Sources

Powdered Nova Scotia dulse, and very high in sea lettuce; sea foods, carrots, pears, onions, tomatoes, pineapple, potato skin, cod liver oil, garlic, watercress; onions, green leek soup, clam juice; nettle tea.

Special Points about Iodine

Indications of iodine deficiency: Claustrophobia/fears; Flabby arms; Pronunciation difficulties; Mental depression.

MAGNESIUM

Essential Mineral Salt

Magnesium: Found and needed mostly in the digestive system. Nerve mineral. Nature's laxative. (W-D)

Mineral Salt Activity in Body

New cell promoter in the body. Relaxes nerves. Refreshes system. Prevents and relieves constipation and autointoxication.

Principal Sources

Grapefruit, oranges, figs, whole barley, corn, yellow cornmeal, wheat bran, wheat coconut, goat milk, raw egg yolk.

Special Points about Magnesium

Indications of Magnesium deficiency: Temper; , Excitement problem, excess passion

IRON

Essential Mineral Salt

Iron: Found in blood. Stored in liver. (O-W)

Mineral Salt Activity in Body

Essential in blood as oxygen carrier. Prevents anemia. Promotes vitality and ambition.

Principal Sources

All green leafy vegetables, wild blackberries, wild and black cherries, egg yolk, liver, oysters, potato peeling broth, whole wheat, parsley, parsnips, spinach, Swiss chard, goat brown cheese, artichokes, asparagus, nettles, caraway, cardoons, German prunes, leeks, lamb's lettuce, white onions, rice bran, romaine lettuce, whole rye meal, salad greens.

Special Points about Iron

Iron foods attract oxygen.

Indications of iron deficiency: Weakness and lassitude; Skin eruptions; Leucorrhea; Tendency for crying; Personal magnetism often fails Asthma problems and bronchitis; Hemorrhages; Anemia;

POTASSIUM
Essential Mineral Salt
Potassium: Found and needed mostly in digestive system. Tissue and secretion mineral. (W)

Mineral Salt Activity in Body
Healer in the body. Liver activator. Strongly alkaline. Makes tissues eleastic, muscles supple. Creates grace, beauty good disposition.

Principal Sources
Potato skin, dandelion, dill, sage, cress, dried olives, parsley, blueberries, peaches, prunes, coconut, gooseberries, cabbage, figs, almonds.

Special Points about Potassium:
Operations need potassium foods for fibrinogen and serum albumen.
Indications of Potassium deficiency: Desire for cold foods, sour foods, and acid drinks; changeable personality.

MANGANESE
Essential Mineral Salt
Manganese: Found and needed mostly in nervous system. Tissue strengthener; for linings of structure. Memory mineral. (W)

Mineral Salt Activity in Body
Controlling nerves in the body. Increases resistance. Coordinates thought and action. Improves memory.

Principal Sources
Nasturtium leaves, raw egg yolk, almonds, black walnuts, watercress, mint, parsley, wintergreen, endive, pignolia nuts.

Special Points about Manganese
Is dependent on iron and phosphorus.
Indications of manganese deficiency: Facial neuralgia; Angry and silent moods; Rectal cramps after meals.

PHOSPHORUS
Essential Mineral Salt
Phosphorus: Found and needed mostly in nervous system. Brain and bone mineral. (D - W)

Mineral Salt Activity in Body
Body and nerve builder. Nourishes brain and nerves. Builds power of thought. Stimulates growth of hair and bone. For thinking processes and intelligence.

Principal Sources
Sea foods, milk, raw egg yolk, parsnips, whole wheat, barley, yellow corn, nuts, peas, beans, and lentils.

Special Points about Phosphorus
Phosphorus and sulphur foods should be eaten together and are controlled by iodine. Excess will cause weak kidneys and lungs. Needs more oxygen.
Indications of Phosphorus deficiency: Loss of patience; Psychosis; Neuroses; Craving excitement; Hermits; Fears and Anxiety;

SILICON
Essential Mineral Salt
Silicon: Found and needed mostly in structural system. Nails, skin, teeth and hair, ligaments. (W)

Mineral Salt Activity in Body
Surgeon in the body. Gives keen hearing, sparkling eyes, hard teeth, glossy hair. Tones system. Gives resistance to the body. Creates a magnetic quality.

Principal Sources
Oats, barley, brown rice, rye, corn, peas, beans, lentils, wheat, spinach, asparagus, lettuce, tomatoes, cabbage, figs, strawberries, rice polishings, oat straw tea, seeds, peelings (watermelon), coconut, lemming cheese, sage, thyme, hops, prunes, bone marrow, raw egg yolk, pecans, cod liver oil, halibut liver oil.

Special Points about Silicon
Silicon helps agility in body for walking and dancing.
Indications of silicon deficiency: Coordination problems; Fungus diseases; Parched lips; Impotence and sexual disability; Feeling of approaching death.

SODIUM
Essential Mineral Salt
Sodium: Found and needed most in digestive system. Gland, ligament, and blood builder. (W)

Mineral Salt Activity in Body
Youth maintainer in body. Aids digestion. Counteracts acidosis. Halts fermentation. Purifies blood. Forms saliva, bile, pancreatic juices.

Principal Sources
Okra, celery, carrots, beets, cucumbers, string beans, asparagus, turnips, strawberries,

oat meal, raw egg yolk, coconut, black figs, spinach, sprouts, peas, Rouquefort cheese, goat cheese and milk, goat whey, fish, oysters, clams, lobster, milk, lentils, highest in raw egg white.

Special Points about Sodium
Intestinal flora needs sodium. Flexibility of tendons needs high sodium foods.
Indications of sodium deficiency: Irritability; restlessness; depression and nervousness; Gloom; Poor concentration; Tender abdominal muscles; Apprehension; Sore cervical glands; Puffiness in face and body; Inactive spleen;

SULPHUR
Essential Mineral Salt
Sulphur: Found and needed mostly in the nervous system. Brain and tissue mineral. (O–D)

Mineral Salt Activity in Body
Purifies and activates the body. Tones the system. Intensifies feeling and emotion.

Principal Sources
Cabbage, cauliflower, onions, asparagus, carrots, horseradish, shrimp, chestnuts, mustard greens, radish, spinach, leeks, garlic, apples, turnip and beet tops, plums, prunes, apricots, peaches, raw egg yolk, melons.

Special Points about Sulphur
Needs iodine to work. Driving force for goals and achievements stimulated by sulphur foods. Excess sulphur: Needs chlorine and magnesium foods. Sulphur drugs: Adversely affect kidneys, liver, and cause blood disease. *Indication of excess sulphur:* Face burning. *Indications of sulphur deficiency:* Fretting; Pouting; Retiring late and rising early; Poor appetite in morning; Extremes of variety and change; Anemic-looking skin;

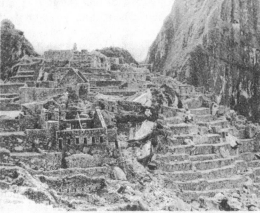

Machu Picchu—the terraces are the first things that are noticed. They were used for the growing of vegetables. Agriculture was the first thing that was recognized as a necessity in all of the past civilizations. In past civilizations these terraces seem to have been built even on the temples and on the pyramids. Vegetables were grown on the terraces and agricultural stores were built all along the pathway to their temples.

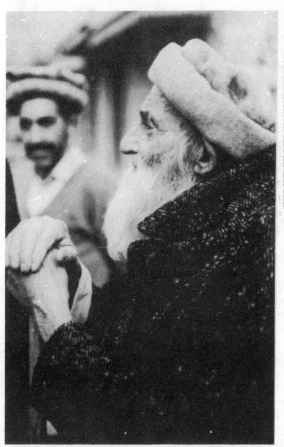

This is one of the oldest men we visited in the Hunza Valley, 120 years of age. He had just spent 8 hours working on a flume made up of heavy rocks but his work was a blessing to him, keeping his body supple and active.

The health food store

FIFTEEN

GOING into a health food store is like entering an entirely different world. It's not at all like the average supermarket or store, and it may be somewhat confusing at first. To begin with, expect one thing: These foods will cost more. Why? All health foods spoil quickly. Natural food does not keep. The beginning of good health is using natural food. Most markets and stores have on their shelves foods that have been made with one purpose in mind- to have an eternal shelf life. That is how they make their money.

Foods that have an eternal shelf life have been overpreserved, overcooked, overspiced, overoxidized. They are no longer what we could call vital foods. Flours that have intact their natural germ life — that is, the reproductive element, the antisterility vitamin which is called vitamin E — can only be obtained from fresh ground whole wheat and fresh ground yellow corn. Flours from whole rice, whole rye, buckwheat, etc., are the type that are health giving, and these are to be found in all health stores. Reading labels is very important in this respect.

Extra labor is required to put up food that is sold in the health store. In most cases it is prepared by smaller firms and in smaller amounts, and the producer cannot compete with others who are mass-producing. For instance, 25,000 bottles of marmalade can sell at a lower price per unit than 1,500 bottles of some health jelly made with raw sugar.

We should never begrudge money spent on food. If you do not buy the best food possible, you will pay a doctor. Doctors are making a living on the shortages found in many of our foods that people eat today, such as vitamin shortages, mineral shortages, enzyme shortages. We are eating half a loaf of bread and expecting to get a whole body from it.

Health food stores market food under many different brands, which may cause indecision to newcomers. If they are shy, they may look around and come out with something they do not really want- perhaps they did not have the courage to refuse the enthusiastic clerk. Clerks do get enthusiastic, because the people who put out health foods take great pride in the genuineness of their products and the fact that they come from natural sources and are invariably organically grown. They have no preservatives in them; no coal tar or other carcinogenic agents are added. These products can bring wonderful results.

However, even enthusiastic clerks in health food stores are not permitted to diagnose or treat. This is the province of a professional physician, and if you are sick, you should go to your doctor for help. If you need therapeutic supplements he will advise you. Health stores usually carry an array of such health supplements.

There are many kinds of people who go to health food stores. A newly acquired knowledge of minerals and vitamins draws some people inside. They may carefully examine the shelves and come out with a big tin with an imposing list of "milligrams" and "International Units"- good value for their money (they think)! Others are so attached to their old way of living that they only want to use the health store to overcome the deficiencies of their diet by using boxes of vitamin pills, mineral tablets, and other supplements — while continuing to eat their coffee and doughnuts. The skeptical customer checks all the brands, is never sure of getting what he needs for his health, and walks out empty-handed. The curious will idly window-shop and go out with a bar of candy which is "chocolate-free." Sometimes people come in for a "wonder food" a friend has recommended. Some are looking for a quick cure and never return if their first purchase does not do the trick after a week's trial.

The only person who will truly benefit

116

from the health food store is the one who goes in with experience and knowledge. Granted, knowledge is something we continue to acquire, but at least we must have some idea of where we are and what we want. The only justification for the existence of health food stores is that they can better your health. He who gets most from them is he who knows most. He has read and studied right living. He knows that the nearer a food is to its natural state, the better able it is to feed his body. He will look first for organically grown fruits and vegetables. He knows that freezing is next best to taking fresh foods. He will look in the cooler for his whole grains and flours. He will buy raw sugar, untreated honey, unpasteurized milk, cheeses, and fertile eggs. His drinks will be chosen from the many herb teas, dandelion coffee, juices, and unchemicalized juice concentrates.

If he wishes to save time making spreads, he knows his health store has supplies of fresh, naturally prepared nut-creams, fruit conserves, and vegetable pastes. He will vary his proteins, using the nut, legume, cheese, and seed counters. Sometimes, for a change, he will experiment with meat substitute products. He will know that such supplements as rice polishings, wheat germ, brewer's yeast, powdered whey, and gelatin are *foods*, and therefore are excellent additions to anyone's diet— and he won't have to worry about vitamin count-downs. The only salt he should buy should be a vegetable powder such as the Broth Seasoning I have created, or a genuine sea salt. Even the health food store will carry a vegetable salt which has an ordinary salt base and this is not good for the person trying to break himself of the salt habit. So again, we say *read your labels*. (Such health aids as blenders, juicers, nut mills, and slant boards may be obtained from the larger stores.)

Of course, the general thing today is to smoke, and to drink coffee, tea, and alcohol. The person who drinks a glass of carrot juice these days is considered a "nut," a "crank," a "health food extremist." But why not drink carrot juice? You'll be better for it. People will buy fruit juices — canned, cooked, pasteurized, and sweetened, and think nothing of it. Why should it be abnormal to prefer the unsweetened kind, the fresh kind, or the concentrates? And why should we not have variety in our diet? If fruit juices are so good for us, why shouldn't the vegetable juices be just as good?

Before we go completely overboard on perfecting our health ideals, there is another important consideration. We live in a critical world, we live in an orthodox community, and even our families may point a finger at us. For peace and harmony, we sometimes have to "make haste slowly."

However, while we are smoothing the way, where will we learn how to get the best from our health food store? Well, the shop itself usually has a good selection of health books packed with knowledge. They may not all express the same principles, but they all uphold the basic truth that natural, unsprayed, unchemically treated foodstuffs are superior.

It's Time for a Change

Anyone who is sick knows it is time for a change. One thing we have to change is our eating habits. Food is not an easy problem to tackle because most of us have well-established cooking habits and our family backgrounds and customs make it very difficult for us to make changes. It seems that we seldom recognize the relationship between our food and our health. We find it difficult to conceive of an actual relation between the food that goes into our bodies and what happens in our toes, or what happens to our hair or our eyes. We do not know that the state of the bloodstream depends upon what we eat. We do not know that what we eat today is going to walk and talk tomorrow. We do not know that what we eat actually becomes the cell structure of the body. But it's true: if we do not change our faulty ways of eating, we can never expect a permanent turn for the better in our health.

A "reform house" which is demonstrating that we really need to reform our ways. They don't call it a health store there in Switzerland. It is called a Reform House.

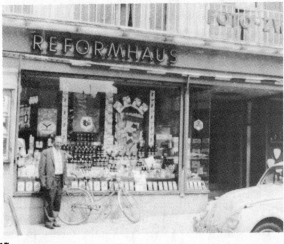

117

Your Life Is in the Label

There are very few people today who give serious consideration to the label on the foods they buy. They may look for a certain brand name or trademark, but they accept with blind faith all articles on the grocery shelf. But if we would read labels it might save our lives.

What Is Your Know-How in Reading Labels?

No selection of food should be made without first thoroughly examining the list of ingredients, which indicates their proportionate quantity, and the inert (inactive) components, if any. You will need a working knowledge of the terms commonly employed. You will also need a working knowledge of the processes involved, the conditions under which it is prepared, the additives the food contains, and the effect of all these things upon its nutritional qualities.

We have found over a peroid of years, for example, that the bleach used in white bread (especially when administered to animals) produces fits, epilepsy, and other nervous disorders. If we must have our food "pure" and white as "driven snow" there are ways that have veen devised of preparing it so that the eye is pleased. If it is a matter of giving us volume, they can puff up the food through the administration of excess heat and certain chemicals. But we get the volume and the whiteness only to the detriment of our health and the filling up of our stomachs with "foodless foods."

We should know what is meant on a label when it mentions as ingredients such items as wheat flour, sugar, raw sugar, fats and oils, eggs, milk products, artificial coloring, and preservatives. If properly labeled, every product containing additives would bear a skull and crossbones symbol, and we would carefully store that product in our medicine cabinets with our other poisons. The carcinogenic factor is inherent in all artificial products of coal-tar compounds, which is the common source of these additives. Consumption of these should be carefully avoided. Methods of processing would soon change if we voiced our objections and refused to purchase these commodities.

Know What's Behind Your Label. We need to learn then, as much as possible about what happens to the contents before they find their way into their attractive containers. Labels are a very important media in the business of selling. But remember, "All is not gold that glitters." Fields and factories should be open for inspection to all, so that we may learn how these processes are carried on. Let us find out some things for ourselves.

The result of our learning to read labels more intelligently will bring us produce in its whole natural state, and it will be labeled to identify production by natural methods.

Such production- and this is the type of preservation that should seriously concern all of us- will preserve the vital life elements in the soil. The less we depend upon those varieties that are subjected to the different manufacturing and packaging processes, the better are our expectations for adequately nourishing the organism.

Learn to Choose "Real" Value. In all commodities, we must depend largely upon the integrity of the manufacturer whose label is on the product. The conscientious manufacturer guards the quality of his products and he labels to assure the consumer that the standard is maintained. We should choose those products that have a reputation for good quality. This should be the primary criterion in our selection of foods. Dollar value is of little importance.

We need first to learn who among those whose products are being distributed in our particular area are the most dependable processors and packagers. Then we should select as often as we can afford them- keeping in mind this is our most important investment.

Demand Better Descriptive Labeling. We also have a right to know the practices of the trade, and should not hesitate to demand a system of labeling that will reveal clearly the operations to which the products are subjected. We have a right to expect our government to establish and maintain controls that will ensure its citizens the highest-quality products, free of any pressure from trade groups or industrial influence. Our best insurance, however, is to demand more and more foods in their natural form, under growers' labels that reflect natural production methods. This will help decrease the consumption of processed foods.

Reading the Label

When you start reading the labels you may not be sure what they mean. Of course, we need to educate ourselves, but here are a few very common ingredients from labels to get you started.

The labels say:	The labels do not say:

Wheat Flour. . This is white flour, from wheat, milled to remove all the vital life elements. The outer coating, bran, rich in mineral content, is bleached to make the flour "pure" white — meaning "pure poison" to the digestive system.

Sugar . . . . This is crystallized stalks of sugar cane. Sugar, in its mineral form, is a rich source of minerals and other nutritive factors. But these are lost by being subjected to prolonged heat and further impaired by bleaching, etc.

Salt. . . . . This is processed to crystallization by extreme heat, leaving a lifeless residue concentrated to such a degree that it is not assimilable in the digestive process.

Eggs . . . . In prepared products eggs have been dried and reduced to powdered form. Generally they are prepared from eggs in which the germ of life necessary to produce the embryo of a chick never existed because of lack of fertility; generally they are the product of fowls never allowed to range on the ground, injected with various antibiotics, and forced-fed concentrated feed which is accessible to them around the clock.

Fats . . . . These are fats reduced to solid form by a process of hydrogenation, which completely alters the fat molecular structure, rendering it unassimilable in digestion. The new fat structure tends to be cholesterol forming and contributes to hardening of the arteries.

Oils (unless labeled "cold-pressed") . . These are extracted from various sources and subjected to heat that alters the minute fat globules, rendering them carcinogenic in tendency.

Special Preservatives, Artificial Colorings, Flavorings . . These are additives, usually of coal tar derivation, that are carcinogenic in nature; flavorings also perhaps having a high alcoholic content.

Vinegar . . . . . . This is distilled, processed quickly by chemicals, as opposed to the slow aging of pure cider or other fermentation. Unassimilable in digestion.

Processed. . . . . As applied to the making of cheese, this is similar in action to that of hydrogenation, which alters the fatty structure, rendering it indigestible.

Food from Animal Sources

Let us consider some of the basic foods. We need to be most particular in regard to food from animal sources. We should accept no compromise on most of these. There are many animal products that only the more robust and balanced of human organisms can handle without impairing their digestive and eliminative functions. Special study is required for knowledge of this important subject. Many new factors and scientific developments enter into the production and processing of animal products, and it is unsafe to assume our customary eating habits may be continued without questioning.

Grains, Cereals, Baked Goods

No class of food is subjected to processing to the extent used on grains. They should come to every consumer's hands whole, just as they are harvested. Destruction of their vital life substance begins with their being fragmented and continues through the processes of grinding and milling that renders them into flour and cereals. Destruction also occurs in the additional processes they go through to make them into prepared cereals and baked goods. Little nutritional value is left in these prepared foods, notwithstanding so-called "enriching" additives, unless they are freshly prepared from whole grains, particularly the sprouted grain.

If you would derive maximum returns for every dietary dollar expended, read the labels of prepared and baked products and compare them with those for natural whole grains. Be governed accordingly. You will soon want to invest in an appliance which will enable you to grind the whole grains in your own kitchen when you are ready to use them. You can learn methods that require only tenderizing, and methods of baking that will ensure greatest nutritive benefits. These will be found so satisfying that you will be able to reduce the consumption of carbohydrates, which generally is far too great for balanced nutrition.

Fats

In processing, fats undergo extensive development so that the natural structure is altered, the fatty elements being subjected to what is known as hydrogenation, making them incapable of digestion. And when something is taken into the body that cannot be digested it becomes harmful to you. Have you learned to select oils which have been subjected only to low temperature?

The furor regarding the cholesterol-forming tendency of these processed fats has made the public more aware of their potential dangers: they increase the incidence of heart disease.

Fruit Juices

For breakfast and other meals as well, children and adults should avoid the various popular beverages which purport to contain fruit or resemble a fruit juice, but are often loaded with additive substances, dyes, sugar, sugar substitutes, acids and oils. Foods containing synthetic food dyes and artificial flavors are particularly to be avoided. A considerable number of dyes which were thought to be entirely safe are now known to be harmful, positively dangerous to health. (From *Consumer Bulletin Annual*, 1962-63)

Ice Cream

Among diary products, the one usually considered the most delectable is ice cream. But ice cream has been reduced in commercial manufacture to the most inferior of foods, containing many artificial ingredients with little nutritive value. When made of natural ingredients it is most wholesome. How can the consumer evaluate the quality except by demanding more explicit labeling?

Canned Foods and Their Effect on the Diet

The container which bears the label should also be seriously considered. The invention of the tin can revolutionized food processing and contributed to extensive changes in the dietary habits of the people. Nowadays, the can opener is one of the most essential kitchen gadgets. The consumption of canned foods is so great that an electrical device has been developed just for this purpose. If the contents are vegetables, they usually are subjected to a cooking process to have greater taste appeal. Prepared and packaged seasonings are added; and they are often immersed in hot fat, which in itself is productive of causes involving metastasis — that change in tissue structure which becomes malignant. Notwithstanding all the evidence and confronted with the increasing prevalence of metastasis, medical science still claims not to have discovered proof of the cause. Why not look in the frying pan or in those foods preserved by artificial means to retard spoilage and to assure a long shelf life? With proper caution on the label regarding the prompt use of any perishable item, the consumer would then assume responsibility for the use within the period designated. The objective should be the quickest possible turnover of all foods, not a long shelf life.

Cleaning Commodities

These factors are not limited to commodities taken internally only. They also apply to those used externally on the skin to keep the body clean and well groomed; also, to the cleaning preparations which contribute to the attractiveness and sanitation of our eating utensils, homes, offices, stores, and shops. Do you know what effects may and do come from the use of detergents? Harsh soaps also can affect the normal health and function of the skin.

Salt

We have both winter foods and summer foods. We should know what the best summer foods are and how to live during the summer. Do you know how to live during the hot weather? It has been discovered that the use of table salt, or salt tablets, replaces salts in the body lost through excessive perspiration. But we should be aware that salt is attracted to certain tissues of the body and can result in hardening of the arteries. Do we have to go from one bad condition to another by taking salt to replace that which has been eliminated from the body? Learn to take care of such conditions in a way that will not cause trouble in the future.

Some Items You'll Want
From Your Nutrition Center

Herb Teas

Oatstraw	Mint
Alfamint	Shavegrass
Huckleberry	Peach Leaf
Strawberry	Fennugreek

Seeds

Safflower	Sunflower
Sesame	Pumpkin
Guatemala squash	

Cereals and Grains

Whole grain wheat	Seven grain
Wheat germ	Barley
Rice polishings	Cornmeal
Brown rice	Oats

Lentils	Millet	Gelatins	Lecithin spread
Soybeans	Peas	Salad dressings	Lecithin granules
Soy milk	Beans	Meat substitutes	Dry cereals

Oils

		Salts	
Safflower	Sunflower	Vegetable salt	Mineral salt
Sesame	Soy	Celery salt	Garlic salt
Peanut	Tahini		
Olive		*Herbs*	
		Paprika	Thyme
Powders		Rosemary	Sage
Dulse	Banana	Basil	Flaxseed
Coconut	Whey		

Breads		*Natural Sugars*	
whole grain	Rye	Honey of many kinds	Date sugar
Millet		Molasses	Raw sugar
		Corn sugar	Maple sugar

Fruit Juices		*Dried Fruits*	
Black cherry	Fig	Apricots	Apples
Concord grape	Pineapple	Dates	Figs
Prune	Pomegranate	Olives	Pears
Apple		Prunes	Peaches
		Raisins	

Nuts

General

Almonds	Peanuts
Pinenuts	Brazils
Pecans	Coconut
Walnuts	Malted nuts
Cashews	

Cherry concentrate or apple concentrate for flavoring, topping on yogurt. Make delicious drinks for the family with cherry concentrate. Cheese of all kinds

Nut Butters

Almond	Cashew
Peanut	

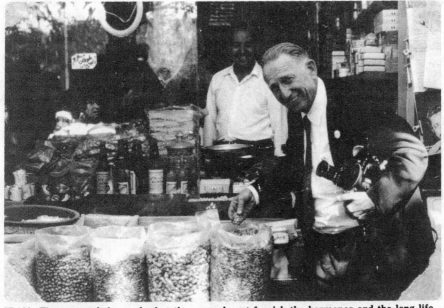

IRAN—The nuts and the seeds that these people eat furnish the hormones and the long life principles for these people.

SIXTEEN

Health tips

BUY A VARIETY of fresh vegetables every day. Find out when the vegetables are delivered to your market so as to get them as fresh as possible. Often markets throw away many tasty tops of vegetables, such as beet and turnip tops. They are worth asking for. When buying lettuce or leafy vegetables, choose the greenest, since they are most beneficial for the bloodstream.

Seasonal Eating. Nature offers different foods during the different seasons. Foods in season are best for you. In the spring we have more fruits, which we need for our bodies' spring cleaning. In the winter there are more fattening and heating foods to prepare our bodies for the cool weather.

Diet. Forget this word when you are living correctly. When you live on good food you are not on a diet. There are many who are on an arthritis-producing diet, and those eating pies, cakes, and artificial sweets are on a diabetes-producing diet. Don't let anyone serve you sickness in the form of foodless foods.

Oils in the Diet. Olive oil or any other concentrated oil or fat is hard on the liver and gall bladder. These are the two most overworked organs in the body. Don't use very much oil in your cooking. Don't use it everytime you have a salad. A sour cream or sweet cream dressing is better for you than an oil dressing. Oils become carcinogenic when heated and must not be used.

Mineral Oil. Mineral oil should never be used. It is a coal-tar product and an irritable drug in the intestinal tract.

Eating To Keep Up The Strength. It is foolish to eat to keep up the strength. If you feel weak without food it is a sign that food is only stimulating you. We must first have strength to digest, assimilate, and carry the food to the cells. Food must be transformed into a structure that has strength before strength can be manifested in the body.

Chewing Starches. Starches should be chewed vigorously and mixed well with the saliva in the mouth. As a suggestion for those who do not chew starches well, eat one bite of celery with every bite of starch and the starches will be chewed longer.

Hot and Cold Foods. Extremely hot or extremely cold foods are not the best foods to eat. When foods are too cold, they may crack the enamel on your teeth and will contract and chill the stomach, slowing up digestion. Hot foods irritate the tissues of the mouth and throat and destroy sensitiveness of the taste buds.

Overeating. You are your own dietician when it comes to eating time. Eat when hungry and eat enough, but do not overeat. No one can tell you these things better than yourself. The natural inner urge guides you. Make sure you eat natural food or your hunger becomes a craving and you overeat because the meals do not supply the body chemicals you need.

Salt. Table salt should be dropped from the diet. We do not need it when we have plenty of greens every day. To change from it, use vegetized salt purchased in health food stores, and gradually use less of this. Or better, learn to flavor foods with vegetable concentrates in powdered form, or herbs.

Eating on Warm Days. On warm days eat more fruits and salads. These are cooling foods. Ice cream, though cold, is not a cooling food. Eat fewer heavy starches and heavy proteins when you are too hot and the day is too warm.

Raw Salads. Raw salads cannot be taken in some intestinal tracts. Cooked vegetables and raw vegetable juice together is the same as eating a raw salad and in many cases eliminates gas immediately.

Egg Whites. Egg whites should always be beaten to a froth and aerated well before eating. An omelet is best when egg whites are beaten well.

Waffles. Waffles used as a starch are permissible when made of whole grain flours and eaten with a little butter and soaked; sweet dried fruits, however, lean toward whole grain cereals, not breads and waffles.

Colorful Meal planning. Meals should be planned with the idea of putting together as many colors as possible. A natural appetite is not stimulated with fried, charred, over-cooked, greasy, colorless foods.

Juices from Vegetables. If you have no vegetable juicer, vegetables may be run through a food grinder, then put the pulp into a muslin bag and squeeze the juices out. Carrots and beets should be shredded or grated first.

Cell Salts. Cell salts are found most abundantly in the peelings or outer layers of fruits and vegetables. Do not be afraid of cucumber peelings. They are not poisonous. Needless to say do not eat orange peelings, banana peelings, and pineapple skins.

Foods and Their Influence on the Body

Fattening Foods.
Good: Nuts (pine nuts are best), avocados, dried fruits, honey, yellow corn, whole grains (well-cooked), cream.

Bad: Heavy denatured refined starches such as cream of wheat, white bread, white rice, pearled barley, etc., white sugar, chocolate, concentrated oils, fat meats.

Thinning Foods.
Good: Citrus fruits (grapefruit and lemon are best), pineapple, tropical fruits, berries, melons, vegetable juices, tomatoes, leafy vegetables, nonstarchy vegetables, skim milk, whey, and health teas such as strawberry, pine needle, etc.

Bad: Spices, stimulating foods, mineral waters, coffee, tea, fried foods, pepper, prepared and embalmed foods, distilled vinegar, patent medicines.

Gas-Producing Foods. Sulphur foods such as cabbage, cauliflower, onions, eggs, etc. Unsoaked dried fruits, fats, fibrous foods, sometimes raw foods (especially lettuce), fried foods, wrong combinations such as acids with starches or starches with proteins.

Constipating and Disease-Producing Foods. Cheese, fried foods, pasteurized milk, candies; all denatured, refined, spiced, concentrated, salted, embalmed, unnatural, or hot foods; all decayed, rich, heavy, hard-shelled, or heavy cellulose foods, such as tops of vegetables and legumes. Canned, burned, fermented, processed food and practically any food wherein man has tried to improve over nature.

Laxative Foods.
Good: Berries (except blackberries), all fruits, natural sweets, such as soaked dried fruits, honey, etc., nonstarchy vegetables. Fruit and vegetable juices, tropical fruits. Whole grains are laxative to those who need them.

Bad: Mineral oil, dynamiting laxatives made from drugs, spiced foods, wines with meals, herb teas that are used just for laxative purposes.

Blood-Purifying Foods. Fruits, berries, vegetable and fruit juices, tops of vegetables, broths, health teas, skim milk, and goat whey. Tropical fruits, nonstarchy vegetables.

Special Health Tips

Comb to Relieve Pain. Many times we can relieve pain by placing a comb in the palm of our hand and holding the teeth of the comb firmly against the tips of the fingers.

A Golf Ball. Because of its curve, a golf ball is a fine thing to be used for exercising the metatarsal arch, working the foot back and forth on it. If we could learn to walk with the soles of the feet turned in, we would find relief for lower back pain.

A Vegetable Skin Brush. This will help bring on relaxation when used on the soles of the feet at night before going to bed. Four or five minutes of light brushing, especially by another person, will bring relaxation.

Spine-Easing Exercise. Walking pigeon-toed a little every day as an exercise is especially good for correcting a curvature of the lower part of the spine.

Charcoal. It is very good in some kinds of indigestion to use an olive oil mixed with charcoal to the consistency of a paste. Old charcoal that has been heated before using is more effective.

Some time ago I was introduced by using charcoal. It is an absorbent and can absorb many times it's own volume in the various gases. It is also antiseptic. It has great oxidizing properties and it is claimed that when taken internally it is excellent for acid dyspepsia, gas and fermentation, heartburn, and cases of colic due to fermentation in the decomposition of foods in the stomach and bowels. It is a valuable remedy and can be used as a poultice over painful areas and as a preventive or curative when taken internally.

Charcoal can be made out of willow, coconuts, soft woods, boxwood, pine, and eucalyptus. Eucalyptus has been used by just placing it in the mouth; it reportedly absorbs poisons from the tonsils. It is also thought that charcoal robs the body of vitamin A, and if it is going to be used for any length of time, you should use a vitamin A supplement. Charcoal mixed with flaxseed has also been used as a poultice for many conditions.

Water Packs. Many times a joint problem may be relieved by wrapping the area in a towel wrung out in cold water, then wrapping with a dry towel to hold in the moisture. This will help to relieve stiffness and pain.

Hot Water Bottle. To make a substitute hot water bottle, fill a bag made of flannel with hot, dry bran.

Flaxseed Poultice. A flaxseed poultice is one of the finest we can use. It can be mixed with warm water, applied as warm as can be tolerated, and kept hot with water baths or an electric pad.

Bulk Elimination Diet. An excellent five day elimination and cleansing regimen has been devised. For the first, three days drink juices of any kind except citrus and take one tablespoon of bulk five times daily. During the next two days eat only fruits and vegetables and juices, and bulk three times daily. On the sixth day return to your regular health and eating regimen, with bulk three times daily until otherwise directed. You may drink water throughout the regimen. Take enemas daily.

Enemas. Plain water enemas are the best to empty the lower bowel. If there is a little inflammation or irritation, use enemas of flaxseed tea, one-half pint to an enema. If it is very thick and heavy, dilute with water. The knee-chest position is the best, on the average, for taking enemas.

A Wisdom Diet

A whole year's experiment was conducted by Dr. W. R. Raymond, nutritional researcher, on a diet regime. During this time he ate nothing but wild rice, Japanese sea greens (for valuable trace minerals that are lacking in land foods), sesame seed meal (for lecithin, amino acids, vitamins, and minerals), prepared with distilled water in a Pyrex glass distillator, and cooked in a Pyrex glass container. He said his health and vitality were never more exceptional than they were during this diet. They surpassed his experience on fruit diets, raw food diets, and so forth. The improvement in intestinal peristalsis and bowel activity was marked.

The Taro Root

Many years ago, I saw a healing take place in a particular lady. She was troubled with a bleeding bowel (colitis). The Seventh-Day Adventist ministry helped her. She had been to the Loma Linda Hospital and she had had the best facilities in the Adventist movement. But somehow or other she came to my office and wanted this bowel taken care of by natural methods. I put her well on the road to recovery by furnishing her with the materials and the knowledge that helped her to get well; and what do you suppose I used for her? I used the remedy that I learned from a Seventh-Day Adventist minister down in the South Seas, where many of these bowel troubles, amoeba problems, and disturbances are so common. It was from this minister that I learned the great value of taro root. It is a starchlike bulb, but has very little actual starch in it, and it is the most soothing thing for the intestinal tract. I used taro root and banana with this little lady.

Many people have used banana in cases of colitis, bleeding, and inflammation of the bowel without success because of its sharp little seeds. Try this: take the middle, brownish vein of a banana, put it between your fingers and work it back and forth a little. The ends of your fingers will bleed!

I found that you cannot use bananas as part of a bland diet unless you remove the seed vein.

What I learned from nature proved to be the very thing that helped most. This lady is now 75 years of age and is still talking about how we helped her 25 years ago by using nature's methods.

Carbohydrates

Carbohydrates are composed of sugars, starches, and cellulose. They produce heat in the body when carbon unites with oxygen in the bloodstream, causing oxidation of the carbon.

The conversion of starches into sugars begins in the mouth, where the process of chewing mixes them with the saliva. Grain and cereal starches are insoluble and cannot be assimilated without this conversion. (That is why your baby should never have cereals or starches until he has the teeth with which this process is made possible). Starch digestion is completed in the small intestine.

Foods containing the least amount of carbohydrates are the most easily digested. They also build a better balanced body. The more ailing a person is, the fewer carbohydrates he should eat.

Cholesterol

Cholesterol is a normal substance found in all bodies; but, of course, it is possible to have too much cholesterol. When we have an excess amount of cholesterol in the blood, it can be deposited in the arteries, causing a hardened tissue that cannot function well. That state can be associated with the disease of the arteries known as arteriosclerosis. This cholesterol is made by chemical changes that occur within the boyd, and it comes from the unsaturated fats we take in. This chemical process is called lipid metabolism.

We need a certain amount of the fatty substances for the maintenance of our body's health, and it takes lipid metabolism to properly develop the fatty substances for our bodies. When blood cholesterol is high, little flat plaques form and settle in the arteries. These plaques attract blood, which sticks to these areas and forms clots.

When doctors find the blood cholesterol high, they try to bring it to a normal level. This can be done by having the patient lose weight. Sometimes he simply needs to change his diet.

The Trappist monks in Canada are a group of vegetarians. They have brothers called the St. Benedictine monks in Georgia who live on a good deal of the meat products. They have tested both of these orders and find that the vegetarian order does not have cholesterol deposits in their arteries like their St. Benedictine brothers, who have a high level of cholesterol.

I believe that cholesterol can be formed in the body by having too many of the fatty foods of animal origin, such as eggs, butter, milk, cream, as well as the fatty meats and fish. The average doctor hasn't practiced nutrition enough to know just how he can control this in his patients, but we who have used dietetic control in cholesterol cases for many years find that diet works very well.

For one reason or another, people nowadays seem to think that fats are needed in order to keep warm or to build the body weight, etc., but this is not always true. It is said that the larger the waistline the shorter the life line. We should avoid overweight, and the many fats, oils, and creams in our diet will cause this excess.

I believe that cholesterol is a disease of civilization. Greens are especially good in aiding the metabolism of fats, and most of us do not have enough of these green leaves in salads and other foods. Many of us would be much better off if we would eat the vegetable fats instead of the animal fats. I believe that cholesterol is the result of poor living, and it goes hand in hand with aging and hardening of the arteries.

To decrease cholesterol excess, it might be well to go on a meat-free diet for awhile, eliminating the use of concentrated fats and oils. If oils are used, make sure that they are unheated. Never have fried foods. Use lots of salad and lots of green foods. Have green teas, such as comfrey tea and dandelion tea. Also use a lot of whey in your diet; it is high in sodium and has a heavy dissolving ability. Lecithin in the diet helps to break down the cholesterol content of the arteries and in the blood. Cocktails made of celery juice, cucumber juice, or spinach in place of the civilized popular cocktails served at the bar will work well.

Find a good healthy way to live; find exercises that keep the liver in a good active condition. A sedentary occupation can build cholesterol in the body. We must find a way of changing our lives, a way to balance our daily routine.

The best food for cholesterol deposits is sprouts! There are four sprouts in particular I recommend for everyone's diet: alfalfa, buckwheat, mung bean, and sunflower seed sprouts. You can grow these very easily in your home.

Percentage Chart for Carbohydrates

The percentage chart which follows is a handy guide to the selection of carbohydrates. You cannot live without eating some of the foods listed in the five percent column. In cases of severe trouble it would be well to select all your carbohydrates from the five percent column. Whenever heavy starches from the 20 percent column are eaten, be sure to eat foods from the five percent column to maintain balance in yours meals.

5 percent	10 percent	15 percent	20 percent
Vegetables	**Vegetables**	**Vegetables**	**Vegetables**
Artichokes	Beets	Green peas	Baked beans
Asparagus	Carrots	Lima beans	Bread
Broccoli	Kohlrabi	Parsnips	Brown rice
Beet greens	Onions		Green corn
Brussels sprouts	Pumpkin	**Fruits**	Potatoes
Cabbage	Squash		Shell beans
Cauliflower	Turnips	Apples	Lentils
Celery		Apricots	Lima beans
Cucumber	**Fruits**	Blueberries	Navy beans
Dandelions		Cherries	Soy beans
Egg plant	Blackberries	Currants	Shredded wheat
Endive	Gooseberries	Huckleberries	Whole rye
Leeks	Lemons	Pears	
Lettuce	Oranges	Raspberries	
Mushrooms	Peaches		**Fruits**
Okra	Pineapple	**Nuts**	Bananas
Radishes	Strawberries		Plum
Rhubarb	Watermelon	Almonds	Prunes
Sauerkraut		Beechnuts	
Sorrel	**Nuts**	Walnuts (English)	
Sea kale			**Nuts**
Spinach	Black walnuts		
String beans	Brazil nuts		Chestnuts
Swiss chard	Filberts		(40% fat)
Tomatoes	Hickory		
Vegetable marrow	Pecans		Peanuts
Watercress			

Fruits

Ripe olives (20% fat)
Grapefruit

Nuts

Butternuts
Pignolias

EASILY DIGESTED FOODS

Vegetables

Artichokes
Beans, tender string
Beets, tender
Butter beans, green
Cabbage, chinese
Cabbage, savoy
Cauliflower, tender
Chard, Swiss
Corn on cob, tender
Dwarf nettles

Okra
Peas, tender young
Romaine
Spinach, tender garden
Spinach, New Zealand
Asparagus
Beet greens
Broccoli
Cabbage, curly
Cabbage, red

Carrots, tender
Celery
Chayote
Dandelion
Leek leaves
Onions, green
Rhubarb
Squash
Tomatoes, ripe

Meat, Fish, Cheese, and Eggs

Cheese, Roquefort
Duck, broiled wild
Fowl, young wild
Game, young
Goose
Liver, from young
   animals

Quail
Squab, broiled
Tuna, broiled
Clam broth
Eggs, scrambled,
   cooked slightly
Gizzard broth

Lamb
Oysters
Oyster broth
Roe
Shad
Whiting

Fruits and berries

Apples, custard
Apples, baked pippin
Apricots, sweet ripe
Blueberries
Brambleberries
Currants, black, ripe
Elderberries
Figs, sun dried
Grapes
Nectarines

Peaches, ripe
Persimmons
Plums, blue damsons
Prunes, sun dried
Strawberries
Tangerines
Apples, mellow
Apples, sun dried
Avocado
Blueberry juice
Cherries, black, ripe

Currants, zante
Figs, fresh
Fruit pudding
Lemon
Olives
Pears
Pineapple
Plums, stewed sweet
Pumpkin
Strawberries, wild

Miscellaneous

Alfalfa bud salads
Clover blossom

Coconut oil

Almond oil

Cod liver oil
Honey

Dairy Products

Goat butter

Whey

Goat Buttermilk

Sprouts

Whey beans, seeds, grains are sprouted, they
are easier to digest than in their original form.

VEGETARIAN PROTEINS

Soy milk powder
Sesame seed butter
Eggs

Almonds, flaked,
   powdered or in
   butter form

Clabbered milk
Lentils

Aged cheese or natural cottage cheese.

Natural remedies

SEVENTEEN

WHEN we consider remedies for the body, the first thing we have to realize is that the body needs food for every single cell. Each cell has its individual activity. They must have different minerals to express differently. A liver cell does not perform the same work as the cell in the gland. The bone cells do not do the same things as the blood cells. Each part of our body is fed according to the "master plan" for mineral and vitamin capacity that is built into these different tissues.

For years we've be using treatment instead of prevention for years. Since early history, records show people going to doctors or healers. The recovered ones stood on street corners and told of their cures and of healing others, then others went home and tried the suggested remedy.

Diseases and Remedies

There are no less than a thousand natural remedies for every disease! In the drug system we have more than 6,000 diseases and more than 28,000 medicinal remedies for these diseases. This is not counting all the remedies we have now for the different diseases in other systems of healing such as Christian Science and psychiatric work. In the realm of mechanical treatments, people have been punched and pulled and massaged and squeezed to a point where every part of the body has been manipulated in every possible means we can think of.

But treating in itself is not the cure. Treatment is not getting at the base of the trouble. For instance, if a person is living on a poor diet of coffee and doughnuts, he could receive every treatment under the sun and those treatments would do no more than manipulate a poor nerve structure and stimulate the circulation of a poor bloodstream. Treatments do not cure disease. Only food and right living will.

Abnormal Foods, Abnormal Bodies

By eating different kinds of foods you can have the kind of body you wish. You can produce any kind of disease you would like — from heart trouble (from lack of vitamin E) to diabetes (through overuse of white sugar and white flour). These diseases are produced from abnormal foods. It should be of paramount interest to everyone, therefore, to get foods that will rebuild and rejuvenate the body.

Food Is the Real Medicine

Natural medicines are found in our fruit and vegetable juices in the color God has prepared — in the apricot, the peach, the tomato, and the greens of our vegetables. These foods contain vitamins and minerals; we call them the block builders. In the vitamin we have all of the ammunition necessary to put minerals in their proper place. There are many things to consider besides food, but let us stay as close to good food as we possibly can. We know that sleep, circulation, pleasurable walks, happiness, relief, relaxation, a proper philosophy, and right spiritual attitude are all necessary requirements if we are to have real health.

Our eating habits must also be good. We cannot eat at any old time and expect the bowels to carry on a rhythmic action for us, even with the best of foods. We must learn to eat slowly and chew our foods well.

Since early history, records show people going to doctors or healers. The recovered ones stood on street corners and told of their cures and of healing others, then others went home and tried the suggested remedy.

A Natural Body Handles All Food Well

Consider what you are doing, especially if you are not well. A well person can take any natural food and find that it is neither too laxative or binding. A natural body handles all foods well. It is only the sensitive, run-down, irritable body that overreacts to laxative foods, such as prune juice and fig juice, while other foods — certain cheeses, milk, and blackberry juice — become constipating.

Stay Young with Sodium

The youth element, sodium, is stored in the body mostly in the joints. When a person says he is getting old or stiff, we know he is lacking sodium. There is no such thing as old age, but there can be a lack of sodium. Sodium is found in okra, celery, and citrus fruits. People sick with acid stomach cannot tolerate citrus fruits; therefore, sodium found in these fruits is of no use to them. They will need to get their sodium in other ways.

When a person has arthritis, hardening in the joints, or spurs on the spine, he needs sodium. Sodium is the dissolver. If sick blood is flowing through the body, it bathes every cell, thereby making the cell sick. Sodium helps to prevent that; it keeps calcium from depositing in the walls of our arteries. When the joints become hard, if you put sodium into the body the calcium in the joints will be drawn back into solution and the joints will become limber again.

As an example, there was a little lady who came to me with her head down below her hips with arthritis of the spine. She had a double curvature with spurs on the vertebrae as large as her thumbnail. She had been told by a doctor that she was going to be in a wheelchair or cast for the rest of her natural life. She came to us, and we increased her sodium intake and put her on a natural diet. In one year's time this lady straightened out; we later had a report from Magnolia Hospital in Long Beach, California, that there was no more arthritis of the spine. She was free from all pathology.

Whey is high in sodium. The whey that we use in the office has 100 times as much sodium as anything else you can use. Taking one teaspoon of this whey means taking something very vital. While I do not believe you can live on this, if you have cheated your body of sodium for years, you had better pay yourself back as quickly as possible. This goat whey can do it.

Valuable Silicon

Silicon keeps the hair and skin from becoming dry. A person who becomes dead on his feet and nothing interests him any more lacks silicon. A dancer has to have a lot of silicon in his body or he cannot dance. Silicon helps nerve messages to travel over the nervous system. If you do not have all of your nerve tissue in good working order you become slow. You cannot bend your finger. You suffer fatigue. You have underactivity in every organ in the body. A tonic that each of us should have is oat straw tea; its botanical name is Avena Sativa.

When a horse has been working hard all day, he comes in fatigued and tired. We do not give him an injection for a pick-up; we give him a tonic — oats. It is the finest thing that I know of for building up the body. Drinking a cup of oat straw tea revives the nervous system. We treat our horses better than we do our own bodies.

Horsetail tea is another herb tea high in silicon.

Manganese

Manganese is a part of the nerve and brain element. A lack of this element is one reason why some women do not have the instinctive mother desire to even produce milk for the child. They do not have the brain and nerve force to do it. One of the best sources of manganese is Missouri black walnuts.

Magnesium. Magnesium is the bowel element we all need. Another food high in magnesium is yellow corn meal. It is far better than white corn meal. For many people, yellow corn meal is better than wheat.

Watch Your Heart. The finest tonic for the heart is plain white clover honey. Take it three times a day, one teaspoon in a glass of water. If you have heart trouble, your disturbance is on the left side of the body. The left side is the negative side. Carbohydrates, starches, and sugars are negative. If the left side is broken down and the negative factors are worn out, the best and quickest way to get this negative side rejuvenated is honey and water.

Potassium

Muscles are made mainly of potassium. Potassium is a healing element, the same as sodium. We need a lot of potassium because our body is made up mainly of muscles. Potassium is found in most of our greens, wild lettuce, dandelion greens, endive, and olives.

Probably one reason people do not have enough potassium is because it is bitter to the taste. But we do need it. Take eight or ten dried olives, steep them in a teapot like a regular tea for about ten minutes, skim off the fat or oil that may have come to the top, and drink. This is a good potassium tea and does wonders for the heart and the muscle structure. Take dried olives and chew them, allowing the saliva to work on them and extract the potassium from them. This is a slow way to procure olive oil, and it is not particularly tasteful, but it is a fine way to get your potassium. Olives do more to revive tired muscle structures than a chocolate bar.

The Brain Food — Lecithin. Lecithin is the brain and nerve food. We should take it when we become tired and fatigued, when we lose our alertness and cannot respond readily and easily to suggestions, when we find a lack of memory. It is necessary to have lecithin in abundance before vitamin B can be held in the body. All the vitamin B that people are taking today is doing very little good, because they don't have enough lecithin to retain it.

If we are using our brain and nervous system to the extreme, it is well to take soy bean lecithin capsules for a short time. In a natural form, lecithin is found best in olives, egg yolk, and avocados. The olives should be ripe and sun-dried. This source of lecithin is better than any we can get in tablets. It takes nearly one quart of soybeans to make a dozen lecithin tablets. It is difficult to get all the lecithin your body needs in this civilized world. Civilization demands more nerve and brain energy than ever before.

Foot Tonic

The health stores sell "Sea Salt." If you use this in your foot baths, it will help tremendously. The bath will break down uric acid crystals that have settled in the feet. The feet have the largest pores in the entire body and the toxins from the intestinal tract will work out through the feet before coming out of any other part of the body. If you want to know what anyone had for dinner, you detect it from the odor arising from his feet — if you know how to tell the difference between odors!

Iodine for the Thyroid Gland

The finest tonic I know for the thyroid gland is produced by painting the soles of the feet with liquid organic iodine. This liquid organic iodine can be brought in laboratories and in the health food stores. Soak your feet in salt water to make sure that the pores are open; then paint the feet with the iodine two or three times a week.

If you take iodine through the digestive tract, many times it will not absorb properly if the system is filled with fatigue acids and toxic materials. Sometimes our bodies need a great deal of iodine, and if we are depending entirely upon the foods we eat for the iodine, we may often fail to get it. But if we will paint the soles of our feet with iodine, in a period of twenty-four hours, even though we sleep, our bodies will absorb and take up the iodine they need.

Sometimes taking iodine into the body by mouth is a shock to the system, and in many cases the body will throw it off. Iodine is one of the elements that the body is very sensitive to and a reaction occurs if we receive an overabundance. In taking a tonic for iodine by mouth, I would suggest that you procure Nova Scotia dulse, since it is probably one of the finest ways of getting iodine into the body. Dulse is a very purple seaweed grown in the North Atlantic; it is very high in manganese as well as iodine.

The most soluble way of getting iodine into the body is by drinking juice. Ask for unsalted clam juice. This juice can be mixed with celery juice or with any of the vegetable juices. We can even make a little clam broth with warm milk. Take ½ cup of clam juice two or three times a week. This will help supply you with they iodine you need.

Raw Facts for Life

Too often we completely destroy our food in cooking, stewing, boiling, frying, and preserving it. Live foods have the germ of life in them, but the germ of life is usually destroyed when we cook them. We receive the greatest good from raw tonics and from foods that require the least amount of heat in their preparation. If we live on crullers, dumplings, and doughnuts, we are going to have a very inactive body. Living on dead foods, like Postum and pigs feet, only means that we are going to end up signing our own death certificates. For strength, youthfulness, and longevity, it is necessary that we have in our bodies the life-giving energies found in live foods.

All the colors that were in raw foods in the beginning must somehow get into our bloodstream for vital energy. The life-giving energy of these juices is what is going to rebuild our bodies. To recharge our tired and failing batteries and bring the blush and bloom back to our cheeks, to have the charm of life and graciousness in our movements, it is necessary that we get all the chemicals and all the minerals back into our body that we burn out in everyday living. It is impossible to build a good body when we are forced to live on the exhausted flours that we have today. These devitalized foods do not have the elements necessary for body building. So many of our breads, breakfast foods, and commercial foods are not conducive to long life and good health.

The germ of life in food is depleted when we pasteurize milk, polish our rice, and mill or bleach our flour. When we look at these food-devitalizing processes in the commercial world today, we can definitely see how some people become insane, ferocious, and even destroy their marriages by eating these foodless foods.

A good thing to remember is the proportion of foods we should have in our everyday living. We should eat four to six vegetables, two fruits, one starch, and one protein daily. Always get the most natural food, the food that is closest to what God made for us. Remember: use simple combinations! When we are sick, take small meals; perhaps more meals a day, but at least a small amount at a time. A weak digestive system cannot take a heavy meal. When babies come into this world, we give them a small meal many times a day.

Tracing the Cause of Sickness. In choosing tonics for the body, we must first consider what part of the body is affected, then look deeper. For instance, a person may have poor hearing, but it can come from a depleted nervous system, so he would use nerve tonics. He may have a depleted hearing because of an excess amount of catarrh has settled in his ears. He would then use catarrhal remedies.

What about Dried Fruits?

Prunes, even though they are acid, have wonderful nerve salts in them. Don't miss them. Most dried fruits have four to six times as much sugar as when fresh. This extra sugar is easy to assimilate and will assist us in putting on weight.

I believe the apricot is best. We have found the one thing necessary in building the blood is iron and copper and the highest fruit in iron and copper is apricot. They are also high in vitamin C, which heals cuts and sores. They are best if they are not put up with sulphur as a preservative. This sulphur is a destroyer of body tissues.

Allergies

The well person does not have allergies. I have tested this fact where allergies to certain foods existed. The patients were no longer affected when they had a healthy body.

Many people under my care who had extreme allergies have successfully fasted to overcome that trouble, especially for hay fever and asthma. People who have allergies are chasing one food after another until finally they get to the place where the only thing that is causing their trouble is camel-hair or dust, and they spend the rest of their lives trying to keep away from dust and the hair of camels.

We are allergic only with a poorly mineralized body. I believe allergies have a lot to do with mineral cravings in the body; they are adjusted through proper eating habits.

It is foolish to include in allergy tests whether or not regular vinegar is bad for you— or pepper, salt, white flour products, and many popular cereals. These things should never go into the human body anyway. We are all allergic to them.

We should avoid the following foods when we have allergies: Wheat and anything made from wheat; anything from a can; all dairy products; citrus fruits, unless organically grown and tree ripened; all sugar and salt; all unnatural foods.

Also, watch for trouble from mattresses, wool, wall cleaners for the home, and cats and dogs.

Proteins Can Stimulate You

There are times when the body is going too slow and we need to speed it up. Food can supply a great deal of this stimulation. Proteins are very stimulating to the body; starches are more soothing. Many people are prevented from sleeping by eating too much protein at night. The protein may cause them to be sensitive, nervous and "on edge." It is better to take proteins at noon and starches at night, especially if you are separating your starches and proteins. We should have vegetables for the evening meal, especially vital vegetable drinks or vegetable salads, since they are very soothing to the nervous system and are conducive to sleep.

Learn from Your Ailments

An ailment can be a tonic to the body. Your ailment can be the best thing that ever happened to you; it may cause you to turn around and do better. It may help you to grow and develop inwardly. Unless you continually develop and grow, you stagnate. When you have gone through a period of disturbance, irritation, or sickness, you seek peace, harmony and health. Disease moves us and so do disturbances and dissatisfaction.

Feeding Our Spiritual Need

We have to consider an ailment from the spiritual side; the spiritual body has to be fed just as your physical body does. We can actually serve tonics to the spiritual mind just as we serve tonics to the physical body. I believe the person who is devoid of love is as ill as the person who lacks calcium in his body. The person with a calcium deficiency does not have the tone in his body and the power to accomplish the things he should do physically. The person who is without love is not well in his spiritual body.

We have a definite process for taking care of the spiritual body, just as we have elements to care for the mental body. There are things we must know and understand mentally in order to be in good mental health. We need to look at the three-fold man and work out tonics for all parts: physical, mental spiritual.

Just What Needs to Be Healed?

I look at our health problems with an all-sided vision. Never look at the healing art in one channel only. The healing art is made up of many systems. We have "mind healers," all kind of physical healers: masseurs, chiropractors, osteopaths, medical men, surgeons—and there is a place for every one of them. I do believe there is a big place for the chiropractor and that he has the greatest scope of any branch of the healing art. The chiropractor, who is the newest baby to be born in the healing system, has a lot to learn in a true healing sense, but he also has a lot to offer.

We must ascertain our greatest need. If we have trouble with those who are handling our finances, we may need an attorney, and he will prove to be the best doctor for the moment. When your doctor sends you to Arizona for your health, you should follow a complete healing program. It is not enough to just go and absorb the sunshine and get the benefit of the dry climate while you go on living on coffee and doughnuts. Wherever you may be, consider that the three-fold man must be taken care of.

Teaching a Person to Live Correctly

Teaching a person to live correctly is far more important than any doctor's treatments. You must decide whether you want temporary relief, or whether a visit to the right doctor is going to be a blessing to you for the rest of your life. No treatment can be a blessing to you if it is in the form of dope, pills, vaccines, injections, or salves. To get absolutely well you must consider starting from the deepest spot within your body and cleanse and work outwards, whether the problem is a boil on the outside or a boil on the inside.

We must realize that all foods are made up of many chemical elements that produce different activities in the body. You may have seen magnesium flares used by policeman in an accident on the streets. When ignited, they flame brightly. Magnesium is one of the necessary chemical elements in our intestinal tract and is required for good action of the muscles. It flares up in the body and creates good muscle tone and moves toxic material along. Other chemical elements may slow down the activity of our gland and muscle structure.

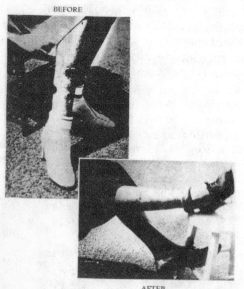

Here is the before and after of 13 leg ulcers that defied treatment over a period of three years. These ran yellow and green pus and we found out after many treatments that plain old green juice, chlorophyll, chopping up the tops of vegetables, mincing them up with a knife, mixing it with pure water, that in three weeks time we had a complete healing of these leg ulcers. When you see these things happening right before your eyes, you believe in the fact that nature does the curing. All it needs is an opportunity.

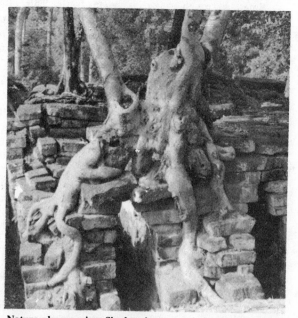

Nature always wins. She breaks up man's inventions, breaking up man's concoctions, breaks up man's buildings. Nature was here before we got here and will be here after we are gone. Let us build with nature so that we can see that nothing is destroyed. Our bodies are controlled by Nature. We cannot work against it.

Know your liquids

I AM OFTEN ASKED what kind of water is best. I don't know what a good water is, from a health standpoint. I don't think anyone does!

I can come to only a couple of conclusions as far as water is concerned. All the old men I've met in my worldwide travels used pure mountain water, and they lived (the last one I saw was 153 years old) without arthritis. No one measured the water to see how much salt was in it, how much calcium, or anything else. But they were long lived, and they were healthy.

How Much Should We Drink?. The amount of water we should drink is determined by the color and odor of the urine. If the urine has a high color and has a lot of odor to it, we need to drink more water. Using a lot of water in soups, juices, etc., will reduce the amount of water we need to drink.

We hear of people curing themselves of some ailment by drinking carrot juice or grape juice or going on a water fast. What was responsible for the cure? Was it the grape juice or the carrot juice or the water? I don't think so. I think the cure came from the body taking a vacation from food. I believe *that* cures.

Water Remedies

Sitz Baths: Water should come up five inches on the body. The feet are never in the water. The baths should only be for the pelvis and the pelvic organs. This is wonderful for congestion in the pelvis and sluggish bowels. These baths are best taken in the evening just before going to bed. However, they can be taken the first thing in the morning before going to work.

The cold sitz bath is an effective, though violent way of stopping bedwetting. Take cold water, sitting in it four to five minutes every morning before going to school or before beginning the daily program or routine. This will help with bladder and prostate, problems in general. A gentler approach is to take two sitz baths every morning. The first for one minute, hot; the second for one-half minute, cold. Do this for five changes, going from one to the other. The treatment should continue for a period of three months.

Foot Baths: Alternate, five times, one minute hot, one-half minute cold.

Other Facts. Did you know water softeners are not really purifiers? They do not kill bacteria or take out mineral or organic impurities. They "do" add salts to the water, so no one on a sodium-free or restricted diet should drink "soft water." Soft water has also been related to irregularity and heart attacks.

Did you know that distilled water is a perishable product and should be consumed in two or three days? The container should be tightly closed immediately after distilling and stored or refrigerated. Before using the stored water, shake the container several times to oxygenate the water.

Our government, scientists, newspapers, television networks, radio stations, and magazines are constantly warning us about the extreme hazards of water pollution. Our sources

Foot Baths—South America
Bathing in waters—both hot and cold has been used in most primitive and natural ways but the result cannot be denied.

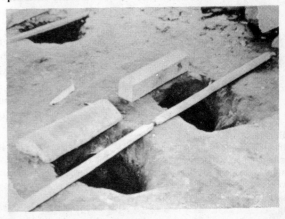

of water supply, such as rivers, lakes, and streams are becoming polluted with poisonous chemicals, insecticides, pesicides, untreated sewage, mecury, cadmium, lead, harmful bacteria, virus, and waterborn diseases. Dr. C. C. Johnson, Jr., assistant surgeon general and administrator of the Consumer Protection and Environmental Health Service of the U.S. Health Service, said, "I'm not exaggerating when I say that a major disaster could occur in the U.S. because of our substandard water systems." (Information from the Pure Water Society, South Sioux City, Nebraska.)

Water Facts. Some interesting and little known facts about water are told by Anthony Smith in his book, *The Body*. He writes:

An average human being doing light work in a temperate climate loses nearly five pints of water a day- and must replace it.
He can take in six-tenths of a pint at each meal without drinking at all because about half of ordinary food is water.
A man at rest is losing over half an ounce of water through his skin every hour.
The maximum possible daily loss and replacement of water ever recorded was about 50 pints.
A 156 pound man possesses 70 to 80 pints of water within his frame, and about half of the water will have been lost and replaced every 10 days.
A woman has less water within her than a man of equal weight.
Even under ideal conditions, a man without food or water will die when he loses 15% of his body weight, usually within 10 days. With water, he can survive for two months!
With water but no food, a 168 pound man can drop to less than 84 pounds and still live.
Without any water, he'll be dead well before he has reached even 140 pounds.

The Wonders of Raw Vegetable Juices. There has been much talk about vegetable juices, mostly quackery and tomfoolery, and I sometimes wonder why we use so many fruit juices and not vegetable juices. Much good can be done through the use of vegetable juices. In order to get the minerals in their original electrical form it is necessary to take the vegetable juices directly from the cellulose, since it gives up its mineral material in the most soluble form. When this is done, a wonderful change for the better is seen in our bodies.

To raise the health level, a variety of juices must be used. The creation and the electrifying of the minerals by the earth and the sun's rays is a preparation especially for our bodies' good.

While I was in the Bircher-Benner Sanitarium in Zurich, Switzerland, I was shown the original juicer consisting of a motor, a grinder, and a pressing machine that old Dr. Benner had made many years ago. Before juicing machines came into their present day use vegetables were chopped finely, the leaves cut crosswise through the veins and arteries to get the bleeding material from the leaf structure; then they were soaked for three to four hours, then squeezed to extract the juice. Originally, the juice was used, with wonderful results, for asthma and many other bronchial and catarrhal conditions.

Proper rest and the use of raw vegetable minerals will rebuild the body. Many doctors are using this system along with nutritional therapy to help many of their patients get well. If a doctor knows his foods, he can vary the juices to help the various systems in the body.

The system can be flooded quickly with raw fruit and vegetable juices and the body will receive therefrom all the needed vitamins and minerals nature has prepared for mankind. Juices can stir up the acid poisons in the body and bring them quickly to the various organs of elimination. Quicker healing will take place when minerals in solution get into the bloodstream.

We can see an example of the benefits of vegetable juices by discussing carrot juice. Infectious conditions of the body respond to the use of carrot juice, since it is very high in vitamin A. It is thought by some that the yellow color of carrot skin is harmful, but we find it is not. This is a pro-vitamin A that cannot be broken down too well by the liver cells, thereby passing it on to the skin to be eliminated. Eyes benefit by the use of carrot juice, but when the eyes are broken down through depletion, it is possible other things are indicated instead of carrot juice. We think of carrot juice for sties, or inflammation of the eyes, especially when there is elimination from the eyes.

If we cannot adjust our eyes well from a bright light to dim light, in a theater for instance, it is a sign we can use more vitamin A. Night blindness, or a glare blindness from auto lights, shows a lack of vitamin A. Many accidents could be prevented if those who are thus afflicted would use more vitamin A. Vitamin A is exceptionally good in all of the tissues needing fortification against infection. All mucous membranes in the body need a large amount of this vitamin. A lack of vitamin A can affect the bladder, the kidneys, the alimentary tract, the mouth, the tonsils, the tongue, the tear ducts, and the eyes. Many nursing children can be given carrot juice during the weaning process. We use a combination of carrot juice and milk together, which makes a fine weaning formula for children three to four months old.

Nursing mothers should drink plenty of carrot juice, since it is also high in calcium, which is a natural resistant to infections. One glass of carrot juice will provide 50,000 units of vitamin A, which is the daily requirement.

The Food and Nutrition Committee of the National Research Council has established a scale for the minimum daily requirement of vitamin A as follows:

	Units
Children under one year	1500
Children one to twelve years	2000 to 3500
Adolescent girls	4500 to 5000
Adolescent boys	4500 to 6000
Adults, men and women	5000
Women during pregnancy	6000
Women during nursing period	8000

There are many tasty juice combinations your family will enjoy. Carrot juice and apple juice makes a wonderful cocktail. Mint may be added for spicing and flavoring. Carrot juice can be made into ice cream. Vegetable juices can be made into aspic salads and gelatin salads. Many vegetable juices can be used as a base in liquefying your combined health foods. Use vegetable juices in cooking instead of water. Some good juice combinations for health in general are carrot and comfrey juice, or beet, comfrey, and pineapple juice. Carrot, soybean, and carob make a good flavor. Carrot juice with flaxseed tea helps an inflamed condition of the bowel. We use a lot of celery juice, sometimes adding a little parsley. All vegetable juices should be used within two or three hours after they have been extracted from the vegetables.

It has been said that many of the juices have a therapeutic value; I believe the greatest value comes in the fact that the minerals in these vegetables can be absorbed very quickly, with very little digestion. Furthermore, I believe that because juices fill the stomach for the moment, they prevent you from taking heavy foods that are not so easily digested. Vegetable juices give the digestive system a rest. Two or three glasses a day can be taken in an ordinary diet regimen; however, two or three quarts a day can be used for cleaning the intestinal tract or for getting rid of mucus or catarrhal problems in the body.

Raw juices can be considered an internal bath. They tend to cleanse and wash the tissues, revitalizing the organs of the body. We need fluids to carry away waste material and the various elements to the tissues. Juices enter the bloodstream in thirty minutes. (Never use tinned juices.)

Going a day, two days, even three days on raw vegetable juices is one of the finest rejuvenating methods there is for developing a new body and cleansing the old one. It is often good to take teas during a juice diet. Shavegrass tea is one of the finest cleansing teas we have, and it also helps to revitalize the body with the proper amount of silicon. Three or four cups should be taken a day.

I do not advise too much of the fruit juices. Fruit juices stir up toxins. Vegetable juices eliminate toxins. For relaxation use vegetable juices.

None of the juices is for any one disease. We do not treat the disease or any one organ. When we have an illness of any kind we are involved with the whole body. You cannot just cleanse one organ, or one part of the body. Every other organ will benefit from and feel the good of a cleansing diet.

During a fast avoid having too many treatments. I believe they interfere with the vital energies of the body. Enemas are the only adjunct we should use to fasting measures. Fasting is a matter of physiological rest, psychological rest, and physical rest. Fasting means *resting*.

Celery and prune juice together are said to be good for the nervous system. Celery juice contains sodium for neutralizing toxins. Use lettuce juice to promote sleep. Beet juice is very good in helping the bile flow more freely through the gall duct. Adding extra parsley to the juices helps the kidneys. Celery and carrot juice are very good for dissolving stones in the gall bladder or the kidneys or any hardness in the joints. The slickage found in comfrey juice is very good for colitis, inflammation of the bowel, and stomach mucosa in the walls of the stomach. One teaspoon of lemon juice five minutes before meals is a good appetite tonic.

Alfalfa juice is the most alkaline of all the juices. Green juices are great blood builders, since they contain chlorophyll, iron, and potassium. A rational balance of vegetable juices is good.

Cucumber juice with whey is high in sodium and is a very cooling drink for the blood. It is also very good in high blood pressure cases. Watermelon and cantaloupe juices are also good summer drinks.

Many times diarrhea is experienced while taking vegetable juices. In most cases it is necessary, as nature is doing a little house-cleaning. To bathe the tissues in your body with these juices will, in time, cleanse them and then rebuild, rejuvenate, and feed a starved body.

Most people lose weight when taking juices. However, in making a new body you must sometimes lose weight in order to re-build.

Make your vegetable cocktails in propor-tions pleasing to the taste. Usually any juice mixed with an equal proportion of another juice will be about right. However, when you mix fruit juices with vegetable juices, as *pine-apple and tomato*, it is best not to mix with starches. Acid fruits and starches do not com-bine. Vegetable juices go best with starches, and all starches should have vegetable juices with them.

There are many combinations of health cocktails you can make. A bitter green taste can be made palatable by adding sweet vege-tables, honey, pineapple juice, coconut milk, or a little sweet cream.

"Cabbage Juice Held Ulcer Cure"

Drinking a quart of cabbage juice daily has proved the fastest cure for uncompli-cated peptic ulcers, it was revealed yester-day to members of the California Medical Association at the Biltmore. The fresh cabbage juice ulcer cure was reported by Dr. Garnett Cheney, San Francisco, who explained that the curative factor in the juice is Vitamin U. Because the latter hasn't been isolated, the vitamin had to be given in the form of one full quart of juice a day. "We have treated 100 patients with the juice and nothing else, over the last two year," Dr. Cheney said, "with somewhat surprising results." *(Los Angeles Times)*

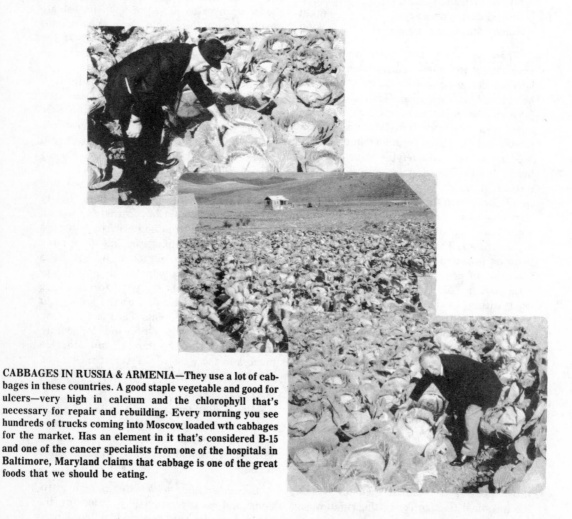

CABBAGES IN RUSSIA & ARMENIA—They use a lot of cab-bages in these countries. A good staple vegetable and good for ulcers—very high in calcium and the chlorophyll that's necessary for repair and rebuilding. Every morning you see hundreds of trucks coming into Moscow loaded wth cabbages for the market. Has an element in it that's considered B-15 and one of the cancer specialists from one of the hospitals in Baltimore, Maryland claims that cabbage is one of the great foods that we should be eating.

HEALTH COCKTAILS

The following listed disorders of the body can best be aided by using a vegetable cocktail or combination of juices as directd. Nearly every disorder responds quicker by adding vegetable juices. Celery, parsley, and carrot juices are good for any condition. They can be mixed any way or can be used alone. The juices suggested for a specific body disorder may be used separately or in combination with each other.

Disorders in the Body	Health Cocktail Suggestions
Anemia	Blackberry and parsley juice; parsley and grape juice
Arthritis	Celery and parsley juice
Asthma	Celery and papaya juice; celery, endive, and carrot juice
Bedwetting	Celery and parsley juice
Bladder ailments	Celery and pomegranate juice. Pomegranate juice is the best for the bladder. Also, shavegrass herb tea
Blood ailments	Blackberry juice, black cherry juice, parsley juice dandelion juice. Tomato juice and desiccated liver
Blood pressure (high)	Carrot, parsley, and celery juice; lime juice and whey powder; grape juice and carrot juice
Blood pressure (low)	Parsley juice, also capsicum and garlic
Bronchitis	Juice of 2 lemons, 3 T. honey to 1 pint of flaxseed tea. Use 1 tsp. every hour. Or bake a lemon, juice ½ of it and add to 1 cup of oatstraw or boneset tea. Then go to bed and perspire.
Cararrh, colds, Sore throat	Watercress and apple juice with ¼ tsp. pure cream of tartar
Circulation (poor)	Beet and blackberry juice; parsley and alfalfa juice with pineapple juice; grape juice with 1 egg yolk
Colds and sinus	Celery and grapefruit juice; water cress and apple juice with ¼ tsp. pure cream of tartar; coconut milk and carrot juice; celery and grapefruit juice with ¼ tsp. cream of tartar
Colitis, gastritis, gas	Coconut milk and carrot juice
Complexion (yellow)	Grapefruit juice
Complexion problems	Cucumber, endive and pineapple juice; 1 T. apple concentrate; ½ glass cucumber juice and ½ glass water
Constipation, stomach ulcers	Celery with a little sweet cream; spinach and grape fruit
Diarrhea, infection	Carrot and blackberry juice
Eczema, scurvy	Carrot, celery, and lemon juice
Fever, gout, arthritis	Celery and parsley juice
Gall bladder	Radish, prune, black cherry, and celery juice; carrot, beetroot, and cucumber juice; prune, black cherry, celery, and radish juice
Gallstones	Beetroot and radish juice; green vegetable juices
Glands (for building)	Pineapple juice with 1 egg yolk, 1 T. wheat germ, ¼ tsp. powdered Nova Scotia dulse — take daily between meals; 3/4 cup carrot juice, ¼ cup coconut milk, 1 T. wheat germ 1 tsp. rice polishings or rice bran syrup, 1 cup tomato juice, 1 T. cod roe
Glands and nerves	1 T. cherry concentrate, 1 tsp. chlorophyll and 1 egg yolk
Glands, goiter, impotence	Celery juice, 1 tsp. wheat germ and 1 tsp. Nova Scotia dulse
General house cleaning	Celery, parsley, spinach, and carrot juice.

137

Disorders in the Body	Health Cocktail Suggestions
Gout...........	Celery juice; combination of celery and parsley juice
Heart	Carrot and pineapple juice with honey; liquid chlorophyll (alfalfa); parsley, alfalfa, and pineapple juice
Hair (to improve) ..	1 T. cherry concentrate, 1 tsp. oat straw tea to a cup of boiling water, steep 10 min. then add cherry concentrate
Indigestion, underweight	Coconut milk, fig juice, parsley, and carrot juice
Infections	Carrot and blackberry juice
Insominia (sleeplessness) ...	Lettuce and celery juice
Jaundice	Tomato and sauerkraut juice, 1 glass every day for a week.
Kidneys.........	Celery, parsley, and asparagus juice; carrot and parsley juice
Kidneys (bladder problems)......	Black currant juice with juniper berry tea; pomegranate juice and goat whey; celery and pomegranate juice
Liver...........	Radish and pineapple juice; black cherry concentrate and chlorophyll; carrot, beet, and cucumber juice
Memory (poor)....	Celery, carrot, and prune juice and rice polishings
Nerve tension	Celery, carrot, and prune juice; lettuce and tomato juice
Nervous Disorders	Radish and prune juice and rice polishings
Neuralgia, neuritis ..	Cucumber, endive, and pineapple juice; cucumber, endive, and goat's whey
Overweight, obesity.	Beet greens, parsley, and celery juice
Perspiration	Celery and prune juice; cucumber and pineapple juice

Disorders in the Body	Health Cocktail Suggestions
Rheumatism......	Cucumber, endive, and goat's whey
Rickets	Dandelion and orange juice
Sinus...........	Sip lemon juice with a little horseradish; sip mixture of cayenne powder in a cup of water
Teeth (poor)......	Beet greens, parsley, and celery juice with green kale
Thyroid.........	Clam juice with celery juice
Vitality (to increase)	1 T. apple concentrate, 1 T. almond nut butter, and 1 cup celery juice
Weight (reducing) ..	Parsley, grape juice, and pineapple juice
Youth (retaining) ..	2/3 cup oat straw tea, 1/3 cup celery, prune, or fig juice, with ¼ powdered Nova Scotia dulse to each cup Cucumber, radish, pepper (1/3 cup each); 2/3 cup concord grape juice and 1/3 cup pineapple juice, with 1 egg yolk

Note: Drink these juices with a straw, or sip slowly, to allow them to mix well with saliva.

If you bathe the tissues of your body by taking these juices you will in time cleanse them, and then rebuild, rejuvenate, and feed a starved body. Don't get the idea you should live on them entirely. Take them with meals and between meals. For the best results, drink at least one pint a day.

NINETEEN

Goat milk – an ideal food

MANY VISITORS who come to our Hidden Valley Health Ranch show great interest in our goat herd. Some taste fresh goat milk for the first time there and find it more palatable than cow milk. Besides its pleasant taste, it is the closest to human milk yet discovered. It is a brain food, is high in chlorine, and is effective in kidney disturbances because it is germicidal in effect.

I have seen the sick virtually revived from a death-bed with fresh, warm goat milk, and could give case after case where the use of milk from a young goat has been successful in transmitting the necessary particles of nutrition to the body. This is because it is easier to digest and assimilate into the bloodstream than other milk.

Goat milk digests in twenty minutes, whereas it takes cow milk from two to three hours to digest. Goat milk is designed to nourish a kid weighing six to ten pounds, about the weight of a human baby. Nature intended cow milk to nurture a calf weighing sixty-five pounds at birth. Cow milk fat globules are five times the size those of goat milk.

Wherever you go, you can find goats. They may be in the minority, but there isn't a section of the country I have visited where I haven't found someone who has a goat, and the reason for having it is for good health.

That health comes in many ways. For young and old alike, goat milk has proved to be the one food that consistently stays down with the most unruly stomach. The most sensitive tissues seem to welcome the administration of goat milk in the diet. The sensitive stomach can use the high sodium content of goat milk. The high fluorin content in goat's milk gives teeth their hard coating and keeps the teeth from decaying. Stomach ailments respond in a short period of time to goat milk and carrot juice. Arthritis, rheuma-tism, and any acid conditions are combated through the use of goat milk. Black Mission figs and goat milk seem to help arthritis symptoms. Soaked and peeled dates with goat milk is a wonderful combination for ulcers of the stomach.

Goat milk is surely a vitality-producing food. Three-fifths of the world today lives on goat milk and thrives on it. It is one of the greatest things known to sweeten the intestinal tract and stop constipation. To develop a sweet intestinal flora use goat whey. This goes well with pineapple juice or any other sweet fruit juices. Goat whey enemas have aided extreme gas cases.

Goat milk is the best food for a baby. It compares in chemical balance to a mother's milk. Nature built mother's milk to nurture, not to harm. Milk balance is necessary for bone structure, glandular balance, good teeth, strong, developed jaws.

Loss of weight can be halted by using goat milk and dried stewed fruits between meals. Using goat whey or skimmed milk will help those who want to reduce. Goat milk is alkaline in reaction because it has a high sodium, potassium, and calcium content. These chemical salts are necessary in the human makeup. Because the goat is so fond of bark of trees and herbs and is a browser rather than a grazer (as the cow is a grazer), we find the milk high in silicon. Silicon is an enemy of tuberuclosis, which is never found among healthy goats or in goat milk, but flourishes among cows.

Milk in general is low in iron; an addition of one or two tablespoons of Blackstrap Molasses helps eliminate anemia. For the run-down system, and when a life is dependent on the most easily digested food, use warm goat milk directly from the goat. The animal energy and the heat seem to have a life force not to be overlooked.

A visit to any goat ranch or a talk with anyone who has goats will convince you of the health-giving properties of goat milk. For those interested in developing a goat ranch or knowing more about goats, send for "Making the Goat Ranch Pay" by Harry J. Smith, Box 42, Bickford Station, Memphis, Tennessee.

The Power of Goat Milk

The story of George Surdel, who lived on nothing but goat milk for over thirty years, is an example of what goat milk can do.

Goat milk saved his life in 1928 when he was near death in the mining town of Christopher, Illinois. He was seriously crushed by a rock fall while employed in the New North Mine.

"The doctors patched me up, but I could not regain my health," Surdel said. "Then a friend told me about goat milk. I tried it and my health miraculously returned."

Surdel's breakfast, lunch, and dinner each consisted of a cup of warm goat milk. He lived exclusively on goat milk — and felt very healthy.

It would be quite impossible for goats to take the place of cows in producing the necessary butter, cheese, cream, and in providing for the great army of milk drinkers. But for babies and invalids, and as a remedy for diseases such as tuberculosis, constipation, malnutrition, rickets, anemia, nervousness, loss of weight, ulcerated stomach, asthma, and other maladies, goat milk holds a unique place.

As a tonic for the weak, for the aged, and for growing children, it is unexcelled, building strong teeth and bones, and firm tissues with power to resist disease.

Dr. Carl Wilson of Palo Alto, California, uses goat milk extensively in his practice and in his home. He says,

1. Goat milk is a far better emulsion than cow's milk.

2. The oil globules are one–fifth the size of those in cow's milk.

3. The reaction of goat milk (cow gives an acid reaction) is alkaline, the same as mother's milk. I have yet to find a case where it did not agree when we had made the proper dilution.

4. The curd in goat milk is small and flocculent, hence easily attacked by the digestive organs. In cow milk the curd is large and dense.

5. When using goat milk there is only two percent curd which precipitates in the stomach, compared with the ten percent when using cow milk.

6. A goat is an exceptionally healthy animal, practically immune from tuberculosis, consequently it gives a healthful milk of uniform consistency. Goat milk has been proven of untold value as a food for infants and invalids who are unable to retain or digest cow milk.

William Lee Secor, M. D., of the Kerrville, Texas, Sanitarium, and a recipient of the Hare Gold Medal in Therapeutics, says;

I am a surgeon, restricting my practices to surgery, but since discovering the value of goat milk in the treatment of stomach and intestinal ulcers, I have not operated on a single ulcer case, and this covers a period of a dozen years.

The Journal of the American Medical Association, the official organization of 100,000 physicians in the U.S., under the heading "Dietetics and Hygiene," says:

"The goat is the healthiest domestic animal known. Goat milk is superior in every way to cow's milk. Goat milk is the ideal food for babies, convalescents and invalids, especially those with weakened digestive powers. Goat milk is the purest, most healthful and most complete food known."

I have been using goat milk for many years and I believe in it because I know what it can do. For babies, growing children, the weak and aged, it is invaluable. Goat milk works its wonders through cleansing and rebuilding abilities. Although it does not contain such curative essences as are found in herbs, its marvelous germicidal, sanitary effects prepare the body for new healthy tissues. However, leaves, barks, and various kinds of herbs are the elements goats crave. Invalids could do no better than to procure a source of good goat milk, for it is a powerful recuperator and rebuilder.

The Best Tonic for Children. I believe the best tonic available for children is raw goat milk. Why? Flourin is a chemical element often missing in our system. Flourin is volatile; it is very unstable. Heat destroys it. Pasteurized milk causes tooth decay for this reason. Flourin is the chemical element that keeps teeth from decaying. Goat milk has ten times the flourin content of cow milk; is alkaline in reaction; and is nearer the human body chemical balance. (America needs a raw milk crusade to protect our future generations.) Diseases are developed in today's youth by current milk treatment. I believe a good deal of infantile paralysis is due to the free use of pasteurized milk. No pasteurized milk has the same vital qualities as raw goat milk. Pasteurized milk is constipating. Calves fed pasteurized milk have been known to die in thirty days. Never use pasteurized or homogenized milk if good health is your goal. Use only raw goat or raw cow milk. Add blackstrap molasses as an iron supplement.

Properties of Goat Milk. The percentage composition of goat milk is as follows:

Water 85.78	Potassium 28.60
Protein 4.55	Phosphorus . . .22.00
Fat. 4.55	Sodium 14.60
Carbohy- . . .4.48 drate	Calcium. 13.88
	Chlorine 13.66
Ash: 0.84	Sulphur. 0.80
	Iron 0.60
	Silicon. 0.28
	Fluorin 0.06
	Manganese . . . a trace
	Iodine . . . . . . a trace

Such a composition makes goat milk an almost perfect food for man, containing all 16 vital elements, and in quantities closely paralleling that of the human body.

It is high in chlorine, known as the "great cleanser" of the body, whose germicidal properties heal wounds and injuries, benefit the bloodstream, and aid the heart function. Chlorine also helps purify the cells. By eliminating decomposed water and impurities it prevents hydrosis and dropsical conditions.

The calcium in goat milk builds and repairs bone and teeth structures, strengthens blood vessel walls to prevent hemorrhaging, builds heartbeat, lengthens the lifespan of body cells, and soothes nerves.

As mentioned, the flourin content is high. Flourin, known as the "antiresistant" element, is successful in clearing catarrhal conditions that have settled in the body. It is reconstructive, healing, and curative to many patients, due to the element balance and overall composition. It acts as a cement, giving hardness to teeth and bones. Fluorin also enters into the skin composition, nails, hair, arterial walls and solid membranes. It is necessary to spleen function, antiseptic and combats anything that threatens the entegrity of bones, nails, or membranes. Oxygen is powerless against fluorin-forti-

fied teeth. Goats have an affinity for flourin foods; they are called the flourin animal. But remember: any heat destroys fluorin completely- pasteurization included.

Sulphur enters nearly all bodyprotein and thus is essential for general well-being. It cools the brain.

Zinc found in goat milk attacks respiratory disorders, helps prevent cardiac abnormalities, epilepsy, neuralgia, and gastralgia.

Sodium, known as the "youth" element, is the star in goat's milk. It maintains body youth, limber, and pliable joints, and counteracts acidosis by purifying the bloodstream. Goat milk is the highest sodium food known. Sodium is necessary to maintain elasticity in walking, youthfulness, brightness, grace, charm, animation, keen wits, liveliness, and general health. We can be old and look young or we can be old and look old. The infirmities of old age creep upon us if our sodium intake is inadequate. Sodium also acts upon the stomach walls and intestinal tract; it is active in the blood, serous and mucous structure, throat walls, pancreas, spleen, alimentary tract, and secretory glands. It helps keep blood fibrin in solution and effects albumin metabolism. Additionally, it is found in joints, bones, cartilage, liver, muslces, blood vessels and brain corpuscles.

Rheumatic tendencies result when sodium is deficient. Burning feet, cold feet, swelling ankles, falling hair, hives, mouth blisters and ulcers, tender scalp, cracked raw tongue, and an ulcerated stomach are deficiency signs. Whey is also an excellent source of sodium.

Animal phosphorus as found in goat milk is essential to the brain. It is virtually unavailable to the vegetable kingdom. In goat milk it is highly evolved and less sublimated. It is easily assimilated. As Dr. V.G. Rocine termed goat milk, "It contains mind stuff." It can't be underestimated for the brain worker or the emotional individual.

Finally, goat milk contains such magnesium, the digestive element; hence, it's easy to digest.

Goat milk contains more vitamins than any other known food:

Vitamin A . . .2,000 − 3,000 I.U.
Vitamin B . . . . 400 −   500 Sherman Units
Vitamin C . . . . 30 −   50 Sherman Units
Vitamin D . . . . . .6 −   12 I.U.
Vitamin G . . . . −   35 Sherman Units

It is important to realize that all the elements of goat milk are vital to the formation of a good life. The human body is wonderfully and fearfully made, an instrument of a million strings. Every part of our bodies has to be nourished. In order to be an honorable individual and to be honored we have to be in good health. We must know our elements, our foods and know what direction we seek in life. If we make the right combination, anything is possible.

All 16 chemical elements are contained in the proper proportion in the milk of goats. Human health depends on securing these elements. So study goat milk and its products. Then combine them with other foods for health building.

Chemistry of Goat Milk. Milk has its own chemistry, consistency, specific gravity, taste, bacterial life, warmth, acidity, alkalinity, and so on. Goat milk differs from cow milk in nearly every respect. It has less protein, fat, ash, and food lime. It has more K_2O, NA_2O, food sulphur, magnesia, silica, chlorine, manganese oxide, and flourin, and more of the hematonic element. Because of the higher evolution of the goat, the brain phosphorus is superior to cow milk content.

Pour goat milk into a glass and pour it out again. You can see through the glass. If you pour cow milk the same way, it clouds the glass. The fat globules in cow milk are much larger, too large for the human system to adequately process. Goat milk is naturally homogenized. In man's attempt to duplicate this process, something went wrong.

Goat milk cholesterol is superior for the human brain. This is attributed in part to the higher percentage of chemical salts it has. Cholesterol is of a finer composition in

Goats are playful, kind, loving and a climber. These elements are necessary as a source for good milk we need in the body. Consider the source for your food and especially millk. Did you ever see a cow on top of a shed?

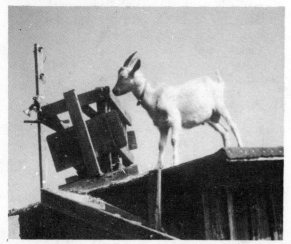

goat milk and thus has a higher value for bone marrow, communication fibers in the brain, nerve structures, endolymph in ears, spinal ganglia, nerve nets, brain cells. There is no better food to be found for man's wonderful thought machine, the brain, than goat cream or goat products.

The fat found in goat milk has 10 fatty principals, the most important of which are olein and myristin, since they favor nerve and brain cells. These fats are more highly evolved in goat milk than most other animal milks. This constituent is entirely unknown to the vegetable kingdom.

Goat Milk for Healthy Infants. Before an infant is born it lives on the mother's blood, which circulates through the fetus. Upon birth it lives on mother's milk. An infant is given its start in life solely through its mother. The vital beginning for bones, organs, and glands lies in the health of the mother during and after pregnancy, as well as many years before conception.

Colostrum, the raw milk secreted for about three days after birth, serves to cleanse the alimentary canal and begins bowel movements in the young. It establishes the high percentage of "friendly bacteria" or acidophilous in the intestinal tract. It is yellow in color and high in albuminoids, nitrogen, potassium, and chlorine.

Many babies suffer from lactic acid indigestion, diarrhea, vomiting, and colic. Often they have been overfed, or sugar has fermented in their systems. Goat milk helps the baby's disposition, especially if the mother is nervous, fussy, angry, or very busy. The goat is a serene creature and not subject to hysteria, fear, disappointments, nervousness, overeating, neurosis or jealousy.

If the mother pursued such adverse habits as drug use before birth, the child would be better nurtured on goat milk. Goat milk often cures a crying, fussy infant and a sickly child. If the mother is disturbed by family situations, miserable and unhappy, plagued by problems, those situations will have an effect on her milk.

Many children have left their moodiness and returned to good health by adding goat milk to their diet. Nature draws enough iron from the mother's system to sustain the child for the first year. Iron foods should be added to the child's diet after the first year. A milk diet sustained for over a year leads to anemia if the diet remains so unbalanced. Milk toast or rye bread or pumpernickel bread is excellent for the small child due to the high content of alkaline salts.

But goat milk isn't just for children. A long, lanky man of six feet two inches tall came to see me at one time. He weighed about 70 or 75 pounds. He was nothing but bones covered by tight skin. He had been to many doctors and they could only conclude that his metabolism was off, his glandular hormone system was not balanced properly, and he was devitalized. It was evident that his vitality was extremely low and circulation was almost nonexistent. He could not digest food, and was thus starving, though he ate well.

He said he would try anything to get well. I suggested he care for the goats and drink warm, foamy goat milk right from the nanny. In two months he gained some 20 pounds or more. In another two months he gained 20 to 25 more. When he left my ranch a trailer was behind his car — with a goat inside.

Goat Milk — Nature's Ideal Food. We are always looking to the source of our food. We look to the soil for the life of the plant, for its elements, balance, etc. We should also look to the type of animal our milk comes from. It must be a healthy animal. The goat is the cleanest of all milk-producing animals, and it is an excellent choice.

There are many vegetarians who will not eat meat because they claim they fear acids and the emotional proponents developed in the meat can be detrimental to the emotional body and even the spiritual body of the person who eats it. Why not consider the loveliness of the goat, the friendliness, graciousness, patience, and love in its temperament? There's no better food, with its fine mental and emotional components, than goat milk.

If warm, fresh milk is used, it requires less gastric juice and pancreatic juice to digest than other foods. It must be sipped slowly. It coagulates in the stomach; but if it is coagulated prior to ingestion it is much easier on the weak or older system.

Goat milk is excellent for the sexual system and the glands in general. It helps those suffering from low vitality, and is charged with sex vitality.

A concentrated goat whey was described b by Dr. V.G. Rocine in his diet programs. He states that extra chemical elements are necessary for those below par and ailing, to obtain balance and to promote health. The Condensed Food Blend, as he called it, is a remarkable combination. The chlorides found in his food blend are needed to a greater extent than other food elements. They form a base in all dietary needs, since all ailing persons are below par in food chlorides and their blood is dechlorinated.

Clabbered milk is still in the raw state, unlike commercial yogurt, which has been heated. If milk is taken alone, gastric juice cannot penetrate the curd formed. Only 90 percent of the nutritional value is able to be assimilated. It is better to take milk with other foods at all time. Never drink milk rapidly; sip it slowly. Do not take it in large quantities because it coagulates in the stomach in a large lump similar to cheese. A high degree of acidity in the stomach favors the formation of such tough curds. A person living on a milk diet alone has blue veins and lacks magnetic qualities. About eight pints of milk would be required daily to obtain adequate iron. A milk diet leads to anemia.

Cream can be separated from goat milk using a simplified physics law. Add water to the milk and the cream will not mix with the water and light milk, The cream will rise to the top. Goat cream is not yellow in color or heavy, as is cow cream. The carotene and the pro-vitamin A have been broken down in this higher evolved animal. Pro-vitamin A is in a form that can be easily handled by the human digestive system.

Full milk contains more water and less butter fat. Strippings contain less water and more fat, with nearly eight times more cream than the full milk. Albumin, sugar, and ash do not vary from full milk to strippings. A lean, dry patient needs the strippings. An obese individual should never eat or drink the strippings. (The strippings are the last of the milk drawn from the goat.)

Pure, Clean Foods for Good Health. Placing cream in a cooler for a certain length of time at 60 degrees to 65 degrees F favors the growth of friendly lactic acid microbes. One can make a delicious drink of buttermilk and juices such as pineapple or other fruit juices. Beat or shake vigorously until the mixture effervesces; drink immediately.

Other pure, clean foods are baked bananas with goat buttermilk, steamed carrots with goat buttermilk, eggs prepared with goat cream and cooked in a double boiler, almond meal muffins, goat ice cream, well-cooked oatmeal with goat milk and cream, raw well-beaten egg white with goat cream. These foods are for all types of people. One man's poison is another man's meat, but not so with goat milk. When you are using a great deal of goat milk or cream, add a concentrated goat whey to attract cleansing chlorine to the bloodstream. For brain and nerve nutrition, add fish roe or fish eggs, and goat cream with goat milk and buttermilk.

To build flesh in lean persons, goat milk, goat cream, goat sour milk, baked bananas, and grated carrots can be advantageous. Of course, breathing exercises after eating and sleeping are highly desirable, in addition, for building the lean body.

A few young, thrifty hens, a few berry bushes, several gentle goats, a dozen fruit trees and nut bushes, and a plot of ground for vegetables would make almost any household independent. Then we wouldn't have to worry about what the manufacturing industry is doing with food.

Wheat, Milk, and Allergies. Today we have gone overboard in the use of milk. Those who crowd out other foods for milk often develop anemia. This runs into many of the mucus, phlegm, and catarrh conditions prevalent today. The proportion is off balance. The U.S. government states that 25 percent of the American diet is made up of milk. Another 25 percent consists of wheat. Looking at God's Garden, this proportion is not correct. No more than five percent should be allotted to milk and wheat — not 50 percent. If the correct proportion was maintained, allergies, bronchial troubles, asthma, and other ailments such as flu would be under control. Doctors support the claim that we use an overabundance of these two products. Cut down milk and wheat products to control allergies. In fact, for a short period of time, eliminate these products entirely. When the body has regained a proper balance, they may be reinstated with moderation. Rely heavily on greens, salads, and other vegetable kingdom foods. Remember to maintain variety.

Remedies for the Human Machine. Warm milk is needed to rebuild the body's vital forces. When people are cold, circulation is under par due to a lack of the vital force found in brain faculties. Energy is necessary to force blood through the body. The creamy globules found in goat cream, which the chemist calls cholesterol, is the best food available for nerves, lungs, bone marrow, optic centers, brain cells, eyes, ears, and general lubrication of the human machine. This fatty substance in goat cream is superior to tonics for tired nerves, crying infants, hysterical individuals, the brain worker and the tired schoolteacher,

doctor, lawyer, or anyone who is "burned out."

Goat milk is exceptionally good for cases of nerve starvation, brain fag, neurasthenia, first stages of tuberculosis, blood diseases, intestinal disturbances, poor nutrition, nervousness, anemia, pneumonia, pleurisy, and many other ailments and diseases. It is not a cure for any disease; it simply aids in building or rebuilding by supplying the essential food elements. Cholesterol and food salts are necessary for curative and rebuilding purposes.

Many people contend that we should not have any milk or milk products due to the cholesterol content that they bring to the body. But in goat milk fat globules are broken down so that the human system can assimilate them and the liver can handle the fat. We need a certain amount of cholesterol in the body or the body is forced to build its own, according to some authorities. The brain and nervous system must have it.

Milk is mainly water, good for summer and good for a weak stomach. If milk is allowed to stand too long after being drawn from the animal — 20 minutes or more — the life principle has fled and nothing but organic material remains. Milk becomes acid upon standing due to germ life that splits up the lactose into lactic acid. When milk is secreted it is alkaline and well adapted to nutrition.

Fresh, warm, foaming milk straight from the goat helps prevent catarrh of the stomach and intestines, hypochondria, hysteria, gastritis, emphysema, lung trouble, acid blood, dropsy, and asthma. Milk in general is healthy if it comes from a healthy animal, if it is not old and acid, has not been treated with salicylic acid, and is not watered down. It also must contain no germs, acids, gas, or impurities.

Milk neutralizes the amount of acid in the stomach and lessens the putrefaction tendency in the intestines. Milk whey is good for the bowels, lacteals, liver, and kidneys. When we take cheese alone, we should add salts found in whey or the drippings from cheese-making. Whey is a great food to correct many stomach disturbances. It is one of the highest sodium foods. Sodium rejuvenates the stomach and the bowel. Always drink whey with cheese. The old men I have met throughout the world take whey from cheese-making. It is their special drink. I believe it helps to keep their joints limber, supple, and pliable.

Calcium phosphate is found mainly in cottage cheese. Goat cottage cheese is a bone and teeth builder, good especially for growing boys and girls and for some almost boneless people having flabby, lymphatic, watery tissues. Such people should have goat cottage cheese. The casein of goat milk contains about 80 percent of the entire protein found in the milk. Being present to the extent of three percent, this is one of the best remedies available for calcium deposits and for dissolving hardened settlements in joints. The cheese of milk is soluble in an alkaline medium.

If there is a deficiency of sodium in the blood tissues and secretions. a milk diet leads to lime hardening, stiffness, arthritis, arteriosclerosis, poor hearing, weak eyesight, urinary ailments, old age symptoms, catarrh, and calculis. This is why all milk and cheese diets call for sodium foods. A high sodium diet cures calcic ailments and diseases, but not other rheumatic ailments. (There are many types of arthritis, rheumatism, hardening.)

Goat cream is good for building weight. It is the closest to the fat in the human body. For this reason, a rounded, well-adjusted body can be built.

When a person suffers from stubborn constipation he should take colostrum pudding to favor intestinal lubrication.

A Profile of the Goat. If man is to live on the milk of any animal, the disposition, health properties, and general make-up of the animal must be taken into consideration. For example, compared to other milks, the atoms of goat milk have a higher vibratory rate and a superior degree of sublimation. They are better organized. The hog contains poisons and obtains its food from underneath the ground; the cow is a grazer, obtaining food from on the ground. The goat stands on its hind legs to reach bark and leaves of trees.

Milk and milk fat differ in various goat breeds. The Saanan gives more milk and less cream. The average Nubian is the opposite in ratio. The Alpine is the middle and the breed I use and recommend to those interested in health building. Stall goats have leaner and bluer milk.

Goats give different milk when fed various diets. Pastures differ in spring as opposed to the winter season. Spring pastures favor fat building. Foods also affect the goat considerably. They have to have unsprayed alfalfa for best results. Comfrey has been found to be a valuable addition to the feed. When we see how green alfalfa in a brown goat living under a blue sky and in harmonious condi-

tions with a favorable emotional environment gives the milk a suitable to man's needs, we recognize that it is surely the work of that Divine Chemist– God.

The goat is the poor or rich man's cow as far as health is concerned. It is a remarkably healthy animal. If the material ingested by the goat is unacceptable, the elimination process is so efficient that it is expelled at once. Goats will not accept an apple a human has first tasted. The instinct for self-preservation is extremely strong. It is alleged that goats eat rubber tires, tin cans, and other rubbish. A goat which is fed properly has a reliable nose for bark, leaves, and herbs. If a goat is hungry, or starving, perhaps it will condescend to nibble at the paper label of a tin can. (Maybe the label contains silicon if it is made from wood.)

A goat pen is much cleaner than a cow pen. Fresh goat milk is of the purest quality, due to their meticulous food habits. There is possibly no cleaner food, providing it is drawn from a young, healthy, well-fed goat. The older goat makes changes. The kid is constantly climbing and playing; its limber joints may be partly attributed to activity. But sodium is the important ingredient. Goats are often seen on barn tops; but you will not find a cow there.

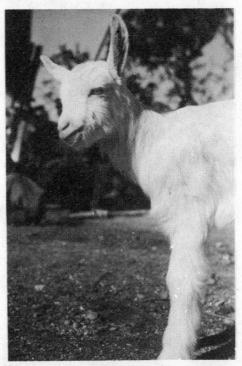

A goat kid—that pliable, supple animal that gives to the person the sodium that is so necessary to keep man's joints supple, limber and pliable.

Man's Separation from God and Nature. Man has turned his back on heaven and follows his own commercial notions. Milk, cream, cheese, butter, buttermilk, and other milk products are acid-forming. But he uses these in his home for himself, his infants, his children, other family members. He feeds his family a Noah's Ark of microscopic "wigglers" to create trouble for the chemical laboratory of the stomach. All eventually become sick. He is the cause of his children's sickness and his own suffering. He calls it destiny and often charges it up to God in his "innocence." Here the heavy doctor bills come in. The milk may be pasteurized to kill the "wigglers" but man does not know he has altered the chemical structure of the milk, the chemical molecules, in the name of efficiency and profit. His children will suffer from poor teeth, bone diseases, and skin ailments later in life. Health begins to take wings; love begins to fly out the window; and he ends up in the divorce court. He blames politics and the President for his misfortunes, his calamities.

He forgets that milk extracted from herbivores should be taken by the process of suction and consumed as it comes foaming from the warm animal. Only then will we obtain the true magnetic qualities necessary for building the body properly. The warmth of this milk will surge through his whole body, giving renewed life. As milk comes from the goat, germs are seldom present. But let it sit and it becomes acid; and bacteria thrive in an acid medium, not in an alkaline medium. Fresh goat milk, cream, butter, buttermilk, and whey are alkaline and curative. Acid milk products are not. As every food chemist knows, kittens, colts, kids, and infants obtain their nourishment directly from Nature's Nutrition Factory according to the plan of that Divine Architect — God.

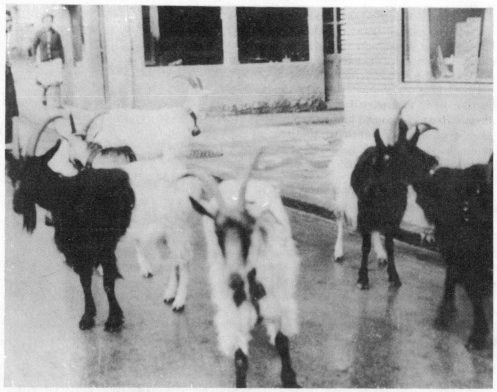

Studying with some of the sanitariums inSwitzerland where they use the goat milk as a cure, Goat cheese was part of their meals and each person developed a wonderful calcium foundation through the use of the goat milk. I have seen many a person taken out of extreme sickness and brought back to good health through the use of goat milk and natural goat products.

Lets learn about foods

THERE are many foods to learn about. Let us learn them all, not just a few. We cannot learn only Greek and Latin and feel we know all there is to know about languages, nor can we learn Sanskrit and French, math and music, and forget everything else. We have to learn more than the specialization the universities are teaching today.

We should learn more of the *universal* sciences that surround us. What is found in the ocean contains iodine, or is predominant in magnesium or manganese. We should know what is above the ocean and what is below it. We should know this from a food standpoint; we cannot study agriculture from only one point of view.

We must learn that we cannot use drugs or any treatment that will drive the wrong elements back into the body. Nature has the upper hand when it comes to healing. Let's see that she has a "free" hand.

God has given us food for every purpose and for every ailment. It is up to us to learn these different foods and how we can remedy specific conditions by their use. We have to learn the different ways to prepare these foods, to cook them less and keep them close to their natural state.

What a blessing it would be to us to learn to use only good foods, get plenty of rest and sunshine, and all the other forms of natural healing. To get a clean body, we must eliminate the old.

Of course, the first bottle of soda pop is not going to harm us. The first cigarette isn't going to produce cancer. It isn't the first eating of any one food that produces a disease any more than the first drop of water will wear away a stone. It is the continuation thereafter that does the damage. Too much fried food, too many dumplings, condiments, or processed foods wears away the good in our bodies.

Some years ago I visited a mental institution. I saw patients served fried foods, mashed potatoes and gelatins made up of 86 percent white sugar, artificially flavored and colored with a coal tar extraction.

Is it any wonder that these people are not recovering? We do not offer them a cure. We do not offer them hope. In the last 25 years, there has been more than a 25 percent increase of population in mental institutions in the United States. This is a *crime*! It has been calculated that 70 years from now, at present trends, there will not be enough sane people to take care of the insane. This may be somewhat of an exaggeration, but it gives us something to think about.

Poor health is on the increase outside of mental institutions, too. Diabetes, for instance, is increasing so steadily that within 25 years every third person will be suffering from it. If we would only realize that we have our life and health in our own hands, and if we could know *where* to seek our health, it would be the most wonderful thing in the world.

In a community just a few miles outside Los Angeles is an animal experimentation farm. On this farm is a hospital for pigs, and there are never less than 500 "patients" of all sizes. There are giants and runts, scrawny pigs, pigs with intestinal disorders, skin disorders, and every other disorder that a pig can acquire. This hospital has learned how to wipe out these disorders almost entirely through proper foods. A long time ago they discovered something that should have been known long before; namely, that pigs cannot live on garbage or leftovers. They have to get good food; whole food. Our hospitals for humans could learn a lot from this animal hospital. We could reduce the population of our hospitals and mental institutions by at least 50 percent by feeding the patients properly.

I have a friend who lives in San Marcos, California, who fasts and feeds his chickens according to the way I take care of my patients: using rest periods, whole foods, natural foods. He gets splendid results. He says it pays, especially when he has over a million laying hens.

Foods That Serve a Purpose

Almond Nut Butter. A teaspoon is good to add to a drink, or a small piece of cheese, the size of a golfball. Proteins of this kind are digested better in these combinations and make good tissue builders.

Many people are so thin because they consume more juices than solid food. They are on too much of an eliminative diet. Add a little protein to any juices or fruit to hold your weight. Dried prunes that have been "revived" contain one of the most wonderful nerve salts available; they act as a laxative and can be added to celery juice or whey for greater laxative qualities. Liquefy if possible. Papaya is good in a laxative drink and is a drink noted for its effect on the digestion.

Celery juice. This makes what I like to term a "dissolving cocktail." It keeps calcium out of the joints or from forming stones, etc. Celery juice is one of the finest food dissolvers we can introduce into the body. Using it with a tablespoon of plain gelatin is one of the finest foods for the joints. This is a high sodium cocktail and is also a protein cocktail. Another wonderful drink is celery juice and whey. It is a cooling drink for that hot summer day.

Bananas. These are a good building food. Thin people can add a little banana or dried fruit or a little soybean meal to the juices to avoid reducing. For those wishing to reduce, this fruit should be omitted.

Gelatin. A good protein to use is gelatin, and it is recommended in a molded form, not in a concentrated powdered form. This gives few calories and at the same time tends to fill the stomach and remove any feeling of hunger. Gelatin can be made with tomato, grapefruit, or apple juice. No sweetening, please. If you are underweight, try using sunflower seed in meal form in your diet. You may add it to drinks if desired; two or three ounces daily will help to put weight on.

Sesame Seed. Sesame seed drinks are wonderful for constipation and for lubricating the bowel. Use a half cup of sesame seed in one cup of water; put in liquefier and run for about two minutes. Take out and strain the hulls out. This uses the inside of the seed, which carries the oil. The oil carries the lubricating qualities of the sesame seed. Anything else can be added as desired in the liquefied drink: fruits, bananas, pineapple juices, dates, etc.

Pomegranate juice. This is good for bladder disturbances.

Food, Your Medicine

Let us look to natural remedies for the relief of many small ills. Here is a list of some foods that can be used, and their values and remedial qualities. Palliative drugs have the power of giving temporary relief from pain and may even reduce the suffering caused from nutritional starvation — but it is food alone that contains the necessary elements to restore a normal condition.

Artichokes have iron, but otherwise they do not have too much nutritional value. The Jerusalem artichoke is one food that diabetic people can take because it contains a natural insulin. To use Jerusalem artichokes as a remedy for diabetes wouldn't be the proper thing to do, but all those who have a pancreatic weakness can handle them much easier than they can potatoes, either white or sweet. I know of no other starch that is better for the body.

Asparagus is a wonderful bulk food, high in chlorophyll. The best way to eat it is to break it off right from an asparagus bed in the garden and eat it *raw*.

Broccoli is a winter vegetable and is high in sulphur. If you don't want it to produce intestinal gas, steam it in parchment paper or eat it *raw*.

Beet greens contain oxalic acid, but not so much as spinach and Swiss chard. Use them raw in salads or steamed. The stems contain more iron than the leaves. They are also good for cooking; to prevent burning of food cooked in stainless steel pans, place some raw beet leaves in the bottom of the pan.

Brussels sprouts, cabbage, and cauliflower are good winter vegetables containing sulphur. There is 40 percent more iron in the green base of the cauliflower than in the bleached head, so make sure to use the greens surrounding the head.

Cantaloupe and watermelon seeds are also useful. The cantaloupe has a "throw-away" seed with real nutritional value. This is one of the finest foods you can eat, because of its high calcium content. Liquefy it in the same manner you do sesame seeds; i.e., with a little water, tea or pineapple juice, and honey, if desired. If you want a wonderful drink for kidney disturbances, make a milk out of watermelon seeds. However, strain off the seed hull material after liquefying either of these seeds to avoid possible bowel irritation.

I know a Canadian family that travels to Florida each winter so that a daughter who suffers from nephritis can have fresh watermelon. This family considers the benefit worth the effort — and it is! There is nothing better for kidney disturbance, nephritis, and Bright's disease than watermelon and its seeds. This is especially so for children. If you can't make annual trips to Florida (I wish I could!) take ten or fifteen watermelon seeds and run them in the liquefier with some liquid and sweetening. Strain off the seed hulls and you'll have a nice drink.

Celery was a food given to the early Olympic games winners as a prize. It was considered the greatest thing they could receive, since it was the one thing that rejuvenated them more than anything else after a long run or some other arduous competitive game. Celery is the most cooling thing you can have in the body. Today it is one of the foods you must be most careful of because it is one of the most sprayed vegetables we have. Brush it well. A wonderful food remedy that can be used in the summertime to keep you cool is celery and pineapple juice together. It replaces the salts lost in perspiration on an extreme hot day. This may be mixed with prune juice, especially for those who need nerve salts to help the nervous system.

Cucumbers are very valuable. Don't forget to eat the peeling, unless it disturbs you. You can get the equivalent value in other foods, especially greens. No drinks are better in summer than cucumber and celery, cucumber and whey, or cucumber and pineapple. In summer they tell us to keep as "cool as a cucumber."

Cucumbers are high in sodium and silicon (in peeling) and are good for the blood. They get rid of pus in the form of rashes, boils, pimples, and carbuncles.

Dandelions should be used for the gall bladder and liver. The finest beverage you can get is made of roasted dandelion root. Learn to use this in place of coffee.

Endive is a wonderful food, very high in potassium. But avoid head lettuce; it has almost no nourishment. It is very gas forming and contains an opium by-product that slows down digestion. Leaf lettuce has 100 times as much iron as head lettuce.

Fish has long been called a brain food, which doctors have called "tommyrot," but from a chemical standpoint we know that our brain and nervous system are built up of vitalin, brain phosphorous, lecithin, and brain and nerve fat. These elements are found in the highest concentration in ocean fish, particularly black bass. While it is not a complete food for the brain and nervous system, it has organized brain and nerve elements that cannot be found in the fruit or vegetable kingdom.

Leeks are classified with onions and are good because of their powerful effect in driving the germ life from the body. All onions have the wonderful effect of ridding the body of catarrh. Onion packs are an excellent remedy for chest conditions. Because of their iodine content, onion packs on the throat are beneficial for thyroid disturbances.

While we are talking about onions, we have to include garlic. One of its best uses is for simple hemorrhoid conditions. Insert a clove of garlic into the rectum each night.

Lemon juice is nature's most powerful antiseptic, used internally and externally. Apply to corns, on scalp, on sores; use it for an eye

All of the chemistry of the earth is displayed for man's use in markets throughout the world. The sulphur foods, cabbage, cauliflower, onions, are here, but are also the potassium foods, sodium foods; this is in Mexico.

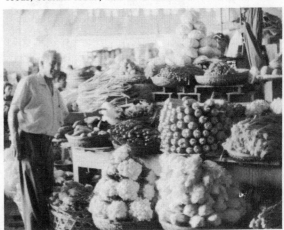

wash; gargle it; brush teeth with it; drink it to purify the breath.

Malva is one of our richest weed plants. It might be called an herb. It is one of our highest foods in vitamin A, an antiinfection vitamin. There are 50,000 units of vitamin A to every pound of malva.

Mulberries favor reduction of high temperatures in the body. Those who are chronically inclined to fevers should eat mulberries. They are also good in cases of stomach disorders, such as ulcers. The heavy coloring in mulberries stains the stomach and intestinal tract so that stomach acids cannot as readily attack the linings. The juices of mulberries reduce the heat of the body without causing excessive perspiration. Mulberries also contain a lot of natural sugar, which we should use instead of the unnatural kinds.

Mushrooms have very little nutritional value. I believe they have an effect on the body and there is some good in them, but they have no real value. Like radishes, they grow fast. A rapidly growing vegetable doesn't have the same value as a slow growing variety.

Non-cooking Cereals are rich in silicon and especially good for bowel activity. The ingredients are usually one half cup of flaked rolled oats, one heaping tablespoon of dried raisins, one heaping tablespoon of dried apples or finely cut apricots, one tablespoon of shredded almonds, and one teaspoon of date sugar. Before serving, soak for ten minutes in two-thirds cups of water and then add fresh fruit such as peaches or bananas; then add cream. Vary the cereal with ground and chopped sunflower seeds, sesame seeds, coconut, and cashews. Add natural supplements or rice polishings, flaxseed meal, and wheat germ for extra vitamins and minterals.

Nuts are all good. The almond is the king, highest in alkalinity. Black walnuts are the highest in manganese, which is the nerve element. Pine nuts are one of the highest in fat content (49 percent). They make a nice salad dressing, best mixed with fruit, especially with apricots.

Papaya is a very good remedy for stomach troubles. Make tea of the seeds; they contain natural papain, which is needed by the stomach as a digestant. Tablets are good for pyorrhea. Papaya tablets disintegrate proteins when they are soaked overnight in the juice. This is why papaya tablets are so wonderful when left in the mouth to dissolve slowly after a meal. They break down toxic protein deposits on the teeth, such as occur in pyorrhea, and should be used after each meal. Following this, use a gargle of liquid chlorophyll, which is a wonderful mouthwash.

Peapods make a wonderful vegetable juice and may be mixed with celery and carrot to make a very tasty drink. Put in soup for flavoring (they may be discarded) or with any vegetable while cooking. There is a lot of value in them.

Pumpkin seeds are an excellent food and a good source of vegetable protein. Fresh pumpkin seeds may be liquefied into a juice or strained and combined with other foods that would impart flavor. Use a suitable sweetening agent.

Radishes are good for gall bladder or catarrhal conditions. Whether they contain much mineral value or not, they add bulk. Black radish and horseradish have a beneficial effect on sinus disturbances and gall bladder troubles. Powdered horse radish is used as a remedy for gall bladder catarrh. Raphenon is an extract that has been developed from horseradish for this purpose.

Red foods are usually the red blood builders. From a remedial standpoint, it is always a food that looks like a gland that will build a gland, or a red food that will build red blood. In fact, green chlorophyll, as found in the tops of vegetables, alfalfa, and other green leaves, contains the greatest amount of iron and is one of our best red blood builders.

Squashes are the mildest vegetable you can have in your diet. When baking squash, leave seeds in for flavoring. Never remove seeds unless you save them for planting.

Turnips are high in vitamin A. They come under the classification of a sulphur food. Since they are so high in this vitamin, they will fight any catarrhal trouble in the body.

Foods to Omit from Your Diet

Rhubarb, cranberries, and plums contain oxalic acid and all dieticians say to leave them out of the diet. Prunes, however, contain a beneficial nerve salt and have a laxative quality, so in spite of having a high acid factor I recommend them, especially fresh prune plums.

When you have any joint trouble, avoid oxalic acid foods such as cranberries, rhubarb, cooked spinach, and cooked Swiss chard. Cranberries may be used for one purpose: to insert into rectum for hemorrhoids and pile trouble. If you must eat cranberries (it doesn't hurt if you use them once a year) don't use too much sweetening. Raisins or apples are good sweeteners, added after cooking. (This applies to all cooking: *add sweetening agent after cooking.*) There is an average of six times as much natural sugar in dried fruits as in fresh fruit.

Know the Unfavorable Foods

Avoid unfavorable foods at all times. One single reckless meal of unfavorable foods may undo the work of a year's careful diet. Be careful of the directions you are taking and watch your habits. Do live moderately, carry out this regime, and you'll be healthy. You *will* see favorable results.

There is something good in everything in Nature. There is a remedy from everything in nature: weeds, skins, flowers, stalks, bark, roots, and leaves.

We should eat foods that do not have many bugs or pests on them. These foods have elements that keep us from getting sick. You seldom see worms in beets or garlic. You will find that if you have a body with all the resistance elements in it, germ life will not live there either.

We have life force, and we must feed that life force.

You will find many remedies in foods, but you will never get well in less than a year, and for some people two years or even five years is needed. The value comes only through persistence.

Food for Arthritis

Alfalfa. Alfalfa-mint tea and alfalfa seed tea are good for arthritic conditions.

Celery and okra. Celery and okra tablets may be used as a remedy for arthritis. Take four of each four times a day. Or, get extra okra and celery juice in your diet. These are very high in sodium, which is what arthritic conditions need. If you have an extreme heart problem, you have to be a little careful, because then we try to withdraw some of the sodium and increase the potassium.

Broth. Take a tablespoon of whey, a tablespoon of lecithin, and a teaspoon of broth powder in a cup of warm water. If arthritis is bad, take two cups a day for three to six months.

Potato peeling broth. Another broth for extreme rheumatism and arthritic problems, excess catarrh in the body, and neutralizing the body's acids is potato peeling broth.

This is a high potassium broth. Use two good-sized potatoes and one and a half pints of water. Simmer for 15 minutes, strain, and drink just the broth. Take one or two cups a day over a period of a month. I have seen many rheumatic pains leave with this.

Veal joint broth. Veal joint broth is a wonderful remedy for arthritis. People who have broken down the joints in their bodies need this joint material if there is going to be rebuilding. Take the shoulder of a young beef and cook the jelly off the bone.

Lecithin, a Wonder Food. In 1952, Dr. Stephen found that injuries to the brain were greatly helped by lecithin. Concussions and traumatic brain weaknesses were improved in a matter of weeks instead of months when lecithin was given in a dry form.

Lecithin is found in all foods that contain cholesterol, is high in fish, and can be made from soybeans. It acts by emulsifying the fats in the body, arteries, and veins by supplying an easily digestible and easily absorbed choline. It also increases the peristaltic action of the intestine. When you feel you just can't carry on any longer, when you feel exhausted, fatigued, and run-down, lecithin may just be the thing to lift you up again. Since lecithin does not have to undergo digestive enzymatic action it is carried directly to the bloodstream, where it can be used for the brain and nerve system.

There are many benefits from lecithin; it provides more energy for the brain and nervous system. It helps in giving us a longer life span because it softens arteries. It helps to cleanse the liver and keep fats in solution. It purifies the kidneys, increases brain power, and is especially good for hardening of the arteries. In taking care of arteriosclerosis, many methods have been tried to get rid of the fatty contents of foods. Lecithin helps to break down these fatty contents. Lecithin adds to the structural material in every cell of the body, especially the brain and nervous cell structure.

It has been determined that when there is a decrease in the intake of lecithin, there is an increase in cholesterol. They are reducing cholesterol with lecithin. Lecithin is also good for dissolving excess oils in the body. Take a tablespoon of granules or two or three capsules of the oil every day. Everyone over the age of fifty should use some lecithin in his diet.

Soybeans. The soybean has been the beef of China. Many a child has been raised to adulthood in the Orient on only the milk beverage made from soybeans. Soy milk is low in fat compared to cow's milk. It is low in carbohydrates, calcium, phosphorous, and riboflavin, but is high in iron, thiamin, and niacin. It is good to add honey to soy milk for flavor. Honey also raises the carbohydrate content. Soy oil will increase fat content and should be blended to give the consistency of cream. It might be good also to use sugar milk to increase the digestibility of the soy.

How to Make Your Own Soymilk. To make soy milk, take one pound of dried soybeans, soak in two quarts of water overnight in a cool place. Pour off the water in which the beans have been soaking. Grind the beans in food mixers or grind very fine. Add fresh, pure water to the mixture. Add three times the volume of soaked beans. Mix thoroughly and put in cheesecloth to filter through the liquid. The milk passes, leaving only the pulp. You can bring the milk to the hot point without boiling. Skim off the surface froth, and cool. Stir frequently to prevent the formation of soy milk skim. If you add other things to the soy milk for flavoring, blend in the liquefier.

Brain Food. When any part of your body is not working properly, go to your brain first. Unless the medulla is fed properly, you will be sick — and will be good only until three o'clock in the afternoon.

To feed the brain properly, we need certain foods to provide lecithin, phosphorous, amino acids, and protein. Raw egg yolk and raw goat milk are the best. Meat protein does have phosphorous for the brain but many people want to avoid meat.

The brain must be well supplied with oxygen. Alfalfa sprouts, vitamin E, and hawthorne berry tea all bring oxygen to the brain.

Brain food can accomplish and do things, but "It is not the food that goes into the man; it is the kind of man the food goes into."

Calcium Tonics

If you lack calcium, you should learn how to make a calcium tonic, a calcium broth, and a calcium soup. One of the finest soups we have is from Denmark. It is a barley and green kale soup called "Grunko." This soup has the highest calcium content of any soup we know. Every mother should use this for her children while they are growing up. Both kale and soaked or sprouted whole barley can be liquefied and served raw, warm or cooked. For additional calcium, use the liquid from boiled egg shells in a broth or use bone meal tablets or powder in fruit and vegetable drinks.

Cramps in Legs

Take a Kneipp bath every day as described elsewhere in this book. Use the calcium foods in broths, soups, tonics, bone meal, kale, barley. Take Vege-Calcium-Lactate.

Cholesterol and Other Deposits

Alfalfa sprouts is one of the greatest remedies available for dissolving cholesterol and other deposits that settle in the arteries. The University of Vancouver, British Columbia, has found alfalfa sprouts great for dissolving the deposits which cause hardening of the arteries.

People who have cholesterol deposits in the body should cut out all oils that have been heated. Oils are concentrated, and the body does not have digestive juices to take care of concentrated oils.

You have to recognize that this body was made by God; it was made a natural thing; and these unnatural ways will give the body trouble. We should have salad dressings without too many concentrated oils. Instead, we should use avocado, nut butter dressings, or yogurt.

The worst of all oils are the commercial oils that have been heated to prevent them from becoming rancid.

Sprouts have been found to be a great dissolver of oil deposits. Sprouts of buckwheat, mung beans, soybeans, alfalfa, and sunflower seeds are all wonderful with a nice dressing such as tomato sauce. Sunflower seed sprouts are a little coarser than most. They need to be picked before they have grown too high or too coarse and then served with tomato sauce or nut butter dressing.

Liquid Chlorophyll. Liquid chlorophyll is a great deodorizer. For bad breath (which usually comes from the stomach) take one-half teaspoon of chlorophyll in a half cup of water before breakfast. Chlorophyll also reduces body odor.

Liquid chlorophyll is also one of our heart remedies. It is high in potassium, high in chlorophyll, and a great blood builder. It relieves and supports the heart.

Dried Olives

Dried olives are one of the highest things in potassium, and the heart needs potassium. You can take ten dried olives, steep them, take off the oil on top, and drink the remaining broth.

Whole Wheat

This is another good remedy for the heart. Grind the whole wheat berry into a cereal form, using one-half cup of hot water. Then put this in a hot thermos bottle, cork it, and leave overnight. This is a splendid heart remedy. Use it every morning for three months.

Hydrochloric Acid Deficiency

Most sick bodies have a lack of hydrochloric acid, the agent needed to curdle clabbered milk is therefore a more available protein for the body than milk, since it doesn't require as much additional hydrochloric acid to break it down. Use lemon juice, some clabber from a previous culture, or kefir for clabbering milk.

Hypoglycemia

There are a lot of people with hypoglycemia who should be taking a pancreatic substance. They should also be taking an adrenal gland substance. Many of these hypoglycemia cases develop mental symptoms. They are sometimes actually classed as mental cases when they should be taken care of as hypoglycemic cases. I believe that many people in mental institutions today could be better taken care of from an adrenal gland and pancreatic standpoint than from a mental standpoint. They need nerve foods. When you feed the nerves, you feed the glands also.

In hypoglycemic cases, I think it is good to have two protein meals and one very small starch meal a day. According to the severity of the case, we might even cut the starches down to a minimum, because the needed carbohydrates can be picked up in vegetables. We might even cut out fruits to avoid the load of sweets they put on the pancreas. Of course, all sugars are cut out. See the hypoglycemic diet in the chapter Special Diets for Special People.

Nerve Depletion

I have a broth I use as a remedy for people who are very sick, very irritable, have nerve depletion, and are on edge. I find it a very nourishing drink for the whole body. Take carrots, celery, parsley, a potato, beets, and maybe beet greens. Chop up very fine and put into a pint or quart of water and liquefy. Then add water, if necessary, to make a nice broth, and simmer for two or three minutes. This gives the least amount of heat, the shortest time of cooking, and keeps the foods as raw as possible, while taking off the acids that can cause a lot of the extreme elimination we find in raw foods. When the broth is just about finished, add a couple of tablespoons of soy milk powder, which neutralizes some of the acids. Strain, and drink the broth.

This is a wonderful nourishing food for the nervous system. It is a very soothing drink for the nervous system, a good building drink, and at the same time an eliminative drink.

Nerve Drink

I have a drink that takes the place of a meal. Many times if I cannot eat, I just ask for my drink. My drink is a glass of raw goat milk, often mixed with a teaspoon of sunflower seed butter, sesame seed butter, almond butter, or other nut butter; a teaspoon of honey; and a nice sliver of avocado. This is a whole meal, and it is all raw. It is a good protein meal, and it feeds the nervous system. This is my favorite.

Prune and celery juice together is a wonderful nerve food.

An egg yolk in black cherry juice works well as a nerve tonic.

Foods for the Liver

I believe that liquid chlorophyll is one of the great remedies in all liver troubles.

An egg yolk with black cherry juice also works well. Black cherry juice helps the liver to produce bile and keep it moving along. Of course, the egg yolk is high in fat, but the black cherry juice neutralizes that effect.

Acid/Alkaline Balance

To get an electrical current, we have to have a positive and a negative. The body too, has to have both an acid and an alkaline. If

ACID–ALKALINE CHART

The following table of foods is from Ragnar Berg of Germany.

Foods preceded by the letters "AL" are alkaline forming

Foods preceded by the letters "AC" are acid forming

Column No. 1
Nonstarch Foods

AL	Alfalfa	AL	Artichokes
AL	Asparagus	AL	Beans (string)
AL	Beans (wax)	AL	Beets (whole)
AL	Beet leaves	AL	Broccoli
AL	Cabbage (white)	AL	Cabbage (red)
AL	Carrots	AL	Carrot tops
AL	Cauliflower	AL	Celery knobs
AL	Chickory	AL	Cocunut
AL	Corn	AL	Cucumbers
AL	Dandelions	AL	Eggplant
AL	Endive	AL	Garlic
AL	Horseradish	AL	Kale
AL	Kohlrabi	AL	Leek
AL	Lettuce	AL	Mushrooms
AL	Okra	AL	Olives (ripe)
AL	Onions	AL	Osterplant
AL	Parsley	AL	Parsnips
AL	Peas (fresh)	AL	Peppers (sweet)
AL	Radishes	AL	Rutabagas
AL	Savory	AL	Sea lettuce
AL	Sorrel	AL	Spinach
AL	Soybean (products)	AL	Sprouts
AL	Summer squash	AL	Swiss chard
AL	Turnips	AL	Watercress

Column No. 2
Proteins and Fruits

AC	Beef	AC	Buttermilk
AC	Chicken	AC	Clams
AC	Cotage cheese	AC	Crab
AC	Duck	AC	Eggs
AC	Fish	AC	Goose
AL	Honey (pure)	AC	Jello
AC	Lamb	AC	Lobster
AC	Mutton	AC	Nuts
AC	Oyster	AC	Pork
AC	Rabbit	AC	Raw sugar
AC	Turkey	AC	Turtle
AC	Veal	AL	All berries
AL	Apples	AL	Apricots
AL	Avocados	AL	Cantaloupes
AL	Cranberries	AL	Curants
AL	Dates	AL	Figs
AL	Grapes	AL	Grapefruit
AL	Lemons	AL	Limes
AL	Oranges	AL	Peaches
AL	Pears	AL	Persimmons
AL	Pineapple	AL	Plums
AL	Prunes	AL	Raisins
AL	Rhubarb	AL	Tomatoes

Column No. 3
Starchy Foods

AL	Bananas	AC	Barley
AC	Beans (lima)	AC	Beans (white)
AC	Bread	AC	Cereals
AC	Chestnuts	AC	Corn
AC	Corn meal	AC	Crackers
AC	Grapefruit	AC	Corn starch
AC	Gluten flour	AC	Lentils
AC	Macaroni	AC	Maize
AC	Millet rye	AC	Oatmeal
AC	Peanuts	AC	Peanut butter
AC	Peas (dried)	AL	Potatoes (sweet)
AL	Potatoes (white)	AL	Pumpkin
AC	Rice (brown)	AC	Rice (polished)
AC	Roman meal	AC	Rye flour
AC	Sauerkraut	AC	Tapioca
AL	Squash (hubbard)		

Non-starchy foods mix with proteins, fruits or starches; and proteins and fruits do not mix well with starchy foods.

elimination has not been good, we may have too many acids. The person who does not exercise enough to produce enough acid in the body becomes too alkaline. A lot of people want to get well with just food alone. But that rarely happens.

The body needs 80 percent alkaline, 20 percent acid. The starches are the acid foods, as are sugars and proteins. The rest of your foods are alkaline. They are the builders. They are the foods for regeneration and rejuvenation. However, you also need some of the acid foods. When you don't have a good balance a variety of serious conditions may invade your body. Exercise helps one to have that balance. We ingest a lot of alkalines, then we exercise. Every time we use our muscles, we produce lactic acid, which neutralizes nerve acids. It also is good for the bowels. A *too* alkaline body is not good for the bowels.

The more perfect you become in your food routine, the more exercise you must do because you become more alkaline. Lactic acid is good acid to have in the body. It gives us the balance we need to keep going. It gives us a good body battery. If you want to recharge your battery, you have to exercise. You can also eat a few of the acid foods, but you make sure that you balance your day's eating.

Some people who are overalkaline take cider vinegar to help balance themselves, but I feel that practice is less than effective. A lot of people have thrown their acid/alkaline balance off, perhaps permanently, by using this apple cider vinegar for too long a time without using more natural means of balancing themselves.

The fruits and vegetables are alkaline as a rule, while starches and proteins are acid-producing. Many of these acid/alkaline food charts are found in *Dr. Jensen's Vital Foods for Total Health*, a cookbook-kitchen guide obtainable in any health food store. One starch and one protein daily, with the rest of the meal consisting of fruits and vegetables, will give us an 80-20 balance.

Using the Acid–Alkaline Combination Chart

For people with weak digestion it is best to make food combinations as simple as possible. Follow the suggestions on how to combine foods. Combine foods found in columns one and two, or in columns one and three. Never combine columns two and three. All foods in column one will combine with all foods in column two.

Fruits. Citrus fruits cause alkalinity. Citrus fruits, when broken down, release an alkaline ash that develops an alkaline condition in the body. Sometimes these acid fruits stir up the acids so rapidly that their effect is considered to be bad. This may be quite the reverse of the real truth! Should the eating of fruits cause you distress, you may be sure you are misinterpreting your symptoms. In any case like that, I would say you are very ill and require the advice of a specialist in natural healing.

But, in general, remember that fruits should be eaten in natural harmony. Oranges and grapefruits, tangerines and lemons, the acid fruits go nicely with other acid fruits like pineapple and strawberries. They do not combine well with the sweet fruits or the dried ones we mentioned, like prunes, figs, raisins, dates, and grapes. Berries and melons should always be eaten alone. There is no more disagreeable suprise for your stomach than watermelon eaten in conjunction with another food.

The subacid fruits mentioned, such as apples, persimmons, pears, plums, peaches, apricots combine fairly well with the acid fruits, but I do not recommend the combinations. The safest procedure is the *simplest* one.

You can use cream, if you must, but never sugar. White sugar is a poison to your system, no matter how much energy you seem to get from it, and brown sugar is like gilding the lily. The fruit itself is plentiful with sugar and you do not need to put sugar on your sugar.

In general, too, remember that sweet milk goes best with the acid fruits, while sour milk, like clabber, yogurt, or even cottage cheese, go best with the subacid fruits. In other words, a glass of milk at orange time is a permissible combination. Again, keep your diet simple.

Columns one and two will combine very nicely, as will columns two and three. Columns one and three never mix. Do not combine acid fruits with sweet dried fruits. Berries and melons are best eaten alone.

Fruits can also be classed in three columns:

Column No. 1	Column No. 2	Column No. 3
Acid Fruits	Subacid Fruits	Sweet or Dried
Oranges	Apples	Fruits
Grapefruit	Plums	Dates
Lemons	Grapes	Raisins
limes	Pears	Figs
	Peaches	
	Apricots	

Good Food Combinations

I would rather you have natural foods wrongly combined than foodless foods properly combined. If it "raises the roof" in the house, forget it. If you are concerned with loss of weight, you may disregard the principle and may combine natural carbohydrates and proteins. Every food contains a certain balance of these elements. Acid and alkaline foods, however, should be taken separately, if possible. Proteins may be used with acid, and carbohydrates with alkaline foods.

Whenever you have a starch, you should have a green vegetable with it. You will not be constipated, nor have a dry stool if you have at least twice as much vegetable material as starch.

With meat or protein foods you should have sulphur food in order to drive the brain and nerve fats into tissue.

Most natural foods are generally good. Have a full variety and you can take care of the whole body as you go along. We need all the elements in proper proportion to build a well-balanced bloodstream.

For the various systems of the body that may be run down or need certain chemicals for repair and maintenance, select your foods for the greatest variety possible, according to the growing seasons. Vegetables as fresh as possible from the garden are best. No amount of nutritional knowledge can compare with being your own gardener. Discover all possible ways of using raw foods. Foods in their natural state are alive and should be our chief source of nutrition.

If you must use fruits and vegetables that have been sprayed, when washing, use a solution of one teaspoon of Clorox to one gallon of water (this is high in chlorine, which is the cleanser, but it is like gas and leaves the liquid rapidly). Allow food to remain in it for five minutes, then rinse in clear, cold water for another five minutes. This is the cheapest and best way of handling the bugs. Try a few drops of a colloidal sulphur.

This is the way we recommend that dried fruits be revived: put into a pan, cover with cold water and bring just to boiling point; immediately remove from heat and allow to soak overnight. In this way, you kill all insects and eggs and will have less intestinal trouble from such causes.

Apples for the Nerves

The apple is charged with malic acid and glucose, both of which are wonderful for the neurogenic aspects of the body. They are wonderful for the nervous system because of the nerve salts they contain. Another excellent food is prunes. Because of their acid, prunes are sometimes not recommended, but I recommend them. Like the apple they contain a high content of nerve salt. Apples and prunes are valuable for growing children because of their benefit to the bowels. They are also helpful in cases of colic.

Fruits for Special Desserts. For a dessert with a high copper content (copper is necessary when building up anemic conditions) use apricots. The apricot whip, made with egg whites and gelatin, is one of the many ways of serving apricots. Homemade sherberts or ice cream prepared in the liquefier make fine apricot desserts. For sherbert we can use a different kind of fruit: strawberries, peaches, pears, or bananas. Ice cream from frozen grapes is not only good tasting but it's good for you. Fresh grapes placed in the deep freeze can be used the rest of the year.

Freezing Cherries or Berries. When freezing cherries or berries, freeze them individually. When frozen, pack them.

Try to Buy Organically Grown Produce

The proper diet must be considered, since everything that goes into the mouth should be a remedy. If it does not nourish the body, it is not a remedy. Nutrition begins with blood building, and the most vital thing in this connection is a diet with the proper amount of protein. Also, we must have nerve fats such as found in egg yolks, nuts, nut butters, and seeds of all kinds. When you want to rebuild the body, think of seeds. All the elements of the mature plant are represented in the seed. There are many ways these can be used in the form of milk substitute drinks. There are four basic types: soy, sunflower, sesame, and nut milks. Soy milk can be made from soy milk powder purchased at your health food store; sunflower seed, sesame seed, and nut milks such as almond and cashew are easily made by putting the seed in water and liquefying it. Tahini, nut butters, or sunflower seed meal may even be blended with an egg beater and made into a satisfactory drink. Add flavorings such as cherry and apple concentrate, dates, or carob powder to your substitute milk drinks as desired. Honey makes a good sweetener. Instead of water, try herb teas or soy milk as a base. These drinks we call catarrhal-eliminating drinks.

Mineralizers and Cleansers

Juices are great mineralizers and cleansers. Bitter tasting greens have necessary elements and palatable cocktails can be made from them by adding sweet vegetable juices, pineapple juice, coconut milk, cream, or concentrated juices such as grape and apple. Everybody can benefit from one or two glasses of juice a day. Try to make them fresh so that the valuable properties are not lost.

The liquefier has been a godsend in the health drink field. Now we can blend delectable beverages from natural ingredients, often incorporating supplementary foods such as rice polishings, dulse, yeast, sunflower seeds, flaxseeds, and wheat germ. We can now make a drink that will pass the critical taste of even a child. Whole fruits and vegetables can be liquefied, as can whole melons, with the seed hulls strained out afterwards.

If you have tooth or gum discomfort or a chewing disability, it may be better to take your meal in liquid form. There are drinks for those who need to stress the protein side of their nutrition, others with a starch nature.

All of our health drinks are suitable for children, but some will appeal more than others. Delicious milks and milkshakes and egg nogs can be made from genuine ingredients.

Although a program dedicated to health has no place for coffee, tea, or cocoa, their fans are not left completely comfortless. We dare not suggest that any coffee substitutes can pass undetected, but out "coffee taste" drinks are thoroughly enjoyable as well as nutritions; herb teas can be zipped up with lemon and honey, and the delicious carob makes a drink that amazes chocolate connoisseurs.

Here are a few "dressed up" drinks for that special party or dinner. Try one the next time you entertain.

Alfa-Mint Tea

1 T. Alfa-mint
1 c. boiling water
Steep five minutes. Sweeten with honey if desired, and serve with a wedge of lemon.

"Iced" Tea

Mix: 1 T. peppermint
1 c. boiling water
Steep five minutes.
Add: 1 T. honey
1 T. orange juice
Pour over ice cubes in a tall glass and garnish with mint leaves.

Broths and Soups for Specific Conditions

The following broths and soups can be used at any time, since as they are made of good food material. However, when your body needs to be revitalized or needs to overcome some special disorders, you may add these broths to your meals. in specific cases, these broths may be taken between meals. These, as all foods, should be prepared and cooked in glass, stainless steel, enamelware, or earthenware.

Veal Joint Broth. Rich in sodium. Excellent for glands, stomach, ligaments, and digestive disorders. Helps to retain youth in the body.

1½ c. apple peelings, ½ inch thick
2 c. potato peelings, ½ inch thick
Small stalk of celery   1 large parsnip
½ c. of okra, use canned 1 onion
if you cannot get fresh,   2 beets, grated
or 1 t. powdered okra   ½ c. chopped parsley

Use a clean, fresh , uncut veal joint. After washing in cold water, put into a large cooking pot, cover half with water, and add the following vegetables and greens, cut up fine.

Simmer all the ingredients for four or five hours; strain off liquid and discard solid ingredients. It should yeild about one-half quarts liquid. Drink hot or warm. Keep in refrigerator.

Vital Broth
Excellent for elimination

2 c. carrot tops   2 c. celery tops
3 c. celery stalk   2 qts. Sparkletts dis-
2 c. beet tops   tilled water
½ t. vegetable seasoning Add a carrot or on-
2 c. potato peeling   ion for flavor if de-
(cut ½ inch thick)   sired

Finely chop or grate vegetables. Bring slowly to a boil, simmer approximately twenty minutes. Just use broth, after straining. Take one cup twice daily.

Fish Broth. Excellent for the nervous system and nerve tissue. It is rich in iodine and phosphorus. (Use only when directed.)

Remove bones from fish, including head, and boil for thirty minutes in parchment paper. Add vegetized salt to taste. Use vitaminized salt, powdered celery, powdered chili, and powdered onions for a delectable flavor.

Potato Soup. Excellent for uric acid, kidney and stomach disorders, and mineral replacement.

Cut peelings of six potatoes three-fourths inch thick and simmer twenty minutes to one-half hour in a covered kettle. Strain off the liquid and drink every two or three hours. Do not make it too strong in a convalescing diet. Celery may be added to change flavor if desired. Add powdered okra it the stomach is irritated.

Potassium Broth. Excellent for poor heart conditions and digestive disorders, for building muscle and skin, and for healing sores.

Steep twelve sun-dried olives for ten minutes in one pint of water. Strain through five or six thicknesses of cheese cloth to catch the oil, since it should not be in the remaining liquid that you drink. Add this to the potato broth if desired or flavor with celery juice.

Calcium Broth. Excellent for bone conditions, lack of tone, and prolapsus. Needed in general throughout the structural system.

Grind egg shells or chicken bones to powder, using them separately or together. Use one-half cup of grindings to two quarts of water and boil thirty to sixty minutes. Strain and add raw celery juice to flavor. Drink one to two cups two or three times daily.

High Sodium/Potassium Broth. For high sodium broth use beets, celery, carrots, and turnips. For broths high in both sodium and potassium, try apple peelings, or better yet, the jelly from veal joints. This veal joint broth will do more for arthritis and rheumatism than all other foods combined. The sodium that has been made from the gelatin of the bones of the animal is virtually the same as that found in the joints of the human body.

More Valuable Health Building Tonics

Oat straw tea is very high in silicon and can be made very pleasant be adding apple concentrate to sweeten.

Egg yolk contains a natural lecithin, one of the finest brain and nerve fats. When added to green juices or cherry it will not upset the liver or cause intestinal distress or cholesterol.

Avocado also contains natural lecithin, and a little may be added to the drink. It can be used in soy milk or raw milk to fortify it with minerals.

A quick energy drink can be made from liquefied yogurt and persimmons. You can even use frozen persimmons. (Did you ever try freezing them? Try it!)

Brain cocktail sounds interesting to anyone. For the brain-building side, put some Missouri black walnuts into powdered form and use a tablespoon of them in the drink. Black walnuts are considered high in manganese, a brain and nerve nutritional supplement.

Wheat germ is a wonderful item to add to our diet. It is high in vitamin E. It develops tone in our tissues and quickens our circulation.

Carob flour is another fine addition and may be added to any of the juices. Splendid for giving a chocolate-like flavoring to milk, soy milk, and sesame milk drinks.

COCKTAILS
(For Pleasure or Therapy)

Cleansing Cocktail

Celery Juice	Parsley juice
Spinach juice	Carrot juice

Vary proportions to suit preference.

Complexion Cocktail

Cucumber juice	Pineapple juice
Endive juice	*Mix to taste.*

Chlorophyll Water
1 t. liquid chlorophyll in a glass of water. (Replaces fresh green juice.)

Jade-ade

¼ c. cucumber juice	¼ c. watercress juice
¼ c. celery juice	¼ c. tomato juice
¼ c. parsley juice	

Green Cocktail

1 c. mint tea	½ c. young spinach

Blend fine in liuqefier.

½ c. yogurt	1 T. lemon juice
1 t. vegetable seasoning	½ t. dulse powder
A little honey	

Blend briefly to mix. Serve in a tall glass with a slice of lemon.

Mixed Cocktail

1 c. oatstraw tea	1 carrot, diced
2 leaves comfrey	3 to 4 dates, pitted
1 T. coconut powder	

Blend in liquefier.

Radiance Cocktail
Whip together: 1 t. raw almond butter
½ c. each of celery and orange juices.

Youth Bloom Cocktail
Whip: 1/3 c. beet juice   1/3 c. spinach juice
2 T. blackberries to smooth cocktail

Mulberry Cocktail
Blend 1 c. fresh mulberries and ½ c. whey.

Whole Melon Cocktail
Juice one melon, skin, flesh, and seeds. Squeeze in a press or strain through a sieve to remove the seed hulls and coarse fiber. In this way the chlorophyll from the skin and all the vital elements of the seeds are used.

Beet Appetizer
2 c. oatstraw tea	¼ slice lemon
1 T. lemon juice	1 t. vegetable season-
1 c. raw diced beets	ing
Sprig of fresh mint	1 t. honey

Blend until smooth.

Aperitif
1 glass tomato juice	1 t. vegetable sea-
1 T. aged cider vinegar	soning
Dash of dulse powder	

Beat together and chill.

SPECIAL DRINKS

Protein Drink
1 c. acidophilous milk	1 egg
1 T. sunflower seed meal	2 prunes, pitted, revived

Liquefy to a creamy drink.

Starch Drink
1 c. soy milk	4 T. cooked cereal
¼ t. dulse	Honey to sweeten
Few drops pure vanilla	

Blend smooth in liquefier.

Meal in a Drink
½ c. mint tea	2 sprigs parsley
1 c. apple juice	2 comfrey leaves
½ c. orange juice	½ c. fresh fruit
1 pitted prune, revived	½ ripe banana
3/4 c. cashew nuts	1 egg
½ c. carrots, diced	2 t. wheat germ
½ celery stalks	

Blend for three minutes. Sip very slowly.

Hercules Punch
½ c. apple juice	½ c. papaya juice
1 t. wheat germ oil	1 t. lecithin granules
1 t. bone meal	1 t. brewers yeast
1 t. skim milk powder	

Blend in liquefier to a smooth consistency.

Nerve Verve
1 c. prune juice	6 radishes
2 t. rice polishings	

Blend in liquefier.

Vitality Drink
1 T. apple concentrate	1 T. almond nut
1 c. celery juice	butter

Blend in liquefier.

MILK SUBSTITUTE DRINKS
(Non-Catarrh Forming)

Many people don't realize that catarrh can be produced from cow's milk, mainly because of the difference between the milk's chemical structure and the body's needs. The body has to take care of this improper balance, throwing off the chemical structure that is not the right balance, usually in the form of catarrh. Here are some substitutes to help you avoid that problem:

Doctor Jensen's Drink
1 T. of any good brand of sesame seed meal or butter
1 glass liquid (may be fruit juice, vegetable uice, soy milk, or broth and water)
¼ avocado
1 honey.
Blend 30 seconds.

Sesame Seed Milk

Seeds and sprouts are going to be the foods of the future. We have found that many of the seeds have the hormone values of male glands and female glands. Seeds carry the life force for many years, often as long as they are enclosed by the hull. Seeds found in tombs, and known to have been there for thousands of years, have grown when planted. To get these seeds into our body in the form of a drink gives us the finest form of nutrition.

For sesame seed milk, take ¼ cup sesame seed to two cups water, raw milk, or goat milk. Place in blender and run for one and one-half minutes. Strain through fine wire strainer or two to four layers of cheesecloth to remove the hulls.

Add one tablespoon carob powder and six to eight dates. For flavor or added nutritional value any one of the following may be added to this drink: banana, stewed raisins, apple or cherry concentrate, date powder, or grape sugar. Your own imagination or taste may dictate other combinations of fruits or juices. Whenever adding anything, run in blender again to mix. This milk may also be used as the basis for salad dressings.

I believe that sesame seed milk is one of our best. It is a wonderful drink for gaining weight and for lubricating the intestinal tract. Its nutritional value is beyond compare, since it is high in protein and minerals. This is the seed used in the making of tahini, a sesame seed oil dressing. This also is the seed that is used so much in Arabia and is used as a basic food in east India.

Almond Nut Milk

Use blanched or unblanched almonds. Other nuts may be used also. Soak nuts overnight in apple or pineapple juice or honey water. This softens the structure of the nut meats. Then put three ounces of soaked nuts in five ounces water and blend for two to two and one-half minutes in the liquefier. Flavor with honey, any kind of fruit, concentrates of apple or cherry juice, strawberry juice, carob flour, dates, or bananas. Or it can be used with any of the vegetable juices.

Almond nut milk can also be used with soups and vegetarian roasts as a flavoring. Use over cereals too.

Almond milk makes a very alkaline drink, high in protein and easy to assimilate and absorb.

Sunflower Seed Milk

Sunflower seeds are the vegetarian's best protein. The same principle as is used for making nut milks can be employed to make sunflower seed milk i.e., soaking overnight, liquefying, and flavoring with fruits and juices. Use in the diet the same way as the almond nut milk. It is best to use whole sunflower seeds and blend them yourself. However, if you do not have a liquefier, the sunflower seed meal can be used.

Soy Milk

Soy milk powder is found universally in health food stores.

Add four tablespoons of soy milk powder to one pint of water. Sweeten with a raw sugar, honey, or molasses, and add a pinch of vegetable salt. For flavor you can add any kind of fruit, apple or cherry concentrate, carob powder, dates, or bananas. You can add any other natural sweetener.

Keep in refrigerator. Use this milk in recipes just as you would regular cow's milk. It closely resembles the taste and composition of cow's milk and will sour just as quickly. Therefore, it should not be made in too large quantities or too far ahead of time.

General Diet Regimen

The following is a general diet regimen that many of my students and patients follow with wonderful, happy results.

Balanced Daily Eating Regimen. Make a habit of applying the following diet regimen to your everyday living. This is a healthy way to live, because, when you follow it, you do not have to worry about vitamins, mineral elements, or calories.

The best diet, over the period of a day, is two different fruits, at least four to six vegetables, one protein, and one starch, with fruit or vegetable juices between meals. Eat at least two green leafy vegetables a day. Fifty to 60 percent of the food you eat daily should be raw. Consider this regimen a dietitic law.

Rules of Eating

1. Do not fry foods or use heated oils.

2. If you are not entirely comfortable in mind and body from the previous meal time, you should miss the next meal.

3. Do not eat unless you have a keen desire for the plainest food.

4. Do not eat beyond your needs.

5. Be sure to thoroughly masticate you food.

6. Miss meals if you are in pain, emotionally upset, not hungry, chilled, overheated, and experiencing acute illness.

Impositions for Getting Well

1. Learn to accept whatever decision is made.

2. Let the other parson make a mistake and learn.

3. Learn to forget and forgive.

4. Be thankful and bless people.

5. Live in harmony — even if it is good for you.

6. Do not talk about your sickness.

7. Gossip will kill you. Neither speak it nor listen to it. Gossip that comes through the grapevine is usually sour.

8. Be by yourself everyday for ten minutes with the thought of how to make yourself a better person. Replace negative thoughts with uplifting, positive thoughts.

9. Skin brush daily. Use a slant board daily.

10. Have citrus fruit in sections only, never in juice form.

11. Have only a limited amount of bread. If you have a lot of bowel trouble, have no bread.

12. Exercise daily. Keep your spine limber. Develop abdominal muscles. Do sniff breathing. Have a daily set of exercises.

13. Grass walk and sand walk for happy feet.

14. No smoking, drinking, spitting, or cussing. Keep away from "spitty" people.

15. Retire to bed at sundown, or 9 p.m. at the latest, if you are at all tired, fatigued, and unable to do your work with vim and vigor. If you are sick you must rest more. Sleep out of doors, out of the city, in circulating air. Work out problems in the morning, don't take them to bed with you.

Food Healing Laws

1. Natural food- Fifty to 60 percent of the food eaten should be raw.

2. Your diet should be 80 percent alkaline and 20 percent acid. Look at the acid–alkaline chart, this chapter.

3. Proportion- Six vegetables daily, two fruits daily, one starch daily, and one protein daily.

4. Variety- Vary sugars, proteins, starches, vegetables, and fruits from meal to meal and from day to day.

5. Overeating- You can kill yourself with the amount of food you eat.

6. Combinations— Separate starches and proteins. Eat one at lunch and the other at supper. Have fruits for breakfast and at 3:00 P.M.

7. Cook without water- Cook without high heat. Cook without air touching hot food.

8. Bake, broil, or roast- If you eat meat, have it. Have lean meat, no fat, no pork. Used unsprayed vegetables if possible and eat them as soon after picked as possible.

9. Use stainless steel, low-heat cooking utensils- It is the modern health engineered way of preparing your foods.

Before breakfast: One-half hour before breakfast, take any natural, unsweetened fruit juice such as grape, pineapple, prune, fig, apple or black cherry. Liquid chlorophyll can be used; take one teaspoonful in a glass of water.

You can have a broth and lecithin drink if you desire it. Take one teaspoonful of vegetable broth powder and one tablespoonful of lecithin granules and dissolve in a glass of warm water.

On doctor's advice you may have citrus fruits such as orange, grapefruit, lemon, or tomato.

Between fruit juice and breakfast, following this program: skin brushing, exercise, hiking, deep breathing, or playing. Shower. Start warm and cool off until your breath quickens. Never shower immediately upon arising.

Breakfast: Stewed fruit, one starch, and a health drink or two fruits, one protein, and health drink. (Starches and health drinks are listed with the lunch suggestions.) Soaked fruits, such as unsulphured apricots, prunes, figs. Fruit of any kind — melon, grapes, peaches, pears, berries, or baked apple, which may be sprinkled with some ground nuts or nut butter. When possible, use fruit in season.

SUGGESTED BREAKFAST MENUS

Monday
Reconstituted dried apricots
Steel-cut oatmeal, with supplements
Oat straw tea
Add eggs, if desired
or
Sliced peaches
Cottage cheese, with supplements
Herb tea

Tuesday
Fresh figs
Cornmeal cereal, with supplements
Shave grass tea
Add eggs or nut butter, if desired
or
Raw applesauce and blackberries
Coddled egg, with supplements
Herb tea

Wednesday
Reconstituted dried peaches
Millet cereal, with supplements
Alfa-mint tea
Add eggs, cheese or nut butter, if desired
or
Sliced nectarines and apple
Yogurt, with supplements
Herb tea

Thursday
Prunes or any reconstituted dried fruit
Whole wheat cereal, with supplements
Oat straw tea
or
Grapefruit and kumquats
Poached egg, with supplements
Herb tea

Friday
Slices of fresh pineapple with
shreded coconut
Buckwheat cereal, with supplements
Peppermint tea
or
Baked apple, persimmons
Chopped raw almonds
Acidophilus milk, with supplements
Herb tea

Saturday
Muesli with bananas and dates
Cream, with supplements
Dandelion coffee or herb tea

Sunday
Cooked applesauce with raisins
Rye grits, with supplements
Shave grass tea
or
Cantaloupe and strawberries
Cottage cheese, with supplements
Herb tea

Preparation Helps. Reconstituted dried fruit: Cover with cold water, bring to boil and leave to stand overnight. Raisins may just have boiling water poured over them. This kills any insects and eggs.

Whole grain cereal: To cook properly with as little heat as possible, use a double-boiler or thermos-cook your cereal.

Supplements: (add to cereal or fruit) Sunflower seed meal, rice polishings, wheat germ, flaxseed meal (about a teaspoonful of each). Even a little dulse, with some broth powder, may be sprinkled in.

10:30 A.M.: Vegetable broth, vegetable juice, or fruit juice.

Lunch: Raw salad, or as directed, one or two starches, as listed, and a health drink. Get salad suggestions from Dr. Jensen's cookbook and food guide, *Vital Foods for Total Health.*

Note: If you are following a strict regimen, use only one of the first seven starches daily. Vary the starch from day to day:

Raw Salad Vegetables: Tomatoes (citrus, lettuce (green leafy type only, such as romaine), celery, cucumber, bean sprouts, green peppers, avocado, parsley, watercress, endive, onion(s), cabbage(s). (s) indicates sulphur foods.

Starches

1. Yellow cornmeal 2. Baked potato 3. Baked banana (or at least dead ripe). 4. Barley (a winter food). 5. Steamed brown rice or wild rice. 6. Millet (have as a cereal). 7. Banana squash or Hubbard squash.
Steel-cut oatmeal, whole wheat cereal, Dr. Jackson's meal, whole grain Roman meal, shredded wheat bread (whole wheat, rye, soybean, corn bread, bran muffins, rye krisp preferred.)

Drinks: Vegetable broth, soup, coffee substitute, buttermilk, raw milk, oat straw tea, alfa-mint tea, huckleberry tea, papaya tea, or any health drink.

SUGGESTED LUNCH MENUS

Monday
Vegetable salad
Baby lima beans
Baked potato
Spearmint tea

Tuesday
Vegetable salad — with health
mayonnaise, if desired
Steamed Asparagus
Very ripe bananas, or steamed,
unpolished rice
Vegetable broth or herb tea

Wednesday
Raw salad plate
Sour cream dressing
Cooked green beans
and/or Baked Hubbard squash

Corn bread
Sassafras tea

Thursday
Salad — French dressing
Baked zucchini and okra
Corn-on-cob
Rye krisp
Buttermilk or herb tea

Friday
Salad
Baked green pepper, stuffed with
eggplant and tomatoes
Baked potato and/or bran muffin
Carrot soup or herb tea

Saturday
Salad
Steamed turnips and turnip greens
Baked yams
Catnip tea

Sunday
Salad
Lemon and olive oil dressing
Steamed whole barley
Cream of celery soup
Steamed chard
herb tea

Salad Vegetables: Use plenty of greens. Choose four or five vegetables from the following: Leaf lettuce, watercress, spinach, beet leaves, parsley, alfalfa sprouts, cabbage, young chard, herbs, any green leaves, cucumbers, bean sprouts, onions, green peppers, pimentos, carrots, turnips, zucchini, asparagus, celery, okra, radishes, etc.

3:00 P.M.: Health cocktail, juice, or fruit.

DINNER:

Raw Salad, Two Cooked Vegetables, One Protein and a Broth or Health Drink, if desired.

Cooked vegetables: Peas, artichokes, carrots, beets, turnips, spinach, beet tops, string beans, swiss chard, eggplant, zucchinin, summer squash, broccoli (s), cauliflower (s), cabbage (s), sprouts (s), onion (s), or any vegetable other than potatoes.

Drinks: Vegetable broth, soup, or health beverage.

Proteins

Once a week: Fish — use white fish, such as sole, halibut, trout, or sea trout.

Vegetarians use soy beans, lima beans, cottage cheese, sunflower seeds, and other seeds, also seed butters, nut butters, nut milk drinks, eggs.

Three times a week: Meat — use only lean meat. Never pork, fats, or cured meats.

Vegetarians use meat substitutes or vegetarian proteins.

Twice a week: Cottage cheese or any cheese that breaks.

Once a week: Egg omelet.

If you have a protein at this meal, health dessert is allowed, but no recommended. Never eat protein and starch together. (Notice how they are separated.)

You may exchange your noon meal for the evening meal, but follow the same regimen. It takes exercise to handle raw food, and we generally get more after our noon meal. That is why a raw salad is advised at noon. If one eats sandwiches, have vegetables at the same time.

SUGGESTED DINNER MENUS

Monday
Salad
Diced celery and carrots
Steamed spinach, waterless-cooked
Puffy omelet
Vegetable broth

Tuesday
Salad
Cooked beet tops
Steak, broiled
or ground beef patties with tomato sauce
Cauliflower
Comfrey tea

Wednesday
Cottage cheese
Cheese sticks
Apples, peaches, grapes, nuts
Apple concentrate cocktail

Thursday
Salad
Steamed chard
Baked eggplant
Grilled liver and onions
persimmon whip (optional)
Alfa-mint tea

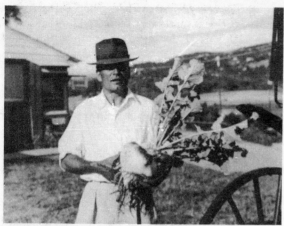

A good-sized turnip but we find when they are planted at a certain time of the Moon you can get big turnips and small tops and vice versa.

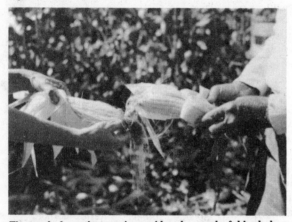

The tassle from the corn is considered a wonderful herb, has wonderful natural herb values used in Cornsilk Tea. It is wonderful as a kidney eliminant and as a diuretic. Indians used so much of this. They found so many things for use in nature and civilization is forgetting these many things that nature has to offer.

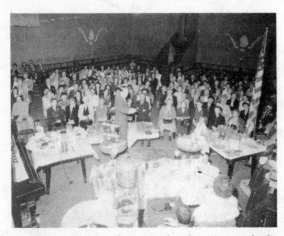

One of my workshops demonstrating how to put foods together, how to combine them, how to cook them under low heat in stainlss steel . . . how to get the most out of our food for the good of our bodies and the best health possible.

Friday
Salad
Yogurt and lemon dressing
Steamed mixed greens
Beets
Steamed fish, with slices of lemon
leek soup

Saturday
Salad
Cooked string beans
Baked summer squash
Carrot and cheese loaf
Cream of lentil soup or lemongrass tea
Fresh peach jello
Almond-nut cream

Sunday
Salad
Diced carrots and peas, steamed
Tomato aspic
Roast leg of lamb
Mint sauce

Vegetarians use vegetarian dishes in place of meat dishes.

TWENTY ONE

Special diets for special people

THE DIET that probably does the greatest amount of good for high blood pressure and for the heart is the Rice Diet. We have known for years that adding more starches to the diet regulated the heart and kept it on a more balanced condition. Many heart disturbances are caused by diverticuli conditions in the descending colon. We learned also that starches take care of much of the gas condition in the descending colon, while too much meat in the diet seems to add to the putrefaction and gas formation that develop in this descending colon.

It would probably be good to have a checkup before beginning the Rice Diet; then have another after three or four days. If the body shows no abnormal signs, such as swelling in the extremities, excess gas, or other abnormal symptoms, continue with the diet. Have checkups every three or four days throughout the diet. We have patients going on this diet in a modified way for many months until the body has been normalized.

The Rice Diet

Breakfast — Stewed fruit and steamed brown rice, using stewed fruit for seasoning. Tea.

Lunch — Salad, and one or two cooked vegetables, if you wish. Cottage cheese one day, egg next day (in the form of egg omelet). Nut butter on the third day. Then repeat.

Dinner — (Evening meal) Vegetable salad, cooked vegetable, steamed brown rice again.

To modify this diet have fresh fruit and protein for breakfast, and salad and vegetables for lunch, with more or less starchy vegetables, such as banana, squash, carrots, or beets. At the evening meal you can have steamed brown rice and vegetables again, or steamed brown rice and stewed fruit (dried fruit that has been brought back to normal again).

We have seen as much as a 60-point drop in the blood pressure in one month's time by using this diet. In addition, overweight people have lost as much as ten to fifteen pounds in one month. It is a matter of mormalizing the body weight and getting the pressure off the heart that helps.

Another good remedy for left-side problems is to use one clove of garlic, chopped up fine with honey. Take this twice a day.

Diabetes

Diabetes is known scientifically as *diabetes mellitus* (not to be confused with *diabetes insipidus*, a different disease altogether) and occurs as the result of a disorder of body chemistry. *Diabetes mellitus* is a metabolic disorder caused by the failure of special cells of the pancreas called the Isles of Langerhans (after the German anatomist who first described them) to manufacture a hormone secretion, Insulin, in sufficient quantity to enable the body to utilize sugar in the normal way. Consequently the sugar content of the blood goes up. When it reaches a certain level, the kidneys are called upon to excrete or leak the excess into the urine. This is why we test the urine for an excess amount of sugar in the blood.

When we do not utilize sugar properly, we have an increased hunger because the body is in need of energy food. The blood sugar is derived from carbohydrate foods — sugars and starches, the starches being converted into sugar by digestion. In the normal person, any excess over immediate needs can be converted into a reserve and stored. In the diabetic this cannot be done successfully and there-

165

fore, the excess has to be eliminated via the kidneys and the urinary system.

In the diabetic person we should try to find out the level of sugars and starches that the body can take. Sometimes starches have to be severely reduced, and many of the sweets and starches that the average person eats can be eliminated altogether. Just how much starchy food can be handled depends on the severity of the diabetes and the amount of insulin being taken. We regulate this with the blood sugar and urine tests.

Who Gets Diabetes? Today diabetes is one of our most prevalent diseases. It is the eighth leading cause of death in the United States and the third leading cause of blindness, and it is increasing at an alarming rate. I personally believe the increase is due mainly to our living habits. There are many more young people with diabetes today than ever before, and it is only in the last 50 years that we have had such an extensive use of white sugar, white flour, and other devitalized products.

Though diabetes does not affect children as often as it does adults, it does appear even in infants. We find that those most frequently acquiring it, however, are between the ages of 45 and 55. Those who have it young usually have inherited the weakness, and many times the inherent weakness is quite severe. Two out of three diabetics are women. It is most prevalent at menopause. Those who are, or have been, married appear to have a considerably higher percentage of diabetes than unmarried women. No one actually knows why, but it could have something to do with the glandular changes that occur during pregnancy. Those changes may affect the way the body uses starches and sugars. In most cases of diabetes, the person has been overweight before the diabetes has been discovered. But the person usually loses weight in the treatment of this disease.

Causes of Diabetes. There are many conditions that set the stage for diabetes to develop. Age can be a factor; hereditary conditions can exist. Also, of course, our habits of living affect our bodies.

Diabetes is found most in the individual exhausted by the mental strain of sedentary office work, who often has great anxiety about work and little chance for physical exercise. It is found more in the overweight person than the underweight. It has been estimated that there are almost a million and

a half people in this country living in ignorance of the fact that they have diabetes.

Recent observations seem to indicate that psychological factors are involved in the onset of the disease. Extreme stress, the loss of a loved one, job difficulties, unrequited love, all these can apparently cause serious stomach upsets in the total health and thus bring on diabetes. Then, too, certain modern drugs have been known to cause temporary diabetes.

Symptoms. One of the chief symptoms of diabetes is the need to urinate frequently. Other symptoms include the condition of extreme thirst (the mouth can be very dry, and the patient may complain of "not enough water"), hunger, loss of weight, easy tiring, the slow healing of cuts and bruises, possible changes of vision, often intense itching in certain areas of the body, pains in fingers and toes, and feelings of weakness and drowsiness.

Diabetes is accompanied by a tendency to develop trouble in the blood circulation in the lower limbs and the proneness to septic conditions, such as boils and carbuncles. Many times a blow to the leg can produce a diabetic ulcer, which is difficult to correct as long as there is an overabundance of sugar in the blood. Consequently, it is important to take care of the feet and skin. Diabetics should do everything they can to take care of the peripheral circulation of the blood. They must give up smoking, since one of the effects of smoking is contraction in the capillaries and the finer blood vessels of the circulatory system. They should keep the feet and limbs warm.

Many other symptoms point to diabetes; for instance, lameness of the back, heavy legs, swollen and numb feet, silent sadness, indifference, gloomy mind, emaciation, impotense, stiffness of the loins, dyspepsia at times, overweight, excessive thirst, desire for stimulants, dryness in the mouth, languor, pain in the kidneys, and hectic fevers.

Insulin. Insulin was discovered in 1921, before which time very little was being done for the victim of diabetes. Insulin has been the lifesaver to the diabetic. It allows him to live as normal a life as anyone else, if the diabetic follows certain rules of diet and provides his body with the proper quantity of insulin daily. However, the only diet restrictions imposed are that he refrain from alcoholic beverages and sweet desserts. But too often since the discovery of insulin diabetics haven't cared for their bodies from a nutritional standpoint. We should not go on following our same way of living or eating the types of foods that can produce diabetes, and just take the insulin to offset the extra sugar produced in the urine and in the blood.

The diabetic should recognize that if he starts eating differently, the body will mold to what he eats. Most people do not want to change their body weight, size, etc., so they do not want to change their diet. Many diabetics come to me with stomach trouble, constipation, and liver disturbances because of the type of diet they have been on.

Insulin is a hormone produced in the cells of the pancreas. When secreted into the bloodstream, it permits the metabolism and utilization of sugar. When there is an overdoze of insulin given, hypoglycemia, or too little sugar in the blood, will develop. This is known as an insulin reaction. Light-headedness, fainting, trembling, sweating, and hunger can develop. In severe reactions, diabetics may lose consciousness. On the other hand, a lack of insulin or too little intake of the substance can cause an excess of fatty acids to pile up. These poison the system, leading to a condition known as acidosis. This, in turn, can lead to a diabetic coma, which can result in death if it is not treated swiftly. The diabetic coma is a rare thing today, but it can occur when one neglects his diet and does not take the proper amount of insulin.

A person who has diabetes and is taking insulin or is under the care of a physician for diabetes should carry an identification card. This should provide his name, address, telephone number, etc., and it should state that if found unconscious or behaving abnormally, he may be having an insulin reaction. The card can indicate that if he can swallow, give him sugar, candy, fruit juice, or a sweetened drink; if he is unable to swallow or if recovery does not immediately take place, call a physician or send him to a hospital at once.

Treatment for Diabetes. There are all kinds of treatments today for diabetes. Various medicines and approaches are used. But to treat diabetes properly, the whole body should be taken into consideration. I believe that in most cases of diabetes the liver is affected as well as the pancreas. We should always look for a kidney disturbance, too. The digestive system should be straightened out so that constipation and bowel disorders are corrected. Each one of these organs helps the pancreas to work properly. In other words, the whole body must be working in balanced order.

There are many diet patterns for the diabetic. However, I think his first consideration should be to find a healthful way of living. The idea of just cutting down on the amount of sugar and starches is not enough. We should find the nutritional balance for the whole body as well. There are very few people who just have diabetes and no other problem.

Most diabetics, when under insulin care, are given a diet that allows coffee and tea. All they have to do is cut out sugar and cream. They are given clear broths, but are not told how to make them or what seasonings to use. They use fat-free bouillons, which in many cases comes from meat that is adulterated and cooked too much. Cranberries and rhubarb are given, as are pickles and other abominable foods that do not build good health in the body. In many cases persons are allowed to have breads, starchy foods, and some sweets, but they are never even told that these should be of a natural type.

Fresh green vegetables are truly the one thing diabetics need to get acquainted with more than anything else. Salads should be eaten at two out of the three meals a day. They are never out of place on the diabetic's table. Vegetables grown above the ground are especially good. We can take the ten percent or 12 percent starchy vegetables to use in most cases, though some need to reduce to a five percent carbohydrate list. A natural insulin is found in Jerusalem artichokes.

When we use a lot of fruits and vegetables, much water is taken into the system, and this is ideal for the kidneys and urinary system. In diabetes we must keep the kidneys and urinary system in good order, because the disease puts a strain on the kidneys. We need to abondon sweetened teas and coffees, and alcohol should play no part in the diabetic's life. Whenever a diabetic person is overweight, he should start in earnest to reduce. Diabetes often starts with people who have been overweight for many years. A curtailment of fats, as well as sugars, would bring a surprising and encouraging improvement.

Foods for Diabetics. In most cases we find that diabetes has been formed and developed from a lack of silicon. The pancreas is a silicon organ. Silicon is found highest in our grains, especially in the bran of the grain. The outside covering of rice, rice polishings, is the food highest in silicon. Rice bran tea, wheat bran broth, oatstraw tea, and shavegrass tea are all wonderful for cases of diabetes. We should have variety in the diabetic diet if we are going to cut out certain foods. Foods high in vitamin B should also be included. These are meats, especially liver and other organ meats, nuts, seeds, unprocessed whole grains, eggs, milk, wheat germ, and brewer's yeast. Cactus Grandifloris, in combination with vitamin B, has been found to be very good. Myrtle berries are also effective in many cases.

Because diabetics are not allowed sugary foods, and corn or other starches, they sometimes turn to more butter, cheeses, vegetable fats, olive oil, milk, creams, nuts, and nut fats for energy. However, we must be careful of these and make sure we use them sparingly. They can be used in various combinations in our soups and drinks, but never in fried foods. Some of the dried fruits need to be eaten in strict moderation, too. A high protein diet plus the fresh fruits and vegetables is indicated in diabetes.

The spleen is mainly at fault in many cases of diabetes. We need more red blood cells. We need magnesium and lime, and a stimulation of the liver and spleen.

Other foods for diabetes are warm water drinks, lukewarm milk with lemon juice, warm drinks made with bran (high in silicon), biscuits made of almond flour, celery soups, tomatoes, and strawberries. Cauliflower and young onions, goat whey cheese, toasted bran breads, veal joint jelly, dried black olives, oatstraw broth, parsley, and chicory are also effective.

Other allowable foods are fish, concentrated soups that are not fatty, spinach, celery, sprouts, celery soup with milk, watercress, lettuce, young onions, tomatoes, cream (sparingly), dandelion, buttermilk, skim milk mixed with warm foods, water at 136 degrees F, grapefruit, lemons (sparingly), sour lemon eaten upon retiring, red currants, pistachio nuts (nuts, however, should be eaten sparingly), boiled mutton, broiled poultry (sparingly), gooseberries, very hot water and milk upon arising in the morning, steel-cut oat muffins, lemon drinks between meals. Lemons, limes, and sour oranges help the liver and arteries and feverish conditions. They should never be taken with a meal. If meat is eaten at all, let it be fresh and from young, healthy animals; broil it quickly and, if possible, take the fluids only. Turnip greens are good.

Diet alone will not overcome diabetes. The mental side of the picture must be also considered and handled. A tired body cannot force glands to produce the proper amount of enzymes, elimination becomes poor, toxic conditions develop, and the whole organic structure of the body can change. If the pancreas is inherently weak, this organ could suffer considerably. Most people do not realize that our nerve energy must be conserved in order to heal any condition, no matter what organ is affected in the body. Prolonged mental tension is not good.

Physicial exercise should be encouraged. It can do the diabetic even more good than it does the average person. He must keep very fit to keep the rest of the body organs working well. The most helpful exercises are breathing, gymnastics to deepen and lengthen the respiratory rhythm, and stretching and flexing to give movement, elasticity, and freedom to all muscles. This helps to metabolize blood sugar more evenly and completely. Outdoor activities should be stressed. A diabetic should shun labor-saving devices, should have a definite plan and principal activity program every day. Don't use a car consistently. Walk—use this to prevent diabetes as well as to try to cure it.

Never become chilled. Simple exercises should be used by the limbs to keep up the circulation in the lower extremities. Keep the skin active and resilient. One of the best methods of doing this is skin brushing.

Other tonics for the diabetic are the fresh thin air at high altitudes, outdoor exercise in the mountains, cheerful surroundings, long walks, internal baths, sponge baths, salt baths, stomach massage, plenty of sleep, nerve tension exercises.

Of course, the best idea in diabetes is to try to prevent it. Most important of all to remember is that neither insulin nor oral drugs prevent the onslaught of other symptoms that cause diseases—mostly heat and blood vessel troubles. We must learn to live correctly to prevent these other troubles that may be coming on. The diabetic seems to encounter these problems earlier and in a more severe form than the rest of us do.

Eleven-day Elimination Regime

There are many eliminative regimes, and they all accomplish about the same results, since the body is given less food, simpler foods, simpler combinations, more watery food— so a greater transition can take place in the cells of the body.

The Eleven-Day Elimination Regime can be used by most persons in fair health and by those who want to overcome the average physical disorder. Those who are weak or feeble, however, should not follow the plan the full eleven days without supervision. Those with tuberculosis should have both supervision and assistance.

Variation as to the length of time and the manner in which the foods are to be taken may be adjusted to suit the history of the patient. For example, fruits, vegetables, and broths can be taken for one day, the next day just fruit can be taken; then you can go with three days straight of vegetables only— or any combination you wish.

Vegetables taken in the form of broths, gently steamed vegetables, and salads are a safer routine for the average beginner than citrus fruits. The Vital Broth recipe as outlined in the broth chapter is especially good.

A hot bath should be taken every night during this diet regime. Enemas may be used the first four or five days, then discontinued for natural movements.

Summary of Eleven-day Diet

First three days: Nothing but water and fruit juices, preferably grapefruit; one glass every four hours.

Fourth and Fifth day: Fruit only, such as grapes, melons, tomatoes, pears, peaches, dried fruit, soaked overnight, such as prunes, figs, peaches; baked apple.

Last six days: Breakfast— citrus fruits.
Between breakfast and lunch— any kind of fruit.
Lunch— salad of three to six vegetables and two cups Vital Broth.
Dinner— two or three steamed vegetables and two cups Vital Broth.
Before retiring— fruit juices if desired.

Rigid adherence to the diet is an absolute necessity for anyone attempting to regain good health. Eat plenty, but not to satiate. The above elimination regime should be followed whenever a person changes from the old ways of living and begins to eat right. Also, it is wise to follow the elimination regime: As a general cleanser two or three times a year; whenever a cold appears; if a fever sets in; when reduction of weight is desired; when hips get too large; when joints get stiff; if constipation is present; if you have any symptoms of catarrh. When you finish the above regime, be sure to always use one of my transition diets.

Transition Diets

After being on a fast or juice diet, it is necessary to come back onto a regular regime gradually in order to get the full benefit from this period without food. We give two transition diets here. Either may be used after a two- or three-day fast or elimination period on ruices with a bulk cleanser. When one has been on a water fast for a longer period, it is advisable to make the transition more slowly as suggedted in the seven-day transition diet.

The Three-day Transition

First day:
Vegetable or fruit juice, one glass every two hours.

Second day:
Breakfast: Steamed dried fruit, or fresh fruit in season.
10:00 A.M. Glass of vegetable juice.
Lunch: Finely shredded carrot steamed for three minutes.
3:00 P.M. Glass of vegetable juice.
Dinner: Finely shredded carrot steamed for three minutes; one cooked vegetable.

Third Day:
Breakfast: Steamed dried fruit, or fresh fruit in season.
10:00 A.M. Glass of juice.
Lunch: One cooked vegetable; fruit or vegetable salad.
3:00 P.M. Glass of juice.
Dinner: Fruit or vegetable salad; one cooked vegetable; cottage cheese.

The Seven-day Transition

First day:
One glass of juice every three hours — ½ pineapple juice and ½ water. (If diabetic, take ½ grapefruit juice and ½ water.)

Second day:
Glass of carrot juice every two hours.

Third day:
Breakfast: Steamed dried fruit, or fresh fruit in season.
10:00 A.M. Glass of vegetable juice.
Lunch: Finely shredded carrot steamed

	for three minutes.
3:00 P.M.	Glass of vegetable juice.
Dinner:	Finely shredded carrot steamed for three minutes; raw fruit.

Fourth day:

Breakfast:	Diced orange and/or steamed dried apricots.
10:00 A.M.	Juice of any kind, vegetable preferred.
Lunch:	One cooked vegetable; a fruit salad.
3:00 P.M.	Juice of any kind, vegetable preferred.
Dinner:	Vegetable salad, sour cream, or yogurt dressing; one cooked vegetable; a baked potato.

Fifth day:

Breakfast:	Diced orange and/or steamed dried apricots.
10:00 A.M.	Juice of any kind, vegetable preferred.
Lunch:	One cooked vegetable; fruit salad; yogurt.
3:00 P.M.	Juice of any kind, vegetable preferred.
Dinner:	Vegetable salad; one cooked vegetable; cottage cheese.

Sixth day:
Same as fifth day except add an egg yolk to breakfast menu.

Seventh day:
Regular diet.

Diet for Hypoglycemia

On arising:	Medium orange, half grapefruit, or juice.
Breakfast:	Fruit, one egg (two slices of ham or bacon, optional), one slice of bread or toast with plenty of butter, milk, decaffeinated coffee or *weak* tea made with a tea bag (not brewed).
Two hours after breakfast:	Four ounces of juice.
Lunch:	Meat, cheese, or fish, salad (lettuce, tomato, raw vegetable, with mayonnaise or French dressing made without sugar), vegetables, one slice of bread or toast with plenty of butter; sugar-free dessert; beverage.
Three hours after lunch:	One glass of milk.

One hour before dinner:	Four ounces of juice.
Dinner:	Soup, if desired (not thickened with flour), vegetables; liberal portion of meat, fish, or poultry; one slice of bread, if desired; sugar-free dessert; beverage.
Two to three hours after dinner:	One glass of milk.
Every two hours until bedtime:	Juice, nuts, cheese, or milk.

Allowable vegetables: Asparagus, beets, broccoli, brussels sprouts, cabbage, carrots, cauliflower, celery, cucumber, eggplant, onions, radishes, squash, string beans, tomatoes, turnips.

Allowable fruits: Apricots, avocados, berries, grapefruit, melons, oranges, peaches, pineapple, tangerines. May be raw or cooked, with or without cream, but *without sugar*. Canned fruits must be without sugar.

Juices: Any unsweetened fruit or vegetable juice except grape juice or prune juice.

Beverages: Weak tea, Postum, Sanka. May be sweetened with saccharine. Sugarless soft drinks, except colas, whiskey, and other distilled liquors.

Avoid absolutely: Sugar, candy, and other sweets, pie, cake, pastries, sweet custards, puddings, ice cream. Caffein and cold beverages. Peas, potatoes, rice, corn, grapes, raisins, plums, pears, figs, apples, dates, bananas. Spaghetti, macaroni, noodles, and other pasta. Cream sauces and gravies made with flour. Wines, cordials, cocktails, and beer.

Stomach Ulcers

Causes of stomach ulcers are many. Chronic constipation is really the beginning of ulcerous conditions, whether they are of the stomach, skin, bone, or any organ of the body. The clogging of the lower colon delays the passage of the food along the stomach tract.

Prolapsed organs cause acid puddles to remain in the stomach, which stagnates food and irritates and inflames the stomach walls. Over a period of years this causes stomach ulcers. Constant purging with drugs is positively harmful in all cases of ulcers.

Many people are constipated. To discover whether or not you are having the proper elimination, swallow a few charcoal tablets before a meal and watch for their elimination. Your breakfast should not stay in the body any more than 13 to 15 hours, your lunch 17 to 20 hours, and dinner 15 to 20 hours.

Blood will not absorb toxins and poisons that are damaging to the body if elimination is regular. A bulky fruit and vegetable diet is nature's own regulator, and we can have this according to the irritation that our stomachs will tolerate.

Dr. Manville of the University of Oregon Medical School placed a number of white rats on a diet deficient in vitamin A, which is not found in devitalized foods. He made a careful note of the effect upon the stomach lining, and he found that nearly two-thirds of all the animals fed on this diet developed dangerous stomach sores. At the end of the test nearly 100 percent of the rats were found to be suffering from ulcers.

Dr. S. Bergman reported after working for years in Abyssinia that most of the natives suffer from ulcers. He traced this condition to the native habit of using pepper sauces at every meal. Most of their meals consist of sour bread drowned in this stomach destroyer that is 50 percent cayenne pepper. Meat, peas, and beans supply the rest of their diet, which is insufficient to counteract the formation of stomach ulcers. *Condiments definitely cause irritation of the stomach.* You wouldn't put pepper in an open sore, would you?

In the past, milk seemed to be the ideal diet for stomach ulcers. However, I am not interested in just allaying inflammation and relieving you of pain; I am interested in building a new stomach. We must try to accomplish three things:

1. Rest the stomach and allay inflammation.
2. Restore mineral and vitamin content to the body.
3. Promote regular elimination of waste.

In severe cases, following a hemorrhage, for instance, it is best to use nothing other than a vegetable alkalinizing liquor. Follow this with a combination of raw goat milk and soaked peeled dates. The milk should be diluted half and half with water, and the dates should be soaked overnight, then peeled before eating. Eat three dates and a half glass of milk every hour and a half. In severe cases follow this regimen for three days, then increase the amount of food to one glass and four or five dates every three hours, with vegetable liquor in between.

Enemas must be taken morning and night. Sun bathe, if possible, every day to build up the calcium of the body. Stay away from bicarbonate of soda, for this only relieves hyperacidity. (When Valentine Ross made bicarbonate of soda for washing soda in 1801, he didn't realize that he was developing one of the worst ulcer-producing habits of mankind.) In severe cases it is best to be under the direct supervision of a doctor.

After extreme inflammation has subsided, you can take soft sweet fruit, stewed fruit mashed through a sieve, well-cooked vegetables, vegetable broths with a little cream in them, spinach toast, raw meat juice from young beef, and an occasional egg. Eat often in small amounts. One food at a time is best. Add one of the above to the regular regimen each day— but don't add everything new the first day. Well-beaten egg whites in food or drinks fifteen or twenty minutes before lunch and supper is good. Also helpful are buttermilk, toast of stale graham bread scalded with boiling water and eaten with a little cream, pigeon (it yields up its phosphates easily), parsley, and diluted parsley juice. When you get to the place where you are having a variety of meals and a goodly amount of food, try the following suggestion:

Eat Every Hour and a Half: No seeds— no peelings— no skins.

8:30 A.M.
Soy milk and dried fruits (steamed or pureed), or milk and dates (soaked and peeled).

9:30 A.M.
Veal joint broth or raw vegetable juice with milk and plain gelatin.

11:00 A.M.
Egg yolk and pineapple juice with beaten egg white on top.

1:30 P.M.
Cooked carrots and veal joint broth or vegetable broth and gelatin.

3:00 P.M.
Stewed peaches or stewed apricots (or water-packed fruit) with milk, if desired.

4:30 P.M.
Prune juice or fig juice or vegetable juice and milk or yogurt and apple concentrate.

6:00 P.M.
Spinach or beet greens pureed and served on soy toast. Baked potato and pureed vegetable.

7:30 P.M.
Vegetable liquor, raw vegetable juice, and soy milk or raw milk.

9:00 P.M.
Milk and dates (date milkshake), four dates to a glass of milk.

Take one tablespoon of gelatin three times daily. Take a duodenal substance every two hours for the first week then reduce to three times daily.

Take daily enemas of one teaspoon powdered whey to one pint of water. Take bulk-forming powders, if necessary.

Later begin to add other things to your diet, such as baked apple with cream or nut butters in fruit or fruit juices. Eat pureed soybeans, lima beans, peas, etc., with any other vegetable during the diet also. Avocados and an omelet may be added at this time also. Use plenty of fruit juices, such as cherry, apple, and prune juice after the diet regimen is underway. No citrus fruits.

Sometimes using a teaspoon of olive oil every two hours will help these conditions. But remember: all this is not a whole remedy and you should be under a doctor's care.

From this limited stomach ulcer diet, gradually work up to a bland diet that is based on the Balanced Daily Eating Regimen. (Choose only bland foods.)

Nervous Indigestion

The mind has an enormous influence over the body. Scientists observed this years ago. Using various animals, such as cats and dogs, they gave them enough barium with their meals that the digestive organs could be clearly outlined. Under the fluoroscope, the animal's stomach and bowel could be observed operating quite smoothly. But the moment the animal was frightened (as a cat might be by the presence of a dog in the room), a marked change would occur. The digestive organs would cease their operations. The normal peristaltic movements of the stomach and intestines would stop— a clear indication of the effect of emotional stress on the digestive tract.

The same thing happens to human beings.

Much of the digestive distress of which many people complain arises from nervous tension. This applies not only to adults, but also to little children. Nervous stress within the family is a common cause of dyspepsia and digestive upsets. Such conditions may be temporarily relieved by taking pills, but they will not be cured by medicines. Only by smoothing out the annoying situation will the condition be fully solved.

Bland Food Diet
(For Colitis, Spastic Bowel, Ulcers, Gas)

A program in which the whole body is fed is the foundation of good health. When we cannot take the foods necessary for health in their normal form and are using the blender as an aid, we must not forget that a balanced daily eating regimen is still required. It is no use living on milk and mush to soothe stomach ulcers while starving the rest of the body. Good health depends on balanced nutrition. When we are sick, we often have to favor a weak organ, but we cannot neglect all the other needs of the body.

Here is a program in which we are following the dietetic law of balanced eating and using the blender almost exclusively. Do not forget that *chewing well* is necessary for a healthy body. Even though the food is liquefied, it must be chewed to mix with saliva.

Using the following foods raw, in liquefied salad form, wherever possible; if necessary, have them cooked and liquefied; or cooked, liquefied, and then strained for severe colitis or ulcer cases.

People on a bland diet usually don't get all the variety that healthy people do. Have daily four to six vegetables, two fruits, one starch, and one protein, with juices or liquids between meals.

Daily Menu

Before Breakfast:	On rising, take any natural, unsweetened fruit juice.
Breakfast:	Fruit (protein or starch)
10:30 A.M.	Liquid or fruit
Lunch:	Two vegetables (one starch), tea or drink
3:30 P.M.	Fruit juice, tea or fruit
Dinner:	Two vegetables (one protein), tea or drink
Fruit Juice Suggestions:	Black cherry, fig, grape, prune, papaya, pineapple. Do not eat starch and protein together. Eat them at separate meals.

Reducing Diets

These diets should be followed for two weeks. Then return to the Balanced Daily Eating Regimen for two weeks. Alternate three or four times according to weight loss.

The meats used may be lamb, fish, lean beef, turkey, chicken. Never have fats or pork. Bake, broil, or roast fish and meat. The fish should be a white fish (one that had fins and scales).

Always use tomato (sliced and ripe—use canned only in an emergency) or grapefruit when you eat meat or fish.

If you do not use meat, then use the other proteins: eggs, cottage cheese, gelatin mold, skim milk, soy milk, soy tofu, lo-fat yogurt.

All vegetables should be from the five percent carbohydrate list (see below).

Drink in-between meals only. This should be one hour before or two hours after meals. Cleaver tea (two cups daily).

Five Percent Carbohydrate Vegetables

Artichokes	Chicory
Asparagus	Cucumber
Beet Greens	Dandelion
Broccoli	Eggplant
Brussels sprouts	Endive
Cabbage	Escarole
Cauliflower	Leeks
Celery	Lettuce
Chard	Mushrooms
Mustard greens	Spinach
Okra	String beans
Radishes	Swiss chard
Rhubarb	Tomatoes
Sauerkraut (not	Turnip tops
canned)	Vegetable marrow
Sea kale	Watercress
Sorrel	
Sprouts (alfalfa,	
mung, etc.)	

Regular Reducing Diet

Suggested eating plan for one week.

Breakfast: One fresh fruit; one or two eggs or cottage cheese
Lunch: Brown rice; one vegetable and salad
Dinner: Meat or fish with tomato or grapefruit, one vegetable (if desired)

Other meal suggestions for regular reducing diet. Skim milk; one tablespoon of sesame seed meal, 1/3 avocado, and one fruit. Liquefy.

Skim milk; watercress or romaine lettuce (liquefy), or salad with fish and tomato. (Or use four - six watercress tablets per meal.) Fruit and cheese. Apples and cottage cheese

You may use rice cakes or Rye krisp once in awhile.

Bananas are a reducing starch. There are four starches that I consider using: millet, rye, yellow cornmeal, and brown rice.

Strict Reducing Diet

Use Only This Menu:
Breakfast: One fresh fruit; one or two eggs
Lunch: Vegetable; salad
Dinner: Meat or fish with tomato or grapefruit

Many people can use this diet for a whole month, others less. It is best to be under a doctor's care.

Vegetarian Reducing Diet
Follow this diet for two weeks. Then, return to the Balanced Daily Eating Regimen for two weeks. Alternate.

Bulk Program for Cleansing

This program is best done under a doctor's supervision. It is a good elimination program to carry out at home any time. You are going to be on juices for the first three days. Acceptable juices are apple juice, pineapple juice, grape juice, and carrot juice. Have carrot juice at 10:00 A.M. and 3:00 P.M. You may have a different juice each time. Apple concentrate or black cherry concentrate can be used. You may use a liquid chlorophyll drink in place of any of the juices at any time.

First Three Days. Do not take any food supplements. Take one teaspoonful of bulk in a glass of juice five times during the day. After each glass of juice, with bulk added, take a glass of water. Do not eat any food. (A good way to mix the bulk with the juice is to put them into a container, seal, and shake.) Take enema daily for six days, as long as bulk is being taken.

Fourth Day.
Do not take any food supplements.

Breakfast: Fruit, fresh in season, or steamed dried fruit.

10:00 A.M.	Glass vegetable juice or fruit juice.
Lunch:	Finely shredded carrots, steamed for three minutes only.
3:00 P.M.	Glass of vegetable juice or fruit juice.
Dinner:	Finely shredded carrots, steamed for three minutes only, and one other lightly cooked vegetable.

Take one teaspoonful of bulk in glass of juice or water, followed by a glass of water, three times daily.

Fifth and Sixth Days

Do not take any food supplements.

Breakfast:	Fruit.
10:00 A.M.	Juice of any kind.
Lunch:	One cooked vegetable and a fruit or vegetable salad.
3:00 P.M.	Juice of any kind.
Dinner:	One cooked vegetable, cottage cheese, and fruit or vegetable salad.

Take one teaspoonful of bulk in glass of juice or water, followed by a glass of water, three times daily.

Seventh Day

Take supplements, if prescribed.
Regular daily eating regimen.

Ask doctor if bulk and enemas should be continued and consult your doctor for further advice any time you have problems with this program.

Cleansing Grape Diet

If America were not squeezing millions of gallons of perfectly good grapes for liquor, thousands of suffering citizens might be cured of various ailments, and many diseases might be prevented, by merely taking an annual "grape fast." For centuries the cleansing property of grapes has been known in Europe, but it is only in recent years, since publishing of *The Grape Cure* by Dr. Johanna Brandt (of Africa) that is has become generally known in this country.

In America it is used as an elimination diet for various ailments. Doctors and patients report that the grape diet eliminates amazing quantities of impurities. If we cleansed the body at intervals, serious diseases would not develop.

In Europe before the war, hundreds flocked to the grape-growing districts of central Europe during the grape season and took "the cure." Several distinguished Americans

went to France every summer and underwent a grape cleansing. A friend of mine was passing on a bus through the French grape-growing districts. She noted a heavy fragrance and inquired of the driver what it was. "It's grapes," he said. "This is the grape season, and every hotel, boarding house and even private home is filled with people taking the grape cure."

Emphasis is being place on the "American stomach." This so called stomach is the result of our tense living. We go at top speed on business and pleasures from early morning until late at night. With most Americans, it is thrills, thrills, thrills!

When muscles are tense, the functions of digestion and elimination are inhibited. The peristaltic movement and all the processes of digestion and elimination are halted. The result is accumulation of poisonous matter in the intestines that will eventually cause disease if the body is not cleansed.

A clean body is a healthy body. A healthy body is not subject to infection, and it is normal in weight. If everyone would take a yearly cleansing, there would be no "bay windows" or big hips, and youth would be prolonged.

California is noted for its delicious grapes. If the benefits of the grape diet were given proper publicity by the grape growers, many tourists would travel to California to take "the grape cure."

Almost everyone can profit by the grape diet. Here's how to make it work best:

Enemas should be taken once or twice daily for the first week of dieting. Don't use laxatives or drugs. If possible have marathon bath or hydrotherapy treatments to aid in elimination. Continue skin brushing and moderate sun bathing throughout the grape cure.

Get plenty of sleep; frequent a congenial environment. Avoid heavy exertion, *but* exercise daily as prescribed and practice slant board exercises twice daily.

Eat three to five pounds of dark-skinned grapes daily. Concord, Fresno Black Beauty, or even Muscat or Malaga grapes are preferable to Thompson Seedless or Lady-finger. Skins and seeds may be eaten, but not too many seeds if any irritation exists. Grape juice may be drunk along with the grapes. Eat approximately five grape meals per day.

If you tire of grapes, change to one day of raw salads or different kinds of fruit. Try a glass of grapefruit juice occasionally. You should enjoy the grapes to reap the greatest good.

Should a crisis develop, get professional advice immediately.

Before going back to a regular diet, first eat raw fruits every other meal for about two days. Next eat raw vegetable salads every other meal for about two days. Next eat raw vegetable salads every other meal one day more unless otherwise directed. In any unusual condition, it is good to be under a doctor's supervision. Then follow my Balanced Daily Eating Regimen.

The grape diet will not make you weak. You should gain strength. However, almost everyone goes through an eliminative process. In such cases, your energy will be temporarily taken away and what is inside and doesn't belong will be cast off, sometimes with miserable effects. But whatever symptoms you may go through, you have gone through them before at some period of your life. What is actually happening is a breaking down of chronic settlements in your body into an active acute eliminative condition. This purification process is the only means of actually making a correction, whether it be through following the grape diet or following any other natural food regimen.

Internal Water Treatment

In the morning water treatment is very effective:

Take two or three glasses of warm water before breakfast as follows: Take first glass of water ½ hour before breakfast. Ten minutes later take second glass of water; the third glass of water should be taken 10 minutes later.

You may use one teaspoon of liquid chlorophyll in one of the glasses of water. Also, in place of one glass of water you may take a health tea.

This water treatment flushes the kidneys and genita-urinary tract. It helps to move the gas and promote a natural bowel movement.

Exercise and warm water should be taken before breakfast. Stay on your regular health-building diet. The water is just in addition to regular meals. This water treatment should be taken for one month.

Table Supplements

Use about a quarter teaspoon a day of Nova Scotia dulse if the doctor advises and you desire (high in iodine). Use one teaspoon

of rice polishings daily high in vitamin B and silicon. Use one tablespoon of wheat germ daily (high is vitamin E). All these can be mixed with morning cereals.

If you are constipated, or your bowels are irregular, use one or two teaspoons each meal of ground flaxseed meal. Be sure you drink water with this; otherwise it will stick in your throat.

Vegetable Juices

Vegetable juices should be taken twice a day, at 10:00 A.M. and at 3:00 P.M. For those on regular health-building regimens, raw vegetable juice is a good substitute for raw vegetable salads if one is desired.

Vegetable juice diets are also good, in some cases. Juices are taken every two hours. Get specific instructions and orders from your doctor. One teaspoon of liquid chlorophyll in a glass of water is equal to one glass of raw vegetable juice.

Special Broth for Sick People

Take four to five vegetables. Liquefy. Bring to a boil. Add soy milk powder and simmer three or four minutes. Strain. This is my special life-giving broth.

Normalizing Weight

If you are concerned with gaining or losing weight, remember it is more important to have a healthy body than to be a few pounds over or under the standard weight chart. No one knows how much you should weigh. The weight chart is made from the average weights of heavy and thin people of the same age. However, no two people are alike. Your parents may be thin or tall or fat or broad-chested or thin-legged or bony or nervous or one of many possible types. The old saying that an apple cannot be any better than the tree from which if fell holds true in than the tree from which it fell holds true in the human family as well. You cannot make a race horse out of a dray horse, neither can you, by diet, change a person's complete basic structure. A good way to determine if you are proportioned right is to stand in front of a mirror and notice the curves of the body. When they are smooth and well rounded, your weight is probably normal. However, when there is a big bulge around the hips or flabby hanging flesh on the arms, your weight is not correct and your health is not good.

Work to normalize the functions of every organ in the body, and the weight normalizes itself. The same applies to gaining weight. Start a "right living" program and nature automatically adjusts you without further assistance.

When you are underweight, do not live on watery and eliminative foods to the exclusion of other foods. When you are overweight, do not indulge exclusively in rich, concentrated foods, even though they are natural.

Overweight

Exercise is the best tonic. Say "No" to the second helping of food. Keep the bowels open, learn to swim—and swim. Take Nova Scotia dulse tablets daily, three or four a day. Take the Eleven-day Elimination Diet. Go on a heavy protein diet. Eat plenty of greens and liquid foods. Stay away from fatty and starchy foods.

Get a high protein supplement to use along with the fruit juice and use that as a meal. Skip one meal a day until you bring yourself down to normal weight, making sure you have a well-balanced diet. Many can get good re sults by eating wisely at breakfast and supper, then eating only one tablespoon of cottage cheese and two prunes for lunch daily for one month. A lunch of just yogurt and fresh fruit is also very good, or select a low-calorie diet from the vegetable kingdom.

Try exercising in a sweat shirt and perspire. If you do perspire a lot, or if the body needs a lot of sodium, take about four okra and four celery tablets with each meal.

For obesity (fluid and hydric), use vegetable broth powder or seasoning, dry food, bran bread, chlorine and potassium foods, a dry climate, and stony soil.

Those with weight problems usually need a chlorophyll supplement. Also use watercress, which is high in potassium salts, and use alfalfa tea.

There are four reducing starches that can help you have starches but will not put on weight. They are rye, millet, rice, and yellow cornmeal. Wheat puts on weight and rye puts on muscle.

An herb tea combination that helps with losing weight is chickweed, licorice, saffron, gotu kola, mandrake, echinacea, black walnut, hawthorne, and fennel.

Epsom salts baths also may be taken once or twice a week to help you reduce unless they prove too weakening. Use about three cups of Epsom salts to the average bath water. Five to seven minutes is long enough or until the body has begun to perspire. Always follow these baths with a cold towel treatment, then with a brisk rubdown. The Epsom salts, plus the water, eliminates toxic wastes as well as weight.

Follow the Eleven-day Elimination Regime. In most cases that gives a loss of weight of from five to ten pounds. Omit all bread and use Rye krisp in its place.

Follow the Balanced Daily Eating Regime after the elimination regime. Eat no more than one slice of bread a day, if you eat bread at all. Drink no milk. When using cream, dilute it with water. Eat only a fruit breakfast and work for the healing crisis or purification process. Use the skin tonic bath. Always leave the table a little hungry. Do daily exercises and eat plenty of fruit and vegetable salads. There are times when glandular foods will help in losing weight.

There is one exercise that works better than all others for losing weight: Before each meal, place both hands on the edge of the table and push away.

Underweight

To gain weight, go through a cleansing process by following the Eleven-day Elimination Regime. Then follow with the Balanced Daily Eating Regime. Play every day. Hike, swim, or exercise, at least one hour daily. Exercising in the open air is a necessity in gaining weight. All trouble, cares, and worries must be forgotten. Sometimes our nervous systems burn up our food faster than it can be turned into sturdy tissue. Picture yourself as the filled-in jovial, "happy-go-lucky" fellow that you would like to be. Get plenty of sleep by going to bed at nine o'clock at night. Cut down mental activity and eyestrain. If you are nervous, use deep breathing exercises.

Place a hot water bottle on stomach each night for entire night. Wear a red flannel belt next to skin all night long (to draw blood to abdomen for better digestion).

Eat weight building foods: bananas, sunflower seed meal, soy milk, and dried fruits with stewed fruit, goat milk, and soy milk between meals. Take flaxseed tea before each meal (one cup).

Weight loss often indicates a vitamin A deficiency. Parsley and carrots are rich in vitamin A.

Typical Meals for Gaining Weight. Baked potatoes with butter, spinach, and other cooked vegetables. Omelet, baked carrots, custard, and salads. Drink a glass mixed with one-half goat's milk and one-half water. Use the Balanced Diet Eating Regime as a base. Use cream on fruits in the morning. A combination of celery, apples, and cottage cheese or goat cheese is a good weight builder; or combine celery, nuts, and dried fruits, such as raisins, dates, and figs. Sometimes glandular foods are necessary to add to the regular meals. Seek professional advice regarding glandular foods.

Never consume calories without vitamins. Ice creams, doughnuts, and pastries may be fattening, but there is nothing healthy about this kind of weight. Get on the regular Balanced Daily Eating Regime with a bias toward the weight-building foods. Have a good whole-grain cereal for breakfast. Put a little flaxseed meal, sunflower seed meal, dulse, and rice polishings on it, and cream or butter. Have a glass of goat milk or buttermilk.

Choose more from the sweet and dried fruits; citrus fruits are for slimming. Take a spoonful of nut butter with them. Have between-meal snacks of nut milk or sesame drinks, using carob, dried fruits, banana, or honey for flavoring. Take a dish of yogurt with fruit. A small whole grain sandwich with stuffed celery sticks occasionally will help. Rich cocktails of fruit or vegetable juices with an egg yolk and other supplements added will help, or a drink of milk with fruit and cheese. On your lunch salad use a cream or oil dressing, sometimes adding an egg yolk. Favor more of the root vegetables, but don't neglect the greens! Choose a cream or legume soup or a soup thickened with barley or whole rice. Nibble on raw nuts, sunflower, and pumpkin seeds at odd moments. Don't skimp on proteins. Drink cocktails with a flaxseed tea base. Before bed a hot carob-milk drink is permissible.

One cup of flaxseed tea twenty minutes before each meal also helps in gaining weight. Rather than use fresh fruit juice in drinks, use reconstituted dried fruits with soybean milk, nut butter, etc. When using raw vegetable juices add one tablespoon sunflower seed meal or one tablespoon sesame seed meal so the drink will add weight to the body.

Weight-gaining is not all food. Get plenty of exercise. Sleep and rest is especially important if you are the thin, worrying type.

Live as much as possible out in the open air and sunshine.

The best weight-building foods are bananas, sunflower seed meal, soy milk, and dried fruits.

Signs of a Good Chemically Balanced Body

Everyone knows what disease looks like. These are signs of health:

General appearance of good health.

Active, alert, vigorous.

Skin clear, smooth, soft, slightly moist, and somewhat pink.

Weight proportionate to age and height; a pleasing carriage.

Hair plentiful, lustrous, having no indication of being brittle or excessively dry.

Eyes bright and clear with no dark rings or circles under them.

Muscles firm and strong. Chest broad and deep.

Tongue pink and not coated. Breath sweet. Posture straight and upright. Nerves steady. Joints limber, free from deposits and stiffness.

Organs working perfectly without sensations of heat, cold, pain, soreness, fatigue, uneasiness, heaviness, swelling, or pressure.

Body willing to do things, can do them, and the person is glad to be alive.

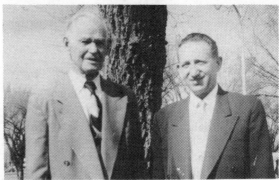

A visit with Dr. George W. Heard in his 92nd year was truly a highlight in my life. Our conversation about natural foods and their relation to teeth confirmed by work with many thousands of patients.

Tonics and remedies

TWENTY TWO

THIS PORTFOLIO is made up for quick reference to the various tonics and remedies. More detailed information on many of these remedies will be found elsewhere in the book.

The doctor and patient must work together effectively. In the very near future, patients will have to have teaching sessions where they are taught how to live correctly because 75 percent of healing lies with the patient, not with what the doctor does for his patients. *The main purpose of my work and teaching is to help a person to have new tissue, not just to control symptoms.* The pathway of life we take determines what kind of a body we have. The body is a servant to the mind and the spirit, to the closeness that we have with nature and the habits that we choose to live by. Every moment of our lives is a remedy or a disease for our bodies. Each moment can either break us down or build us up.

Absent-Mindedness—Brain Tonic

Good for people who are suffering from dizziness, lack of memory, and poor decision ability. Fish broths, and the use of the slant-board. The nerve and gland tonics. Make sure that the transverse colon is in good position.

Acidity

Celery and celery juice; yellow dock tea.

Alcoholism

Take rice polishings, the B vitamins, and have a good nutritional program.

Anemia

Anemia calls for quiet deep breathing, proper diet, mountain air, pleasant companions, and release from all emotional strain. Anemic persons lack cobalt, which is found in the highest amount in the skin of the almonds. The best tonic is blackberry and parsley juice, black fig juice (mission figs) and an egg yolk, black cherry juice, all greens, and a higher altitude are also very good for anemia.

Chop vegetable leaves fine and soak in distilled water for a couple of hours. Strain and just drink this liquid all day long instead of water.

Also good are watercress, parsley, grape juice, wheatgrass, and chlorophyll.

Anemia indicates an iron deficiency problem and can be caused by too much cow milk. Pernicious anemia needs folic acid and almond skin (contains cobalt). Use red bone marrow and bone meal. (See chapter on blood.)

Appetite

To curb the appetite, take a tablespoon of flacked banana 20 minutes before eating.

Arthritis

One of the best remedies for arthritis is using the whey of milk. Another good remedy is black mission figs and raw goat milk. If possible, get the derivative from pure cane sugar — this has the antiarthritic factor in it. Lecithin is found to help the pains of arthritis and needs phosphorous to combine it with body. We have also used cherry juice and a cherry drink in arthritic cases for many years. Cherry juice is claimed to be a wonderful preventative for hardening of the arteries. Avoid citrus fruits. Other good remedies are papaya juice, aloe vera juice or poultice, calcium with phosphorous (bonemeal), and a vitamin D supplement as in cod liver oil.

Arthritic joints

Arthritis is in the joints and tendons. Rheumatism is generally in the muscles. For arthritic joints, use one-half pint of alfalfa seed tea per day. Use turnip juice diet.

Arthritic cracking joints

This indicates a sodium deficiency. If

joints are stiff use a hot carrot and wild thyme compress or Epsom salt compress; also try an Epsom salt bath. Massage "Oil of Juniper" into the joint.

Veal joint broth replaces lack of calcium in the body. Also eat green kale and barley broth, bone meal, vegetable soup, nut butter. Add flaked yeast or wheat germ to any of these. Try one teaspoon cod liver oil three times daily.

Arthritic fingers

For people who have arthritic fingers, exercise them where calcium will grate against calcium in the joint structure. When exercising in room temperature, it is best to put them in hot Epsom salt water, allowing the heat to relax the tissues and exercise the hands in this water and not in the air. Doing this ten minutes every day will prove to be a great remedy.

Backaches

One of the finest things to use is sheepskin. This remedy is used in Australia and New Zealand. You can lie on this sheepskin bed. Use one that is bleached and white. Do not get the colored ones.

Bad Breath

This is usually from a bad stomach and poor digestion. It can be handled best by liquid chlorophyll. It also helps to chew cardamon seeds or anise seeds. Whole cloves can also change the atmosphere of the mouth.

Bad breath indicates a deficiency of sodium foods. After you have eaten garlic or onions you can free your breath of the odors by chewing vigorously a small amount of fresh, uncooked parsley. Be sure to swallow the parsley after thorough chewing.

Bad breath has formed the basis of thousands of lines of advertising matter. Its technical name is now a household word, but parsley alone is the safe, satisfactory remedy to be used in an emergency.

Bedwetting

The Sitz bath is one of the most wonderful remedies for bedwetting in children. By sitting in cool water for four or five minutes, and then up to ten minutes, will help to revitalize the bladder and the pelvic organs.

When we start out using the bath every day, it is best to use water that matches body temperature. Each day get a little cooler until the person is able to sit in cold water. You can start in with one minute the first day and finally increasing the length of the stay in the bath. Four or five minutes should be the maximum in very cold water

Bee Stings and Bites

Your own saliva will often take care of this problem. All animals lick their sores and wounds. Also, you can squeeze out the venom and rub in raw onion juice, or use plain mud, or a tomato, onion, or celery poultice. Press an old-fashioned watch key firmly over the spot to force out the venom before rubbing in raw onion juice, or moisten earth and apply as a poultice and secure with a bandage.

Bleeding Bowel

Use chlorophyll, either taken by mouth or as an enema.

Blood Pressure

High blood pressure: This usually indicates too much meat. Use garlic, parsley, and watercress. These have been found to be effective in bringing the blood pressure down. Garlic has been used to kill germs and parasites in the intestinal tract. Combination of capsicum and garlic is very good.

Use these foods for one week and eat nothing else: rice, barley, potato, and yellow cornmeal; dried fruits of all kinds and other fruits such as citrus; vegetables of all kinds fixed in any way; garlic oil capsules. Also, the turnip diet is sometimes very good for high blood pressure; use a skin brush; make tea of comfrey leaves and roots; drink black cohosh tea; go on the rice diet or a fast under close supervision. Stay away from high altitudes and dry climates.

Low blood pressure: Use a high protein diet, protein and tomato combination, amino acids, sunflower seed meal, rice bran syrup, cucumber juice to thin blood. Get exercise.

Blood, Purifier

Use burdock and nasturtium juice.

Blood, to Build

Use calcium and iron foods.

Boils and Pus

Take silicon supplement and iron supplement. Use potato peels as potassium broth; use potato pack; use aloe vera juice or poultice. Boils may be brought to a head by using onion poultice. Bran packs contain silicon and are very good on boils, pimples, and eczema. Boils and acne indicates sulphur deficiency.

Felon (A painful abcess on a finger or toe near the nail): Use vinegar poultice, put finger in lemons, or use a lemon poultice. (Stick the finger in a lemon, tying it on and keep it on all night.)

Bone Tonics

Take green kale soup, green kale raw juice, barley broth, raw goat milk, goat cottage cheese, Biost.

Bone disease (structure): Use organic calcium, organic iodine, and clay packs. Take calcium foods.

Bone fractures: Use comfrey internally and comfrey poultice externally; use sulphur foods and calcium foods.

Bone knitter: Poultice combination of comfrey, golden seal, and slippery elm.

Cartilage problems: Take sodium and chlorine supplements.

Breastfeeding

Babies store iron from mother in their blood in the last few days of breastfeeding to provide for the next six months. Using one tablespoon of molasses in milk is a wonderful drink for the young children to make up iron deficiencies. To increase lactation use a diet with greens, chlorophyll is a good source of iron. To stimulate and increase mother's milk, use borage and alfalfa. If breast becomes caked, use hot and cold application of tomato poultice.

Brown Spots on Hands and Skin

This is often caused by malfunctioning of liver and can be helped by taking a calcium supplement. Also, rub aloe vera juice on spots.

Bruises

Take vitamin C supplement. Use strong tincture of cayenne pepper with an equal amount of glycerine to remove discoloration, then hot packs and cold packs or use comfrey packs.

Burns

Use salt water or moistened salt. Also try a flaxseed (or linseed) poultice.

Car Sickness

Massage web of hand between thumb and finger for five minutes.

Catarrh Tonic

One-half lemon in one-half glass of water with one-half teaspoon of pure cream of tartar, ten minutes before meals for one month. Practice balanced living.

Choking

Raise the left arm above the head as high as possible.

Circulation

Use foot baths, skin brushing, exercise, pleasurable activities; walk barefooted in the sand. Dwarf elder root tea is the best for all elimination organs. Use vitamin F; take iron foods.

Clay Packs

We have used mositened clay for various conditions in the body and have had very good results with sprains, arthritis, eyestrain back of neck tension, over the abdomen for extreme gas, and for many skin disorders. Bentonite is one of the finest of all clays if it is possible to get it. It is mined out of the ground and is one of the finest healers. The Luvos mud was used extensively by Father Kneipp and in many of the German sanitariums.

Colds and Coughs

Take hot drinks, sage tea, baked lemon in hot water, vegetable broths, enemas daily, and lots of rest. If a cough develops, use the onion and honey cough syrup recipe: Over a chopped-up onion pour one tablespoon of honey. Let stand four hours. Use one teaspoon of the juice every one-half to one hour.

Try onion packs on the neck and chest: slice a large onion, place in small pan, cover tightly (use no fat or water). After onions are hot, simmer in own juices. Put hot onions in muslin bag or cloth and fold to cover area to be treated. Prepare second onion pack. Use alternate packs until pack cools (about five minutes) and continue application for one-half hour a day.

Herb teas to try include a combination of comfrey and fenugreek; thyme; angelica; violet; and comfrey leaves and roots. Or flood the system with onions and garlic for two days, along with vegetable broths.

Cold Sores (Canker Sores)

Usually called stomach sores, these may well be from stomach upsets. Take a maximum dosage of calcium lactate tablets, three times a day over a period of a couple of months. Cold sores are also a sign we are lacking in vitamin B. Many times we can use a rice bran syrup to overcome this vitamin B deficiency.

Colic

Chamomile tea is a wonderful tonic for all ages. It is a tonic and an antispasmodic and can be used in nervous conditions caused by the digestive system. Colic often indicates need for a chlorine supplement. Other herb teas: fennel; aniseed; lovage; mint; savoy-rue; and caraway, both as a tea and as a poultice.

Colic and Cramps

Ginger can be used to help expel gas in cramps and colic and can even be given to children. Peppermint and spearmint tea can be used interchangeably; both are especially valuable for children.

Colitis (Ulcers of Bowel and Stomach)

Take flaxseed tea drinks — one cup ten minutes before each meal. Also good are taro root and seeded bananas, mental rest, ease of mind, inward calm, soft foods, and raw vegetable juices with a little milk or cream in them. Take agar for bulk. Flaxseed tea enemas with liquid chlorophyll added work well. This problem indicates a need for sodium foods. Use comfrey juice and golden seal tea.

Constipation Tonic

Prune juice and lemon when mixed together make a good drink — mix ¾ prune juice with ¼ lemon. Fig juice is a good drink; goat whey or cow whey help to eliminate constipation. Roughage helps some people by adding raw salads to the diet. Never eat starch unless you have vegetables with it. Use aloe vera juice and yellow dock tea. Constipation indicates a need for magnesium, potassium, and sodium foods.

Diabetes

See chapter, "Special Diets for Special People."

Diarrhea

Parch a pint of rice until brown, then pour it over a pint of boiling water. Let it steep and then drink all in one day. Take one to three pints of hot milk five to six times a day, *eaten* with a spoon. Sometimes using rice with cinnamon helps, or sage with boiled milk.

Taro root is a very easily digested starch, soothing to the bowel. Use it especially where bland foods are indicated, or where diarrhea or any bleeding of the bowels has occurred. Taro root is one of the wonder foods of Hawaii.

Digestion Problems

Digestion begins in the mouth. Chew the food very well. Good digestion needs vitamin D from the sun and can be helped by walking in warm sand, then cold water. After meals take savoy and thyme. Use mint and huckleberry tea.

Dysentery (Chronic)

Use yarrow herb tea.

Dyspepsia

Indicates a sodium deficiency. Can be caused by fried foods.

Ear Problems

Hearing sensitivity indicates a calcium deficiency. Infections: use chamomile tea to wash. Ringing in ear indicates a manganese deficiency; also use chaparral tea. Rushing sound indicates manganese and phosphorus deficiency. Buzzing may indicate anemia, high blood pressure, emotional strain, indigestion, or gas in bowel. Use nicotinic acid, vitamin B as found in rice bran syrup, vitamins A and C. Deafness in the morning indicates fluorin deficiency. For an earache use balm herb. Treat the bowel. A drop of garlic juice in each ear is also very good. For general ear infections, the combination of echinacea, golden seal, poke root, and capsicum is very good.

Wax: To remove wax accumulation use glycerine. It is the only oil that mixes with water. Put warmed glycerine in an eye dropper, drop it into the ears, and leave overnight — it will mix with the dissolved wax. In the morning, fill eye dropper with warm water and drop into ears to rinse clear.

Eczema/Scurvy

A homemade ointment for eczema: Use garlic oil or garlic powder mixed with lanolin, or liquid chlorophyll mixed with lanolin. They should be saturated into one another. Go on elimination diet; cleanse the bowel;

use raw vegetable juices. Take air baths; fast. Try a bath using oat straw tea (one gallon to each bath). Use yellow dock tea, vitamin F, tomato packs. The body needs potassium foods. Use lemon and sun-dried olives, watercress, tarragon.

Epilepsy

As in all illnesses, sufferers of epilepsy should be under a doctor's care. This problem can be aggravated by a flickering from movies and TV. It can be caused by bleach in white bread. I have found certain things to be very important: do not use salt. Salt will bring on fits. Epilepsy can sometimes be helped by supervised fast, by using boiled parsley roots, by drinking valerian root and tea.

Eye Tonic

Take carrot juice if the eyes are infected. If eyes or the optic nerve is broken down from strain, use nerve tonics. The best tonic for the eyes is submerging the eyes in cold water two or three times a day. The eyes are an extension of our nervous system and the brain; you must therefore feed the nervous system and the brain in order to feed the eyes. For meat, eat the glands of animals rather than their muscles. We learn something from the meat-eating animal. He does not eat the muscle structure of the animals but leaves that part to the carrion and he eats only the internal organs, such as the stomach, glands, liver, and heart. These are structures that are much better organized in their chemical evolvement; we can use that material to our advantage much better. There is less toxic materials to these inner organs than there is to the muscle structure itself. Much more uric acid is found in the muscle structure than in these internal organs. To use only the muscle structure we are getting only part of the chemicals that our body could use well. Using the brain and the tripe, we find we get some of the most vital mineral elements for our body. Using cod roe is wonderful for building the nervous system.

Other eye foods: Take barley water, oatstraw and caraway teas, goat milk and cheese; Roquefort cheese, blackberry juice, veal joint broth, white fish, leafy vegetables, grapefruit juice.

Night blindness and light sensitivity of eyes: Indicate vitamin A deficiency and potassium deficiency.

Weak eyes: Indicate iron deficiency.

Vision problems: Indicate possible vitamin B deficiency.

Eyes poor in strong light: Indicate a manganese deficiency.

Blood vessels in whites of the eye: Indicate strong drugs, local irritation, or dissipation.

Bluish tint in white of eye: Indicates venous congestion or disease of the genital organs.

Upper eyelids veined or swollen: Indicates heart lesion.

Lower eyelids veined or swollen: Indicates Brights: disease or kidney problems.

Under surface of lower eyelid pale: Indicates anemia or chlorosis.

Whites of eyes red and inflamed: Indicates arterial tension, high blood pressure or dissipation.

Eyeballs, aching: Indicates fluorin deficiency and sodium deficiency.

Eyelids and ankles puffy: Indicates kidney problems.

Styes on eyelids: Indicate intestinal toxins, wrong diet, overeating; a need for glasses; a lack of silicon, calcium, magnesium, and vitamin A.

Protruding eyes: Indicate a toxic thyroid; brain and nerve depletion; deficiency of vitamin A, phosphorus, iodine, chlorine, and sodium.

Dilated pupils: Indicate vitamin B deficiency and fatigue.

Pupils, unsteady and glittering: Indicate too much sulphur.

Dark rings under eyes: Take sulphur foods.

Black spots before eyes: Take sulphur foods.

Discharge from eyes: Use malva juice.

Eye diseases: Use sage flowers.

Eye pack: Use warm goat milk and boric acid mixed in water.

Eye bath: Pour carefully strained chamomile tea over eye. Also drink this herb tea.

Eyes inflamed: Cold application of potato poultice, mashed or liquid; drink flaxseed tea.

Eyestrain: May indicate stomach problems.

Eyes inflamed and watery from smog and smoke: Use one drop of sterilized raw linseed oil from flaxseed in each eye. Eyes need plenty of sleep before midnight.

Cataracts: Indicates excess calcium. Need sodium, iron, sulphur, and phosphorus foods. Use purple lens for glasses.

Glaucoma: Indicates a sodium deficiency, calcium excess, is out of solution.

Fasting

General Rules: Avoid extremes and always fast under close supervision by your doctor. Fast until hunger leaves and then fast until hunger returns.

Fatigue

Indicates iron and phosphorus deficiencies. Take vitamins E and C, and perhaps more protein. Use a slant board.

Energy depletion: Rebuild energy by sun's reflection (sunbath), and by drinking warm goat's milk (fresh from goat). Use proteins, six to eight desiccated liver tablets per day, two vitamin E, four capsuls of soybean oil extract, extra vitamin C, chlorine. In the mornings eat a good lunch; midday eat a good supper; at night eat a good breakfast. Exhaustion in morning indicates too much food at supper. As a builder of resistance, use bone marrow. Hard physical work needs iron, calcium and silicon foods.

Energy herbal pickup; Try a combination of gotu kola, ginseng, and capsicum.

Vitality tonic: Use apple, almond nut butter, and celery juice.

Do not stimulate your body with food or drink when tired. Lie down for ten minutes and you will refresh yourself.

Feet

Hot Epsom salt foot baths are very good.

A hot and cold water foot bath is also good. Spend one minute in hot water and one-half minute in cold. Do this eight times.

Brush soles of dry feet with skin brush. Walk barefooted in sand or in grass daily. Never wear damp socks, damp shoes. Change shoes daily. Do not wear the same shoes all the time. Do not lace shoes too tightly as it can hinder the circulation; never buy too tight a shoe or too short a shoe. Make sure that each shoe fits the foot properly as no two feet are alike.

Sun bath for feet: Feet should be sunned daily.

Callouses on bottom of feet shows a need for calcium.

Athlete's foot: Indicates a manganese deficiency.

Bunions: This can be helped by walking in sand. You can also twist the big toe up and down and in and out in circular action; taking hot Epsom salt foot baths daily and massaging the bunion with wheat germ oil will help.

Carbuncles: Indicate iron deficiency.

Sore feet: This may be relieved by using a tomato poultice.

Ingrown toenails: It is best to cut a V-shaped piece out of the top of the toenail. Cut in towards the center of the nail and let the edges grow. File down the cut edges until smooth. You can keep the nail moist with castor oil. Be sure to walk in the sand or grass each day.

Burning Feet: Use magnesium. May be relieved by a tomato poultice.

Corns: Apply linseed oil to cover them, or tie a piece of lemon over them and leave overnight. Scrape them off in morning.

Cold feet: Indicates iron deficiency and fluorin deficiency.

Swelling: Take nettle herb tea.

Sweating feet: This can be caused by the inactivity of the skin and by indigestion. The proper diet, plenty of iron in the intake of foods, and the skin brush will help, brushing body area and also soles of feet.

Rawness between toes (and fingers): Indicates a manganese deficiency.

Heel pain: Indicates ovary problems.

Fertility Problems

Often indicate vitamin B_1 (thiamine) deficiency.

Many people do not understand that the ovaries of woman and the testicles of man, as the procreative glands in the body, need the same nourishment; however, they are of a different vibratory rate, which develops them into the male and the female— with the different hormones such as the testoterones and the estrogens. When God created man and woman or when there was a separation from the original creation of man, the ovary was placed on the inside of the abdomen while the male glands were placed on the outside. With this natural creation a heat is generated for the ovary that allows it to become different in its activity and expression than the male testicle. We are finding that to have the response as much male and as much female as possible, it is necessary that we keep the heat and the temperature of these different glands as God intended. Many men today are wearing what they call "jockey shorts." These keep an extreme amount of heat around the testicles. With many men just changing from the jockey shorts to the boxer shorts, which permit a cooler environment around these glands, permitted conception where no conception had taken place for many years. In other words, the ovaries of the female need warmth to perform their creative function and the testicles of man need a cooler temperature for fertility.

Fevers

Can be caused by too much silicon. Silicon accelerates the vital processes and facilitates the removal of wastes and toxins from the body.

Cold water towel bath: Bathe only one part of the body at a time. Dry, then do another section. Keep the body covered except for the area being bathed. Use a cool enema; use hot water bottles on the feet. Give no food and drink unchilled grapefruit juice only. Herb teas to use include catnip, fenugreek, parsley seeds, and sorrel.

Flu and fevers: Combination herb tea of fenugreek and thyme.

"Feeding" a fever: Eat nothing during a chill or fever. Drink water or grapefruit juice until the fever has subsided, all pain is gone, and food is desired. Then eat only fruits and vegetables for a few days.

Flatulence/Gas

Sodium foods are excellent remedies for flatulence and gas. Well-beaten egg white in vegetable broths helps gas in many cases. A dry diet is often indicated. Chinese cabbage is good for gas, but try no other varieties of cabbage. Lemon juice in milk can help. Other good remedies are Japanese seaweed, spinach on toast, parsley tea, endive, apricots, okra, celery (okra and celery are available in tablet form), peppermint tea, evaporated sea salt in hot water, milk for putrefaction, and catnip tea. Four drops of oil of peppermint to a cup of hot water will help. Good herb teas are peppermint, chamomile, catnip, sweet flag, anise, caraway, cinnamon, dill, and fennel. Also good are a buttermilk acidophilus cul-

ture, whey, a vegetable diet of simple combinations, dry graham toast, soybean toast, a salt and hot water solution, and magnesium sulphate. If you get gas at night, you may have simply eaten too much food for supper.

Fungus

White iodine will help to kill fungus under fingernails. One of the best natural remedies for fungus is aloe vera, a plantlike cactus, which grows more abundantly in Florida than elsewhere. Apply a piece of aloe vera around the infected finger, bandage, and leave on overnight. (A book has been written on the remedial uses of aloe vera, published by the University of Florida at Jacksonville.)

Gastrointestinal tract

To change the intestinal flora, two of the finest remedies are acidophilus culture and yogurt. Gastritis indicates magnesium deficiency. Gastric ailments need sodium phosphate.

Gall Bladder

Black horseradish is one of the finest remedies for gall bladder disturbances. Sodium and magnesium supplements. Yellow cornmeal is very good. Raphanon is used for draining the gall bladder and is found in radish. Dandelion tea is helpful.

Gall bladder and liver: In cases of constipation, to encourage bowel movement and to help the gall bladder to drain, use beets: Mix one cup finely shredded raw beet, two tablespoons Virgin Cold Pressed Olive Oil, and juice of one-half lemon. Take one teaspoonful of this mixture every one and a half hours during the day for three days. Continue this program three days a week for one month.

Sluggish bile needs sodium foods.

Biliousness: Use juice of two lemons in water with honey. Use sodium sulphate.

Gallstones

Formed from deficiency in sodium and sodium sulphate, from excessive nitrogenous supply, from excessive lime diet. We find that milkweed or bitterroot is a good tonic and a slight laxative. Teas of cornsilk, slippery elm, celery, and parsley are all good. Use goat milk; hot celery broth three to four times per day; vitamin A from carrots; finely shredded beet; olive oil.

Glands

Take seafoods that have either been ground up or made into broth along with parsley juice. This must be mixed with love and joy, happy surroundings, fraternal companions, a soothing environment, light reading, good music, hobbies that fit us.

Use vitamin E, such as adding wheat germ in food and adding one fourth teaspoon powdered Nova Scotia dulse to pineapple drinks.

The glands need iodine and silicon; inactive glands need sodium foods; swollen glands need fluorin.

Adrenals: Are depleted by tension, anger, and hatred. To stimulate, use borage herb tea; need trace mineral tin; use parlsey juice.

Lymph gland system: Needs chlorine foods; herb teas of blue violet, lemon grass, and chamomile.

Pituitary problems: Indicated by fleshy, paunchy hands; use watercress.

Thyroid gland: Needs iodine. Use lettuce and watercress juice; boiled parsley roots and watercress; combination of Irish moss, kelp, parsley and capsicum; clam juice with celery juice or vegetable broth, Nova Scotia dulse tablets, iodine painted on the feet; neck exercises.

Goiter: Put hot oak bark compress over swelling. Use vitamin C. (See recipe for *Hormone Tonic*, this chapter, which is very good for all the glands.)

Good gland tonics: Oat straw tea helps to rejuvenate the glands. Also, take one teaspoon of sesame powder or one teaspoon of sesame seed butter every day.

Gravity Problems
Indicates calcium deficiency.

Hair
One of the best remedies for the hair is alfalfa. If you take alfalfa tablets, you help your hair; if you take alfalfa tea, you help it more; if you use alfalfa sprouts, which are very high in silicon, you will help it the most. For a good growth of hair you must have a relaxed scalp, which will allow good circulation to hair root. Long hair brings serenity and balances us magnetically. Short hair increases nervous tension. Use the slant board to increase circulation and massage. The hair needs blood and greater circulation. It is controlled by the pituitary gland. Cherry juice helps the hair, as do herb teas of oatstraw, caraway, rosemary and sage.

Dry hair: Needs iodine, clam juice drinks; silicon is very important; Nova Scotia dulse (two or three tablets, two or three times a day); North Atlantic fish, lecithin granules, parlsey tablets.

Loose, falling hair: Use beaten egg yolk with one-fourth teaspoon sea salt. Apply to the scalp. Leave on for 20 minutes and then rinse with apple cider vinegar. This is your shampoo, using iodine and silicon supplements.

To help scalp circulation: Eat onions, horseradish, and sulphur foods; eat honey, celery, and Concord grape juice.

Scales (psoriasis): Indicates a silicon deficiency.

Dandruff: Rinse hair with rosemary tea.

Fungus: Soak scalp with a combination of sheep fat and garlic oil. Let soak for 20 minutes, then shampoo with Castile soap.

Graying hair: Use parsley juice, one-half glass daily, mixed with celery, pineapple, or apple juice; one or two tablespoons of black strip molasses daily is also helpful. Use thyme extract as a concentrated rinse to help give hair back its natural color.

Baldness can come from demineralized starches. People partly bald have grown heads of hair by rubbing garlic oil well into scalp night and morning. Or pour equal parts of rosemary, bay rum, and olive oil into a bottle, shake well, and rub into the scalp well each night and morning. Baldness indicates an underactive thyroid, and indicates a lack of lecithin, sulphur, iron, and silicon. Also use inositol and vitamin F.

Hands
For detergent hands, massage the hands under heat lamp before going to bed each night. Use camphor ice and unrefined petroleum jelly, the yellow color.

Cold hands and feet: Use sage tea, raw cucumber, and parsley juice. Cold fingers indicate lack of vital energy.

Fingernails: Cracked nails indicate a silicon deficiency. White marks on nails indicates a deficiency in calcium. Add calcium foods. Blue nails indicates a venous condition. Big moons on fingernails indicates good circulation, good oxygenation. A lack of the big moons reveals poor circulation in the extremities.

Hay Fever
Indicates too many starches and proteins. Avoid devitalized foods; alcoholic drinks; refrain from smoking. Indicates an iron deficiency and also needs a chlorine supplement. Use juice made of celery, endive, and

carrot. Use papaya juice or papaya tablets and vitamin F.

Headaches

Dull, heavy, persistent headaches indicate problems with skull bones and periosteum. Headaches can also bring the following symptoms, which are actually caused by digestive problems: confusion, dullness, eyesight problems, hearing problems, bad dreams, insomnia.

Emotional. Indicates excess sulphur
Extreme: Indicates a silicon deficiency.
Frontal: Frontal burning, bursting, head pulsing, and stomach pulsing, indicates sodium deficiency.
Migraine: Use neck traction and stretching.
Head pain at base of skull: (heat and inflammation) too much silicon. *Acute:* Use rue or marjoram tea.
In lower forehead: Needs magnesium spearmint poultice on forehead. Use squaw herb tea. A hot mustard bath for the feet helps.

Heart Troubles

Hawthorne berry tea is the most valuable of all the remedies, especially for elderly people. Hawthorne berry has an affinity for oxygen. Also good combined with capsicum.
Arteriosclerosis: Use whey and vegetable broth; use chlorine foods.
Heart palpitations: Use borage; use valerian root.
Heartburn. Mix one-half teaspoon of lemon, two teaspoons of celery juice— use in water; potassium broth made from olives; chew olives that are sundried; take sodium.
Heart muscles (to strengthen): Take vitamin E, liquid chlorophyll, whole wheat formula in thermos bottle, rice and dried fruit, vegetable diet, lecithin capsules three times a day.
Whole Wheat Formula in Thermos Bottle: ½ cup fresh ground hard northern wheat; 1½ cup hot water.
Put in thermos bottle, cork tightly, and let stand overnight. Use as a cereal in the morning every day for three months. Heart troubles often indicate an iron deficiency problem. Needs whole wheat as a food. Use only natural starches. Use honey.

Urinary-prostate tract cleanser: Herb combination: Kelp, black cohosh, hydrocotyle asiatica (gotu kola), licorice, golden seal, lobelia, capsicum, and ginger.
Nephritis (Inflammation of the Kidneys): Watermelon seed tea is one of the best. Crush two teaspoonsful of the dry seed through the grinder or mortar pestle. Steep the ground seeds in a cup of warm water for an hour. Stir and strain. Drink one cupful four times a day. Basil and marjoram have a wonderful effect on the kidneys and the heart.

Leg Cramps

Apply hot and cold packs to the legs. Try sand walking, bone meal calcium, and cod liver oil — one teaspoon three times daily. Calcium foods which are found in our grains are good; barley and kale broth is very high in calcium. Eat sodium foods. Leg cramps sometimes indicate prostate problems.

Left Side Problems

Usually need more starches in the diet.

Liver

Liver problems are indicated when the white area of eyes becomes blue. Take iodine, silicon, sulphur, and iron foods. Use dandelion greens in the diet. Take black cherry juice— one glass three mornings in succession. Good herb teas: slippery elm, woodruff, and sage. For toxicity, use chlorophyll. For enlargement, use sodium sulphate. Combination to help liver and gall bladder: one cup finely shredded raw beets; two tablespoons olive oil; juice of one-half lemon. Dose: one teaspoon every half hour for three days.
Tonics: Black cherry concentrate and chlorophyll; carrot, beet, and cucumber juice; and radish and pineapple juice.
Herb combination for liver disorder and cleanser: dandelion, red beet powder, liverworth, parsley, horsetail, birch leaves, lobelia, chamomile, blessed thistle, angelica, gentian, golden rod, and golden seal.

Longevity Tonic

Foods that have been grown in mineralized gardens; lots of raw foods or raw juices in the diet. A peaceful heart filled with love.

Lung Troubles

The pine tree has been used as the substance for helping the lungs for many years. It is good to go to the ozone areas where the pines give off an ozone that helps the lung structure. Leaves, pine cones, and pine needles have been put in buckets over hot coals and the person has inhaled the fumes. Many people have claimed results by putting pine needles in a pillow and sleeping on it all night long. See other chapters for the various lung disorders.

Malnutrition

Symptoms are headache, burning eyes, apprehension, pessimism, nausea, and bloodshot eyes. Solution: Get back into God's garden.

Memory Problems and Lack of Concentration

Take Missouri black walnuts with apple cider; lecithin, vitamin B, wheat germ, and foot baths. For these problems, especially after the age of 50, after an operation, or after some emotionally depleting experience, add ribonucleic acid and lecithin to the diet. Use the maximum dosage as given on the bottle or whatever you are taking. This also helps with longevity and helps take care of wrinkles.

Menopause or Change of Life

Try an herb combination of one ounce each of goldenseal, pulsatilla, motherwort, tansy, and blackhaw, and one-half counce of arrach. Place these in one-half quarts of water and simmer until only two pints remain. Strain and cool, taking a water glass of the mixture in an equal amount of water, between meals three times daily. This should be taken two to three months, even a year, until all symptoms begin to disappear.

Hot flashes: It might be good to use an extra amount of vitamin E, sometimes as much as 1,000 to 3,000 units a day for awhile, and then start reducing it until there are no more hot flashes and hot sweats. Also take two Nova Scotia dulse tablets, three times a day. If this does not control these symptoms, seek a doctor's care; he will have to control it with a glandular supplement.

Menstrual Disorders

Elderberry tea is very good for ovarian problems and menstrual disorders. Include iodine foods in the diet, and seek good bowel management. Health drink: Black cherry juice, one egg yolk, one-third cup oat water, and one-half teaspoon Nova Scotia dulse powder. For pain use dill as a tea. For irregular periods, use chlorophyll; sweet marjoram tea. Stimulant: Rosemary tea, sage tea, and saffron tea.

Stoppage: Geranium tea and shepherd's purse tea.

To increase: Sage tea, red clover; horehound leaves, rue and rosemary leaf teas. In general, foot baths and Sitz baths are good, and use the slantboard.

Organ tone: Raspberry leaf tea.

Chlorosis (anemic conditioned characterized by greenish hue of the skin in menstrual disorders): Use balm herb.

Mouth

Cracks in the corners and a sore red tongue indicate need for riboflavin. Dryness of mouth indicates an iodine deficiency; dryness of lips indicate a silicon deficiency. Blisters indicate need for sodium foods. For bad breath or coated tongue use chlorophyll, chew parsley sprigs, eat raw apple between meals. A good mouth wash is shavegrass tea. For mouth ulcers, use sorrel herb tea.

Potassium broth to help muscle weakness is made mostly from greens, adding carrots, celery, and potato for flavoring. Simmer for 20 minutes and then strain off the bulk of the vegetables. Just drink the juice or broth.

Multiple Sclerosis

This is not an easy thing to handle through nutrition; however, we have found that raw vegetable juices, bean sprouts, raw egg yolk, and a diet under strict supervision of a doctor are beneficial, as in all ailments.

Nasal Drip

Use golden seal tea.

Nasal Passages (to open)

Take a peppermint or spearmint cluster, squeeze it, and rub your hands together, then smell your hands. What it does for them, it will do for your entire body. What it will do for the nasal passages alone is unbelievable.

Muscle Weakness

The muscles need iron, potassium, sodium, and chlorine foods. Potassium foods are especially good for building, power, and structure. Learn how to make the potassium broth and take it often. Twitching muscles indicate need for chlorine. General weakness indicates iron deficiency.

Muscle spasms: Use flower of rosemary tea.

Sprains and strains: Take hot Epsom salts bath.

Prolapse organs: Caused by hot foods and drinks overrelaxing intestinal muscles. Can be helped by using a stiff-legged walk on all fours. See slantboard exercises.

Nerve Tonics

Nervous people will find that vegetables are more soothing to their nerves than fruit.

Drink more vegetable juices than fruit juices until the nerves become more steady. Citrus fruits especially tend to keep the nerves on edge; however, this should be temporary, as no healing is complete without the fruits. Take smoked black cod, finian/haddie steamed, fish broths, pineapple juice, one egg yolk, one teaspoon of rice polishings. Warm drinks are very good for tension in the body.

Brain and Nervous System: Stew an ounce each of vervain, valerian, skullcap, and mistletoe in two quarts of water for 20 minutes. When cool, strain and drink half of a small cup three times a day. Eat plenty of onions, raw, if you can digest them, preferably green onions with tops. Egg yolk may be used in liquefied drinks. Wheat bran tonic (called the "staff of life") contains 16 chemical elements and is one of the finest nutrients.

Neuralgia and Neuritis

For neuralgia (acute pain in a nerve) or neuritis (inflammation of a nerve or nerves), use celery juice, okra and celery tablets (two of each with each meal), bone meal, veal joint broth, gelatin, raw apple and celery juice combination; or cucumber and endive juice with whey powder. Herb tea: Motherwort.

Nose Bleeding

Use liquid chlorophyll, one teaspoon in a glass of water three or four times a day; or use gelatin two or three times a day. For frequent occurrences of nose bleeding, make veal joint broth and use over a period of time.

Nose, Red

A red nose indicates a sulphur deficiency. A tendency to pick nose indicates a silicon deficiency.

Pancreas

Needs iodine, silicon, zinc, and colloidal sulphur. If inactive, indicates sodium deficiency. If disturbance exists, eat no bread and use more natural starches and Rye Krisp.

Pellagra

Symptoms are headaches, weakness and depression, reddening and itching of skin, cramps in legs, giddiness, and insomnia. Tongue is red and ulcerous. Use vitamin B complex and turnip greens.

Perspiration

If burning and profuse, indicates manganese deficiency. Cold sweat indicates calcium deficiency and too much potassium. Hot and cold sweats indicate calcium deficiency. General problems need sodium.

Summer foods to use when perspiring freely: cucumbers, okra, celery, strawberries, and vegetable juice. Use one teaspoon of vegetable broth powder in a glass of water. Take celery powder or four celery tablets or four okra tablets with each meal. They are high in sodium. Use silicon and potassium foods and elderflower tea.

Juices: Celery and prune; cucumber and pineapple. Sage is good for night sweats; to bring on a sweat, use red raspberry tea.

Pets

Quite a few people bring their pets to me or write asking if I know of something that would help them. I have found that the use of garlic and grass juice cleans up many a sick animal. The combination of kelp, alfalfa, and dandelion conditions the coat and skin and keeps fleas off pets.

Poison Oak

Poison oak rash is caused by an oil and can spread merely by touching the affected area. Do not take a hot shower; this will really tend to spread it. Keep sunshine, air, and heat away from it so that the oil does not penetrate. I have found no natural remedy for poison oak, but one of my patients says he successfully uses brown laundry soap; another uses impatiens leaf tea; and yet another swears by buttermilk and sea salt, applied as a paste to the affected area.

Pruritus

An itching of the skin with no visible cause. Use horsetail extract.

Psoriasis

Use a blood root extract to paint the affected areas.

Ptomaine Poisoning

Use caster oil with hot lemonade. Check in 20 minutes. Thyme herb tea is very good.

Radiation Exposure

Will often cause vitamin A deficiency. Also use vitamin F.

Rheumatism

Rheumatism is generally in the muscles. Uric acid rheumatism gets better in hot weather and sunlight and worse in cold, damp, windy weather. Chronic building rheumatism is benefited by a sodium diet, heat, salty hot applications, internal use of salty water.

Local vapor baths with massage help thick joints, swollen bones, stiff limbs and muscles, and chronic rheumatism. Vapor baths should range from 98 degrees to 140 degrees. They can be made in many ways, for instance, little stones can be put into boiling water, the person being covered with blankets, and bricks that are hot can be sprinkled with boiling water, or these baths can be taken by means of a steam cap. A vapor bath increases the body temperature, moistens the skin, draws out oil from the skin and tissues. It elevates body temperature rapidly from one to three degrees in ten minutes. In one-half hour it may raise body heat temperatures from three to eight degrees. This increases the rapidity of breathing and pulse but not depth of breath or volume of pulse. It leads to oppression at first, but afterwards to a larger pulse and a deeper breath. Then clogging takes place in the vital organs, and the head feels full. There is a pressure upon the eyes, vertigo, dizziness, sluggishness, and pressure in the head. Carbonic acid in the system, sluggish blood action and heart action, or general hyperemia is the result. After the bath has acted such symptoms disappear but the man has lost in weight.

Use a high sodium, low calcium diet. Get warm food, hot drinks, protein foods, a warm climate, and exercises. Use figs and goat milk.

Try a poultice of mustard, whole wheat flour, and egg white, or a comfrey poultice. Herb teas: Parsley and nettle.

Rickets
Use dandelion tea and orange juice. Get vitamin D from sunlight.

Right Side Problems
Usually need more proteins in the diet.

Saliva
To increase saliva, take a date seed and suck on it one hour a day. Spit out accumulated saliva.

Sexual Disorders
Sexual disorders in both male and female are best treated by diet, exercise, and hygiene. Nearly all sexual diseases are caused by indiscretion either in habits or diet or both. A heavy meat diet is not good, nor are highly seasoned foods or an overabundance of sugar and white flour. This is considered a dietetic error.

We must have hygiene in the way of cleanliness; and rest is very important. Lewd dancing and racy dressing can be potent causes for sexual disorders. Many times if we get away from red coloring in dresses, rooms, etc., and turn more to the greens, the blues, and the purples, we will be less tense. Reading novels of a sensual character and witnessing pornographic movies should be dispensed with. The mind must be kept right and thinking right. These prevent sexual disorders.

Constipation can cause problems. Doctors should be consulted to see if there are any mechanical disorders. Use a lot of the alkalinizing foods. Take potato peeling broth; stay away from stimulating foods such as beef, carbonated drinks, and condiments. Use a lot of chlorophyll and green in the diet. Exercise, the proper balance for the day, a good hobby, good companions, true friendships — all help these conditions the most.

Sinus
To clear the sinuses of congestion, breathe deeply while walking. Take sage, rub between hands, breathe into nostrils to open up passages. Carry a few bay leaves, inhale aroma while walking. Put some fresh horseradish on tongue and take some deep breaths to help to drain the sinuses.

Sleeplessness/Insomnia
See special section in "Vitality Through Brain and Nerve Force."

Skin
For care of the skin, see chapter, *"Beauty Starts with the Skin."*

Smoking
How to break the smoking habit: Take a pinch of chamomile leaf tea when the desire to smoke arises. Ask any doctor about the evil effects of coal tar from cigarette smoking. They all know that it has a direct effect on the lungs and irritates ulcers of the stomach. Smoking is one of the greatest factors that makes Buerger's disease worse, which is additional proof that smoking never did any good for the body. All doctors know that coal tar products from paper and tobacco are carcinogenic in their effect; in other words, they are cancer-producing. I sincerely hope this will help you to quit.

Spine
For good care of the spine:
Walk 50 steps per day with arms folded.
Walk 50 steps with toes turned in and arms folded.

Walk 50 steps with toes turned in, arms folded, and head turned to the left.

Walk 50 steps with toes turned in, arms folded, and head turned to the right.

Pain and tenderness indicate need for silicon. For lumbago (rheumatic pain in lower back), use hops poultice.

Spleen

The spleen stores fluorin and uses large amounts of fluorin. Eat plenty of the natural fluorin foods. Inactivity of the spleen indicates a need for sodium. One of the best herbs for the spleen is sassafras tea.

Sterility Problem

There are various laboratory examinations that may be given to disclose whether or not one is sterile. There are ways of telling if the fallopian tubes are blocked. Childless couples might consider these tests. We always take care of both husband and wife when dealing with sterility. Use Sitz baths, slant board exercises, mountain climbing, walking, pelvic and abdominal exercises. Use a great number of correction exercises, including weight lifting exercises as taught in gymnasiums. Get lots of vitamin E as found in wheat germ oil, taking one tablespoonful three times a day. If you don't use weight lifting exercises, use vitamin E capsules (high potency — 100 units) three times a day. A combination of vitamin A, E, and F are very necessary as is phosphorus.

Male hormones are found in date seeds; female hormones in citrus seeds. A good male rejuvenator herb combination is ginseng, damiana, echinacea, white willow, gotu kola, saw palmetto, sarsaparilla, periwinkle, chickweed, golden seal, garlic, and cayenne.

Stomach

For nervous stomachs, use two tablespoons of powdered papaya in one quart of water; sip slowly throughout the day. In the morning drink water.

Tonic: Take cream celery broth, using just the stalk of the celery.

Excess acidity: Chewing licorice root may help to allay the symptoms of an extreme acid stomach.

Irritations: Take raw goat milk and soaked dates. See other sections of book for more information.

Stomach cleanser: Liquid chlorophyll taken in the morning is a splendid cleanser for the stomach. Most people have an idea that bad breath always comes from the mouth, but in most cases it comes from the stomach. A stomach that is in a fermentation stage usually gives off bad breath, and liquid chlorophyll is one of the things that will help it.

Belching stomach: Peppermint tea.

Stomach ulcers: Use celery juice and sweet cream; and spinach and grapefruit juice. See *Ulcers,* this chapter.

Tapeworm Remedy

In one of my books we have a picture of a tapeworm close to thirty feet long we eliminated from an intestinal tract with garlic and onions. Germ life cannot live with this combination.

At one time, I studied with a San Francisco doctor who had many clever means of going back to nature for remedies. This doctor did not believe in many of the modern methods of healing. We called upon a patient suffering from a tapeworm. He was put on an exclusive garlic and onion diet for three days. The fourth day he was given an enema of powdered garlic and water, then a severe herb laxative. To climax this strenuous treatment, he was seated in a tub of warm milk. The entire tapeworm was almost immediatly eliminated.

The efficiency of this method will be easily recognized by any physician, who knows that ordinarily the tapeworm is cut off through the elimination perhaps only six inches at a time. When this happens, the tapeworm continues to grow and reproduce. If you do not want a tapeworm, put milk at one end and garlic at the other. It may sound crude, but it is most effective.

Teeth

Tooth decay: To attempt to control this by fluoridating water is a poor remedy, especially when we are not told how to get organic fluorine into our bodies through foods.

People are getting breakdown of teeth from the pampered luxury foods. Sweetened devitalized foods are also responsible for tooth decay. If we do not learn to stop breaking down our bodies before resorting to remedies, the remedy is going to be worse than the disease. It is possible that ten years from now we will look back and be sorry for fluoridated products, for the flourine can accumulate in the body tissues and eventually cause problems that will be worse than teeth decay.

Toothache: This can sometimes be helped with a ginger poultice. Indicates a calcium deficiency. Use balm as a tranquilizer, and catnip tea.

Help for the gums: In preventing trench mouth and in taking a papaya tablet and put gums, or tartar of the teeth, take a papaya tablet and put it on each side of the mouth and hold there for half an hour. This papaya will eat up all toxic material that has settled there and destroy all tissues that are not live tissues. It is one of the greatest mouth cleansers that we can put in the mouth. For gingivitis (inflamed gums) use a yeast supplement. Use a chlorophyll mouthwash. Take sunflower seeds. Pyorrhea indicates a chlorine deficiency. Bleeding gums need a natural fluorine supplement.

Tooth Problems: Needs vitamins A, C, and D, calcium, phosphorous and fluorine foods, and sometimes iodine. Use beet greens, parsley, celery and green kale juice.

Television
Exposure to excessive television rays will often cause a vitamin A deficiency. Much research is being done today about the effects of these rays.

Tension
This sometimes indicates too much salt. Relaxing herb teas: Thyme, catnip, and skullcap. Use tension exercises for relaxing. Consciously relax fifty times per day while recalling and visualizing a beautiful restful scene, a beautiful flower, or painting.

Throat, Sore or Hoarse
Indicates sodium deficiency and is aggravated by iron deficiency. Use alfalfa juice (high in chlorophyll). Use barnett herb tea. If sore, gargle lemon or unsweetened pineapple juice.

Tongue, Coated
Your tongue is a mirror reflecting the condition of your intestinal tract. When it is coated it shows that the intestinal tract is in a state of acute elimination and is overloaded with toxic material. A change of diet is indicated and a change of living habits should be started. Study ways of cleansing the intestinal tract to stop this self-intoxication.

Tonsils
If swollen, use eucalyptus, honey, and onions. Mix the juice. Swelling is caused by excessive proteins and acids from stomach, and it is something that must be taken care of. If the problem is suppressed it will usually result in appendicitis. Use ½ teaspoon of chlorophyll to ½ cup of water 3 times per day.

Tuberculosis
For tuberculosis there is a thirty-day garlic cure that has been used very successfully. It calls for taking the cloves of garlic, chopping them up fine, and using this for all meals for thirty days. Garlic packs may be used for the chest. Also take garlic enemas of finely chopped garlic in warm water. A person can use any amount of this. After using it a few days, a person doesn't mind the odor or the taste and can eat garlic like apples. The Bircher-Benner Clinic in Zurich, Switzerland, uses this remedy.

Ulcers
When you want a healing of any mucous membrane, put a teaspoon of chlorophyll into a cup of flaxseed tea. Take three times per day. Freshly pressed green juices make a liquid chlorophyll. If you buy liquid chlorophyll, be sure that it is made from natural sources such as alfalfa. This type is usually quite concentrated. Avoid the commercial type chlorophyll, which is made in a copper vat from electricity.

Ulcers of the stomach: Rest in higher altitude, and eat a smooth diet, soothing broths, puree of soybeans, and baby lima beans in broth form. Also good are barley broth, rice broth, sauces made from dried fruits that have been soaked well or cooked slightly and pureed, raw goat milk with soak-slightly and pureed, raw goat milk with soaked, peeled dates, uncooked whole goat milk cheese, okra powder, one to three tablespoons gelatin daily, cabbage juice, vitamin A, comfrey juice. Slippery Elm food is one of the finest remedies we have. It can be used as a breakfast cereal and mixed with other cereals, such as millet, and used each morning. It can also be taken at night before going to bed. mulberries; use woodruff tea, internally and as a wash. An herb combination system builder for ulcers is golden seal, capsicum, and myrrh gum.

Ulcers and sores: Need an iodine supplement and sodium foods.

Mouth and throat: Use sorrel tea with honey.

Peptic ulcers: Use alfalfa tea.

Leg ulcers: Use poultice of pine needle oil with olive oil on cotton; apply every twenty-four hours; and fast. Use poultice of green curly cabbage and oat straw tea. Use chlorophyll salve with lanolin.

Veins
Study the chapter, "The Blood: Fluid of Life and Rejuvenation."

Phlebitis — milk leg: Veins appear blue, indicates too much milk, not enough magnesium. Use buckwheat supplement, which contains rutin. Use apple packs.

Venous congestion (thrombosis): Indicates an iron deficiency.

Varicose veins: Do not cross legs. Elevate feet on pillow four to six inches while sleeping. Take a warm bath before retiring. Use Epsom salt compress. Massage upward on legs with olive oil. Use vitamin E supplement; use oatstraw packs at night for thirty nights; use the Kneipp baths, foot baths, barefoot walking, Sitz bath. Put feet up in the air frequently. Herb tea: Oatstraw.

Voice.

If weak, needs the sodium foods and a good strength-building regimen.

Stuttering: This often happens when left-handed children are forced to be right-handed.

Vomiting.

Needs sodium sulphate.

Warts.

As in all these remedies, work with the guidance of your doctor. Several things can be done: use nitric acid; put vaseline around it; apply silver nitrate; use green papaya, take thick material from papaya and apply to warts.

Weight Problems.

See the various sections on Underweight, Overweight, and special diets under "Special Diets for Special People.

Worms

Garlic enemas: Garlic capsule put in rectum every night for one month. Too much sugar produces these conditions. Herb teas: Rue, sorrel, gentian. For children: Wormwood tea with strawberry or carob.

Tapeworms: Soak and grind pumpkin seeds and make a paste with honey. Give four ounces of castor oil several hours after eating three tablespoons of paste. Give this after fasting for two days. Have patient sit in warm milk or warm water when evacuating. Use garlic and onions, and see special section about garlic and onions. Also see *Tapeworm Remedy* this chapter.

X-Ray Burns

Use aloe vera poultice.

Youth/Longevity Tonics

Get lots of greens in our diet; also berries, figs, goat milk, a lot of outdoor life, changes in climate, living in rooms where the air is constantly in motion, cultivation of the affections, development of the interests, making sure that your mental attitude is working for the higher good of all mankind. Lift others; do not drag on others, when you drag on others you are a care to others. When other people look up to you, it represents a youth influence.

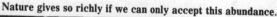
Nature gives so richly if we can only accept this abundance.

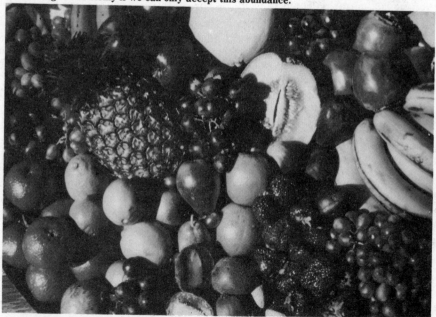

Healing with herbs

TWENTY THREE

HERBS are the greatest healers of all and I feel everybody should get acquainted with them. They have a particular property in the root structure that draws to them the chemical elements, vitamins, and minerals necessary to change certain conditions in the human body. Herbs also carry a radiant, vibratory force that benefits our bodies. They are an easily found natural remedy. Study how to use them in teas, tonics, tinctures, infusions, extracts, etc. Many homeopathic remedies are made from herbs and can be obtained from herb stores or homeopathic remedies are made from herbs and can be obtained from herb stores or homeopathic drug stores.

Herbs have been part of our culture throughout history. Herbs were used in China long before the time of Christ. They are still being used in peasant homes in Europe. Visit the people of any country and you will find that they have their favorite little herb tea or their favorite way of doing things with the herbs in the garden. I believe the regular diet should always be supplemented with herbs.

HOW TO MAKE HERB TEAS

Use one heaping teaspoon of your favorite tea to two cups of water. Bring the water to a boil in a glass or stainless steel pot, add herbs, and let stand until cool. Then strain it and use the remaining liquid as tea. It can be taken cool or warm. Add whatever flavor you wish (such as a little honey). You may refrigerate it and use throughout the day. This recipe will work for most teas.

Catalog of Healing Herbs

Alfalfa leaf. Stimulating for kidney , bowels, appetite, and digestion. Highly alkaline. Use for peptic ulcers.

Alfalfa seed. Rich in silicon. Liver cleansing. For arthritis and similar pains.

Alfamint (Alfalfa mint): Rich in minerals and vitamins. Good for arthritic conditions, digestion. An antacid — very alkalinizing. Alfamint should always be on your shelf. Alfalfa is one of the greatest alkalinizers we can put in the body. Mint is a gas driver. It is great for toning up the intestinal tract. Both are very high in chlorophyll.

Angelica. Use for bronchial problems, colds, indigestion, colic.

Balm. Helps to soothe nervous headaches, toothache, hysteria, earache, chlorosis.

Balsam. Balsam tea with ginger can be used to help expel gas. It is also used for cramps and colic. Can be given to children.

Basil. For circulation and catarrh problems. A stimulant.

Bay. Used as a skin tonic for skin problems. A stimulant.

Blueberry. Tea made from blueberry leaves is a specific for hypoglycemia.

Blue violet. Leaves and flowers are good for lymph gland drainage, catarrhal conditions, severe cough, healing sores. High in vitamin C; the leaves are especially high in vitamin A.

Borage. Used for palpitations, hysteria, adrenal problems; to increase mother's milk.

Buchu. Good for the kidneys, genito-urinary tract, uric acid gravel, and the lungs. Stimulant and diuretic.

Burdock. Used to reduce weight and is a blood purifier. A renal cleanser.

Burnett. Used for throat infections and to control hemorrhages.

Catnip. Carminative, diaphoretic, and tonic. Relaxes nerves. Used as a tranquilizer. Relieves fevers, pain, flatulence, and colds.

Chamomile. Aids digestion. Clear complexion. Good for flatulence and gas. Soothing for colic. Discharges catarrh; soothes inflammation; has potassium and calcium. A wonderful tonic for children and all ages.

Chickweed. For acne and a good all-around tonic.

Chicory. Is used to help jaundice. Roasted chicory is a good and healthful substitute for coffee.

Comfrey leaves. Rich in minerals. Tonic for fevers, kidneys, bladder; internal healing; used as a poultice for swelling problems and for gout. As a tea for hemorrhage problems.

Comfrey root. Gets toxic material out through the lungs, loosens colds. I believe that comfrey root and the leaves are one of the finest herbs you can use. Comfrey is very high in protein and has a mucilage in it that makes it very good for the intestinal tract. It is very high in chlorophyll, iron, and potassium. Used for milk-giving animals, it raises their milk production. As a remedy, the leaves are wonderful in packs. I have seen the root used in intestinal troubles and to control hemorrhages. The leaves and roots are wonderful in catarrhal problems, high blood pressure, asthma, bronchitis, and colds. A combination of comfrey leaves and fenugreek is wonderful in catarrhal problems. Comfrey root also gets toxic material out through the lungs and loosens colds. The leaves are good for the kidney and bladder.

Russian comfrey has been used effectively as a poultice for open sores.

Cornsilk. Kidney and bladder; genito-urinary tract; mucous linings. rich in magnesium. Dried cornsilk is a wonderful kidney tea, especially for one who has a tendency to have gravel in the kidneys and gall bladder. It helps to dissolve the gravel and break it down. down.

Curly cabbage. In Germany, they use curly cabbage, chopped up fine, for varicose ulcers, milk leg, phlebitis, ulcers of the leg.

Dandelion. Purifies blood; contains iron. Rich in calcium. Diuretic. Good for cold , dyspepsia, diabetes, tuberculosis, rheumatism, arthritis, kidneys, gall bladder, liver. Dandelion tea is especially good for the gall bladder and the liver. Leaves and flowers help the bile to flow.

Elderberry. For catarrhal conditions, colic, diarrhea. Good for the blood and the kidneys. Elderberry tea is a fine tonic for ovarian problems and menstrual disorders and the sexual orifices. Use leaves and berries for teas. Blossoms may be used in omelets. Can be used to lighten freckles.

Eyebright. Tonic; astringent; clears and tones; for gastric trouble and eye beauty.

Fennel. Used for gas problems and colic.

Fenugreek. Soothes mucous surfaces; for ulcers, poor digestion, fevers, very healing. If you have a weakness in the bronchial tubes, comfrey and fenugreek used half and half helps remove the catarrh. Fenugreek tea is used for drug poisoning.

Figwort. For blood clotting problems.

Flaxseed. Demulcent; for constipation; enema for bleeding bowel. High in silicon and vitamin F. Flaxseed tea with one teaspoon of liquid chlorophyll three times per day is very good for stomach ulcers.

Garlic and onions. I observed while visiting Armenia that they wrapped garlic in comfrey leaves and dried it for the wintertime. The Armenian people also use it in a soup. I asked a mother why she used it, and she told me that it helped her children to be free from colds and kept her husband on the job without any sickness.

In Russia they have discovered an antihistamine reaction from garlic extract. Is it possible that we can get something of a remedial action from these herbs and these foods? When I look at all the herbs and foods, I think that garlic and onions are the two best and most powerful of them all.

Garlic is a remedy for high blood pressure and hypertension. It has powerful antiseptic properties.

For asthmatic contractions and bronchitis: An onion pack on the chest is splendid for loosening asthmatic contractions and works well in cases of bronchitis and catarrhal congestion of the chest. Place clove of garlic under tongue. Leave all night for those who have asthma attacks.

For gland congestion: I have seen the onion pack work well on growths on the neck caused by thyroid disturbance. I have seen it work on lymph gland congestion where the lymph nodules on the neck have been enlarged.

For tuberculosis: In the Bircher-Benner Clinic in Zurich, Switzerland, they use garlic and onions for 30 days to get rid of tuberculosis.

For worms: Garlic has been used for getting rid of worms in children. You can take three or four garlic oil capsules three or four times a day for three days, and you will find that most of the worms will leave the body. Worms cannot stand garlic. No person can either! Eat as little food as possible during the treatment.

For tapeworms: For tapeworms, give garlic for a period of three days. It takes about three days for the garlic to permeate the bowel and the body; then the worm really

194

starts to crawl. We use a heavy laxative, and have the patient sit in warm milk. Do not have any air between the bowel passing and the milk, because if you do, the worm will cut itself off. The worm comes in three to six-inch sections, and if you do not get the head, it keeps on reproducing.

Garlic enemas for worms: Use garlic oil or garlic powder in one quart of warm water, using one teaspoon of either. You may also take onions and garlic for three days by mouth. Repeat in 27 days and repeat again in another 27 days.

Geranium green leaves. Astringent.

Golden seal. Stimulates gastric juices, speeds up and aids digestion. For all mucous membrane problems. For colitis, catarrhal discharge problems, nasal drip.

Golden seal is better when mixed with other herbs. It appears to be a catalyst to make all the other herbs work better. You will find that both alfalfa and shavegrass will work better when they are mixed with golden seal. Try first for correcting any condition of the body.

Hawthorne berry. Hawthorne berry tea is one of the finest remedies for the heart. It acts as a support. This remedy comes from a sanitarium in Germany. Hawthorne berries have an affinity for oxygen and bring oxygen to the brain, too.

Hops. A bitter herb for soothing sleep.

Horsetail. Diuretic. High in silicon and calcium.

Huckleberry. Antispasmodic. Very good for the pancreas and for diabetes. It helps in the digestion of starches and is used in cases of high blood pressure and diarrhea.

Hydrastis. Very good for indigestion.

Juniper berries. Father Kneipp used one or two berries a day in a tea and built up to 15 berries on the tenth day; then down to two a day. This really cleans the kidneys. Juniper berry tea is also good for liver and blood cleansing, weak stomach, foul breath, gas, urethral infections, bladder stones, and as a stimulant.

Lavender. Good for nervous headache, both blossom juice and as a tea.

Lovage. For indigestion, colic, scurvy, and as a diuretic.

Marigold. Used for scarlet fever. Helps to smooth scar formations on skin.

Marshmallow root. Combine with slippery elm for skin.

Nasturtium juice. Is used for itching skin, as an antiscorbutic, and as a blood purifier.

Oat straw. High in silicon. Soothes, stimulates, tonic, mineralizer, potent solvent.

Oat straw tea has been used for years for all kinds of skin troubles. Psoriasis, pimples, acne, and postules. It is one of the greatest remedies for getting silicon back into the body. Silicon lives in the skin and is stored in the skin. If you use two cups of oat straw tea every day for a year, you will see the benefits to the skin, hair, and nails.

An oat straw tea pack is good for various problems such as varicose veins. Oat straw is a potent solvent, and it soothes as it stimulates. Oat straw tea is one herb tea you boil. This takes the silicon from the oat straw shaft. Oat straw is also a good gland tea to rejuvenate the glands.

Papaya. Digestion of protein, dyspepsia, stomach weakness, pyorrhea. Hold papaya tablets in mouth to dissolve tartar on teeth.

Papaya tea helps to digest protein. If you do not have hydrochloric acid for the stomach, then use papaya tea. If you have papaya seeds, dry them and use them for tea. Use a tablespoon of the seeds to a cup of hot water. If you want to simmer the mixture for just a moment, you will get more of the papain out of it. Papain is found more in the leaves; pepsin is found more in the seed. Some people use the seeds as a spice by grinding them up real fine, but I would suggest that the benefits will better come out as a tea.

Papaya-Mint. The mint adds a nice flavor and is also a digestant.

Parsley. Best diuretic; also an aperient. Rich in iron and manganese. Parsley root, when dried, makes a wonderful tea for the kidneys. It is also good for gallstones, diabetes, jaundice, and rheumatism. Is a good stimulant.

Parsley seed tea is used for fevers.

Parsley juice is used for genito-urinary tract infection, urine retention, iron deficiency; boiled parsley roots are used for epilepsy, adrenal deficiency, and thyroid deficiency. Eat parsley with onion and garlic to get rid of odor.

Pennyroyal (mint). Combined with ginger helps to expel gas and helps with colic and cramps.

Peppermint. Antacid; aids digestion, circulation of blood; eliminates toxins; rich in manganese. Peppermint and spearmint can be used interchangeably. Both are good for colic and cramps, especially soothing for children.

For flatulence, use four drops of oil of peppermint to a cup of hot water.

Persimmon leaf. Very high in vitamin C.

Pine needle tea. High in vitamin C.

Primrose. For sense of well-being, poise, and calmness.

Raspberry. For poor circulation. Tones female organs; aids confinement period.

Red clover. One of the wonder herbs. Rich in iron and vitamin C. Cleansing tea for drug deposits; used for diarrhea.

Rice tea. Is used for congestion, acute head pain, nausea, fainting, difficult breathing, stomach cramps, colic, worms. Also used as a sedative. The juice is used as a disinfectant.

Rose hips. High in vitamin C. Used for kidneys and bladder; bladder stones.

Rosemary. Very soothing to the brain. Combined with rue, it is a very good disinfectant.

Rue. Used for nausea and head congestion.

Sage. Virus eradicator, cleansing, blood cleanser, astringent (gargle) clears complexion, a sedative; used for eye diseases; good for heart, liver, and kidneys; strengthening. For longevity and memory problems. For a menstrual flow stimulant, use red sage tea. Helps to combat night sweating.

Sarsaparilla. Rich in iodine; purifies blood; good for rheumatism. It is said in the herbal field that sarsaparilla has the equivalent of the male hormone, testosterone. It is generally used for building up and maintaining the vitality of the body. Sarsaparilla taken three times a day in an eight-grain capsule will help the mental alertness and the physical strength and helps to feed the glandular system.

Sassafras. Purifies blood, spleen, liver; digestant; reduces catarrh.

Savoy. Is used for lethargy, colic, digestion problems, tonsillitis, bee stings, and an herb bath.

Saw palmetto. This is one of the finest herbs for the prostate gland. For sexual impotency it can be combined with damiana and kola nut. One ounce each of these dried herbs, simmered in two pints of water until one pint is left. Strain and cool. Take a wine glass full of the mixture after meals.

Senna. Purgative; cleanses digestive tract; relieves constipation.

Shavegrass. High in silicon. Good for kidneys, bladder, gas, varicose veins, mucous membranes.

Shavegrass is very high in silicon, which is one of the elements we need most in our bodies. A lack of silicon shows up in rashes of the skin and in the nails.

Shavegrass tea is one of the finest I have found in my experience. It removes toxic material efficiently from the body. It is good for people who want to reduce and take some of the water out of their system through the kidneys. We have found that it is not irritating, and it does not seem to overwork the kidneys. It is especially good in all ulcer injuries, skin conditions, psoriasis, wounds, and sores. Before or after the tea is used, you can use the leaves on wounds and sores by wrapping it around with a wet cloth on the ailing sections of the body.

Slippery elm. For inflammation of mucous tissues, colitis, diarrhea. Slippery elm can be used in the form of small chips. Pour one pint of boiling water on a half ounce of chips and let it stand for one-half hour. You can then take as much as desired and sweeten it with various natural sweeteners. It has wonderful, healing virtues and is also high in nourishing value. It is as good as any cereal. It counteracts acidity and soothes the membranes of the stomach and intestines. An inflamed organic state is relieved by the use of this food.

In cases of duodenal and stomach ulcers, slippery elm is unsurpassed. The kidney and bladder are improved through its use. The weakest stomach can take it. It is digested when probably no other food can be tolerated. For troubles of the bowel and stomach, it can be mixed with rice gruel.

Slippery elm combined with marshmallow root is very soothing for the skin.

Sorrel tea. For ulcers of mouth and throat use sorrel tea with honey. A stimulant; is

Ecuador—Huancaya Indians—Their own herb market.

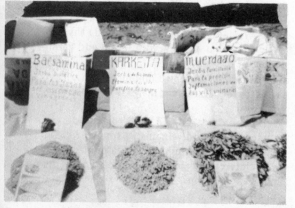

used for catarrh, fever stomach, blood problems, worms, and as a refrigerant.

Spearmint. Diuretic. Contains iron. Good for nausea, vomiting, flatulence. Antidote to feverish conditions.

Strawberry. Diuretic. High is sodium and iron. Good for liver; blood purifying; heals mucous membranes. With woodruff is used as a cleansing medicine.

Uva ursi. Diuretic. Useful for kidney complaints.

Valerian. Natural tranquilizer, relaxes nerves; relieves despondency, pessimism, head congestion, coughs, insomnia. Valerian root tea very soothing for epilepsy. Use one-half cup of warm milk, one-half teaspoon of molasses, and one-half cup of valerian tea for a soothing tranquilizer.

White oak. Rich in iodine and potassium. Used for diarrhea, dysentery, bowel problems, and for enemas.

Woodruff. For duodenal ulcers, internally, and as a wash. Used for liver, kidney, and abcesses. With strawberry leaf tea is used as a cleansing medicine.

Yellow dock tea. For acidosis, eczema.

The Oriental Favorites

Fo Ti Tieng. Fo Ti Tieng is known in Chinese medicine as the elixir of life. It is said that the Chinese herbalist, Li Chung Yun, who died at the age of 256, used this herb in particular.

This herb is found only in certain jungles in the Far Eastern tropics. We refer to *Nature's Medicines* by Richard Lucas in which he states that he has found Fo Ti Tieng to be the finest of all herbs, tonics, and nutrients. It appears to have no equal in the treatment of general debility and decline—digestion is strengthened, other foods are better absorbed, and the process of metabolism increases. Experiments have found that the leaves and seeds energize the nerves and brain cells.

Ginseng. Ginseng has been used in the Far East for centuries for its restorative and vitalizing effects. It is known as the panacea for all diseases.

Dr. G. W. Crile, a physiologist, said, "Ginseng emits an ultra-violet type of nitrogenetic radiation that has a beneficial effect on the sexual and other endocrine glands. When these glands are stimulated, they increase hormone-producing activity."

It is believed that Ginseng overcomes disease by building up general vitality and strengthening the endocrine glands.

Gotu Kola. Gotu Kola is known for its rejuvenating qualities and is a brain food, not a stimulant. One or two leaves a day can bring a natural, progressive return to good health.

Gotu Kola is used to lengthen the life span and is used by religious groups in India to develop spiritual powers. It is known as a food for the brain and is similar to Fo Ti Tieng and ginseng. Legend has it that the long life of the elephant can be attributed to the use of Gotu Kola.

Nature never breaks her own laws.—Leonard Da Vinci

Nature has a remedy . . .

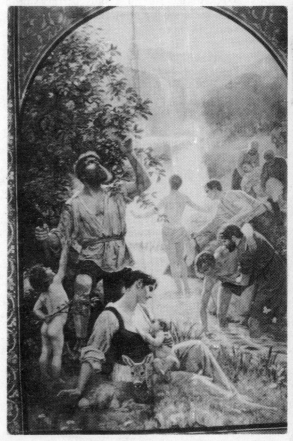

197

Herbs and spices

TWENTY FOUR

IN ancient days herbs and spices were not only used for flavoring but were also used in foods as a general preventive therapy. There was no refrigeration in those days, and food spoiled quickly. People found that they felt better when they added the herbs and spices, which, of course, also offered a great variety of flavors. Their medicine was taken with their foods. At one time in our history the spice market influenced world commerce in the same way that the oil market influences ours today.

Today using herbs and spices as seasoning and flavoring is a custom that is so universally accepted that we think only of these properties and have forgotten the original purpose. You will note that most of their healing properties relate to the stomach, aiding digestion, relieving gas, and so forth.

Allspice. Sauces; steamed puddings; pumpkin, raisin, and other pies; fruit salads and fruit cups; spiced cakes and cookies.
Healing properties: Wild allspice is used as a fever-breaker in colds.

Aniseed. Used whole or crushed in fruit and vegetable salads, cakes, breads, and rolls.
Healing properties: Comes from the anise plant native to Egypt. Very good for stomach upsets and baby's colic.

Basil. Salads: tomato, mixed greens, cucumber, cheese and fruit; sauces; vegetables; egg and cheese dishes.
Healing properties: Basil is of the mint family. For stomach flatulence and gas.

Bay leaves. Vegetable and tomato soup, tossed green and vegetable salads, French dressing, potatoes, carrots, dessert custards and creams.
Healing properties: Soothing to the stomach; relieves flatulence.

Caraway. Cheese dishes; coleslaw, cucumber, potato, and tomato salads; crushed in salad dressings; vegetables.
Healing properties: Use for stomach gas and colic, hair problems, and vision problems.

Cardamom. Cardamom cakes, cookies, and breads; with honey to flavor fruit, whipped cream; with spices in pies, puddings, and desserts.
Healing properties: The spicy seeds of this East Indies herb are used medicinally for soothing relief to digestive system.

Cayenne (Red Pepper or Capsicum). Adds color and wonderful taste to vegetables, broths, soups, meat and fish, cheeses, salads.
Healing properties: A well-known natural stimulant, has less reaction than many and can be used constantly with no ill effects. It increases the power of all organs, arouses the secreting organs, helps the digestion. Whenever a stimulant is indicated, we find that you can use it with utmost safety.

Celery seed. Breads; butter and spreads; dips, ground in egg and cheese dishes, vegetable juices, salads, and salad dressings; sauces; vegetables.
Healing properties: Celery seeds, leaves, and stems are especially indicated for stomach disorders of all kinds.

Chervil. Egg dishes, sauces, soups, salads.
Healing properties: An herb of the carrot family. Can be used as a poultice for bruises.

Cinnamon. Good in beverages— hot spiced fruit drinks, hot "chocolate," eggnogs, milkshakes, spiced tea, or fruit punches; desserts and puddings; fruits. Use whole in hot drinks.
Healing properties: Astringent; stimulant; as a tea, soothing for intestinal tract.

Cloves. Whole in fruit punches, when cooking fruit; ground in spiced cakes and cookies, egg dishes, sauces, and vegetables— beets, sweet potatoes, and tomatoes.

Healing properties: Used as an anesthetic; for gas/flatulence; oil of cloves for toothache.

Dill. Seed: Cream cheese dips and spreads, butter, vegetables — cooked green beans, cabbage, squash, and turnips.

Herb: Rich sauces, appetizers, vegetables as above; salads— avocado, cucumber, vegetable, coleslaw; soups.

Healing properties: Used for hiccoughs and as a sedative.

Garlic. Appetizers; salads — green and vegetable, potato; dressings; sauces; soups; entrees; butters. Now available as salt, powder, and chips.

Healing properties: Cleansing, purification, high blood pressure. See other sections of book for its many healing properties.

Ginger. Grind in tiny quantities in vegetables, salads, savory rice, and most Chinese recipes.

Whole dried: Some cooked fruits.

Ground: Ginger cookies, cakes, and puddings; fruit sauce, winter squash, glazed carrots, onions, and sweet potatoes.

Healing properties: Can be used to help expel gas, in colic and cramps, and can be given to children in mint (pennyroyal) or balsam teas.

Horseradish. Sauces, dips, spreads, salad dressings, vegetables.

Healing properties: Is a stimulant for sinuses, mucus, and phlegm problems. Bruised horseradish is used as a poultice for sciatica. Gets the bile flowing, clears out the gall bladder and the liver.

Mace. Whole: In cheese sauce, cooked apples, prunes, apricots, fruit salads, sauces, and marinades.

Ground: Breads and cakes, "chocolate" puddings, fruits, and vegetables.

Healing properties: Mace is made up of the hulls of nutmeg. Cleansing and detoxifying.

Marjoram. Soups — spinach, onion; cream sauces; egg dishes; vegetables — mushrooms, carrots, peas, spinach, zucchini.

Healing properties: Is used as an antiseptic, a stimulant, purifier, headaches, irregular menstruation, and skin diseases.

Mint. Appetizers; fruit and gelatin salads; coleslaw; vegetables— carrots, peas, potatoes, zucchini, cabbage; mint sauce; fruit, gelatin, and ice desserts; beverages— hot and iced teas, "chocolate," fruit punch.

Healing properties: Digestant, antispasmodic, diuretic for vomiting, asthma, colic.

Mustard. Whole: Salads — coleslaw, salad greens, vegetable and potato salads; vegetables— cabbage, buttered beets.

Ground: Salads, dressings, sauces, butters, vegetables.

Healing properties: A stimulant for sinuses, croup, coughs. Poultices are used with whole wheat flour and white of egg for rheumatism and hot foot baths for headaches.

Nutmeg. Beverages — milkshakes, eggnog, spiced hot drinks, hot "chocolate"; breads, cakes, pies, desserts. Fruits— grated over applesauce, compotes, mincemeat.

Healing properties: One-half nutmeg crushed and steeped in a cup of hot water is good for insomnia. Helps indigestion and nervous stomach. The aroma of this warm spice soothes a headache. Must be used in small doses. Has a narcotic effect in doses too large.

Oregano. Vegetables — zucchini, eggplant, tomatoes; hot sauces.

Healing properties: Aids digestion and is soothing to stomach.

Paprika. Appetizers, cheese, salad dressings, sauces, butters. Adds color to foods.

Healing properties: Stimulates appetite.

Parsley. Salad dressings, sauces, cheeses, fish, meats.

Healing properties: Best diuretic. Contains iron and manganese. Helps kidneys, gallstones, diabetes, jaundice. Fresh parsley helps eliminate food odors.

Pepper (black). *Do not use.* This is 17 times more irritating to the liver than alcohol.

Saffron. Adds color to rice dishes, vegetables, and sauces.

Healing properties: Antispasmodic; used for scarlet fever.

Sage. Soups — cream and chowder; salads; vegetarian stuffings; vegetables— lima beans, eggplant, onions, tomatoes.

Healing properties: An antiseptic. Used for eye diseases, longevity, memory problems, as a blood cleanser, astringent (gargle); for menstrual flow stimulant use red sage tea. Helps correct night sweating.

Savory. Soups — bean and lentil, consomme; salads — mixed green, vegetable, potato; sauces — horseradish; vegetarian stuffings.

Healing properties: Savory is a very aromatic herb of the mint family. It is so pleasing to taste and smell that the phrase "a savory meal" came from this herb.

Tarragon. Mixed green and fruit salads; sauces; egg dishes.

Healing properties: Soothing for eczema and scurvy.

Thyme. Tomato salad, aspic; tomato juice; sauces; vegetables — onions, carrots, beets.

Healing properties: After meals, aids digestion. An antiseptic for ptomaine poisoning. Helps to relieve phlegm and mucous, bronchitis, whooping cough. Is a good relaxant and can be used in bath.

Turmeric. Salad dressings; cream soups and chowders; for coloring; scrambled eggs.

Healing properties: A stimulant and carminative. Helps to remove phlegm and mucus; has protective value to the gall bladder.

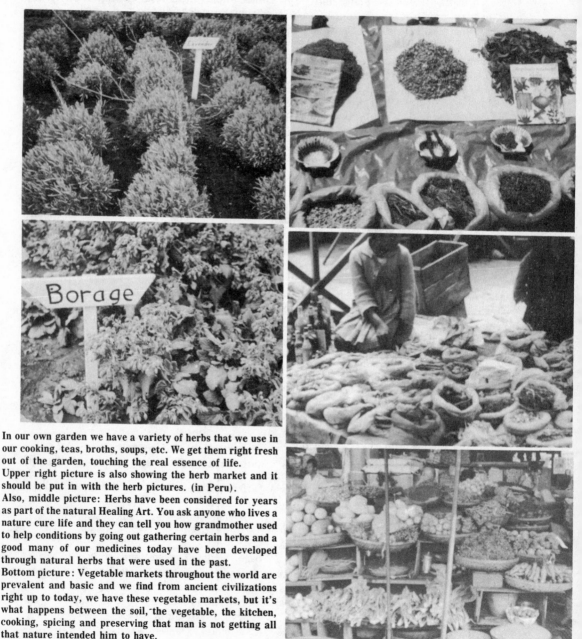

In our own garden we have a variety of herbs that we use in our cooking, teas, broths, soups, etc. We get them right fresh out of the garden, touching the real essence of life.

Upper right picture is also showing the herb market and it should be put in with the herb pictures. (in Peru).

Also, middle picture: Herbs have been considered for years as part of the natural Healing Art. You ask anyone who lives a nature cure life and they can tell you how grandmother used to help conditions by going out gathering certain herbs and a good many of our medicines today have been developed through natural herbs that were used in the past.

Bottom picture: Vegetable markets throughout the world are prevalent and basic and we find from ancient civilizations right up to today, we have these vegetable markets, but it's what happens between the soil, the vegetable, the kitchen, cooking, spicing and preserving that man is not getting all that nature intended him to have.

TWENTY FIVE

Balance – key to health

I BELIEVE that balance is the most important thing in the world. We need eight hours of work a day, eight hours of sleep, and eight hours of recreation.

One of the greatest secrets as far as remedies are concerned is to find out what we should be doing during our recreation time. You do not need to know what to do while you are sleeping; you leave that to God. As far as work is concerned, you usually leave that to the boss. But recreation is something that belongs to you. This is your creative time; this is the time you do what you really love to do. If you do not do the things you love to do, you cannot balance out the things you have to do.

In rebuilding the nervous system and brain, get away from what you have been doing during your working time. Go in another direction. If you have been working with certain brain centers and have had to be serious, critical, analytical, you should go from all that seriousness to humor. In your spare creative time, you will be ready to do the things that make you feel good. You should sit down and come to know what you want to do in your spare time. Most people don't have any spare time, and there are others who are afraid to use their spare time for doing something good. There are times when you should use your spare time to do nothing.

If you do heavy thinking at work, do light thinking in your spare time. If you keep your nose to the grindstone, so to speak, don't come home and practice heavy music—practice light music. Read a light book, don't read a heavy, brain-taxing book. This is how you use your spare time to compensate for what you do at work.

Use Your Recreation Time Properly. If you want to recreate any of the mental faculties that have broken down in your body, you should get off of them and leave them alone. Don't touch them, and they will recreate by themselves. The only time your mental faculties break down is when you overdo them. Sometimes a good trip will help. It is just a matter of dropping and letting them go. A variety of mental activities is another cure.

People are looking for new cures today, new diets, new ways to gain health. Try finding some of the old fundamentals — the good old water cure, a good food, unsprayed, clean and unadulterated. Stick to that, and your body will throw off a few things you don't need; it will take care of things. You don't need to worry too much about it.

Life Is Simple. I believe in the words of Emmet Fox who said, "Life is very simple but not easy." It is difficult to do nothing. It is difficult to do the simple things in life and the simple things are what get you well and keep you well. The complicated things are confusing and enervating. I have seen people drive fifty miles for a quarter pound of lecithin and waste more nerve energy than the lecithin could ever give them. The trouble is that everyone wants to cure everything with diet. I have seen more acids produced in the body with mental attitudes than all my potato peeling broth would ever neutralize. We must put this whole health program together. Find the simplest things you can do and then work with this simplicity. We have become so complicated that we cannot even unravel ourselves.

Belief—A Spiritual Remedy. There are times when you work on a physical job and become so physical that it is time you thought of spiritual things in your spare time. Few people are paid to meditate or to think on spiritual things in this age of ceramics, money, and tobacco.

The proper spiritual things can relax a

person and help him to let go and let God "speak." They can give us a new mind with new thinking. There is absolute peace and harmony in spiritual thinking. There are no tensions, no sicknesses in spiritual thinking.

<u>One Lives on His Beliefs</u>. Sometimes faith in a remedy that may have no virtue of itself will help a person, because one lives on his beliefs. If a belief relaxes a person and gives him hope and peace and harmony, his needs will be met a lot better than with the parsley I can give him.

In India they place tiger's claws around a child's neck when the child has a fear of the night — and the child has no more fear at night. The Minister of Health in India gave me a pair of these claws — one cannot buy them since they are only for the prince or the maharajah in India.

People in the Virgin Islands have a worry stone with a niche they rub with the thumb to give them a feeling of protection.

In Russia, they believe the fat of a bear's left hind foot has healing properties. If you have enough faith, this will help you.

Some of us work all day long on a job we must get done, but we don't like to get it done, so we are living in resistance. But the spiritual word tells you to resist not. The resistance of unpleasantness is killing more people than unpleasantness itself, because in resistance you can kill yourself. One person out of every seven in this country is taking tranquilizers, and he takes them because of the resistance he has to life.

As remedies, we should be thinking again about meditation, quietness, being alone, getting acquainted with ourselves, doing the things we love to do, and associating with

Resting, relaxing, a moment of recuperation.

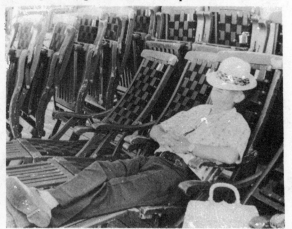

wonderful companions that uplift us and make us feel fine. We find that good friendship, good scenery, beauty, and country living are very relaxing and will help us to let go. We need green surroundings and a beautiful garden.

<u>Sit and Don't Do Anything On Purpose</u>. Don't be afraid to sit and do nothing. There is a time we have to let the rest of the world go by; there is a time when we have to loosen our families and let our children go. These are healing things and healing remedies.

<u>Other Mental Remedies</u>. There are some people who try to overaccomplish, try to overdo, try to do too much during the day. This has to be stopped. The remedy is in quietness and in solitude and meditation. A life of all thinking can break a person down.

There are some people who are meant to have more money than others, because they have a mind for money. Don't try to compare yourself with other people and expect to have the same amount of money they have. Learn to accept what is possible in your life, and learn to live within a budget that you are capable of earning.

<u>Get on the Healing Path</u>. First, a program is necessary. There is an old saying, "Plan your work and then work your plan." Remember that getting well is a path in life. You must go on a certain path. The path to good health is rough and must be followed. Certain paths are good as far as the health is concerned. Therefore, you *must* take the healing pathway.

<u>Rest Before You Become Fatigued</u>. Fatigue is one of the things we must learn to overcome. It is necessary to learn to rest while you are still rested; don't wait until you are tired and worn out before you rest. It is not a matter of seeing how far we can go, but of stopping when we are supposed to stop, realizing our body's limitations.

A splendid way to completely relax is simply to lie down! Act like a rag doll. To do this, lift one leg and let it drop; then lift the other leg and let it drop. Then tip your head to one side and then to the other side. Lift one arm and let it drop; then lift the other arm and let it drop. Lift both arms and just let them drop.

Say to yourself, "At the count of ten, I will be more relaxed." When you reach ten, say, "I feel relaxed." If you are not completely relaxed, say, "I will do it again, and I will be more relaxed than ever at the count of ten." When you arrive at the count of ten, you will be completely relaxed. I have reduced the count to five, so that at the count of five, I can go into complete relaxation.

Variety is a great cure as far as mental activities are concerned. I feel one of the greatest remedies possible from a mental and spiritual standpoint is forgiveness. I think another thing is to bless problems so that you can get rid of things that mentally bother you. It is the only way to gain absolute freedom from painful thoughts. To get rid of your problems, learn to bless them, be grateful, and be thankful. One of the finest things I know in the way of relieving the mind is to forgive and forget. These are remedies for that sick, tired, weary, burdened body. So let this be the beginning.

Live Happily. Most of us have burdens. The burden we would like most to rid ourselves of is the troubled mind. I would like to give you an untroubled mind, but that is something no one can give and no one can buy. It is something you gain for yourself: you meditate; you go into quietude. You will discover an untroubled mind is something you will have to feel once and know what it is, and then you will want it. Your mind can make you well, if you will only accept it.

Soul Communication. Most people when they wish to rest think about going to bed, but you will find that there is such a thing as absolute rest in divine communication. In soul communication, you can recuperate. Very few people have met souls who can help them. Most of us work with souls who irritate us and we have to endure it because we cannot cure it. This situation takes its toll. Like the little drop of water on the stone, it takes many years to wear away the stone, but it *will* erode in time.

Understanding Can Bring Happiness and Success. In working with our weaknesses it would be nice if we were trained in consciousness. We should be trained to prevent rather than to cure. For instance, if a mother and father both have pancreas weakness, then what chance has a child to have a good one? What happens when two pessimists get married? The reason we have so many divorces today is that with the personalities we have, either we click or we don't. I saw a man the other evening whose wife wanted a divorce because she thought he had gone

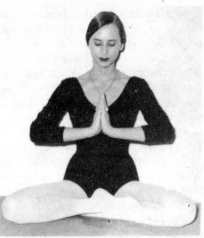

Mrs. Janssen of Sydney, Australia, who is one of the great teachers of Yoga, in one of her Yoga postures and what great work she is doing for the vegetarian and for the physical art of Yoga.

"nuts." He was always out in the garage working on his inventions — crazy little inventions, such as how to make a better faucet — but to him they were the great things in life. She blamed him for fiddling away the time that he should have been spending with her. If she could only accept the fact that he was a man who had to invent things for his self-expression, then they could overcome the misunderstanding and be happy together. (Personology can help with this situation. See the next chapter.)

When you marry you must both be interested in each other's work. I see so many people going through life just hanging on together. "It is my duty to hold on." "We stay married only because of the children."

The wife should admire her husband- look up to and respect him for the position or job he has and for the money he brings home to her. Then it makes no difference whether the man is a plumber, a musician, a doctor, or a ditch-digger; he will do well. If she is dissatisfied with him no matter what he does, he can't go to his work feeling happy, and he will never be a success. There are many women who keep men from becoming successful.

Mental Temperament Should Decide Vocation. Why is it that 90 percent of the people are reportedly misfits in their jobs? Those people who have jobs where they can live with joy are the ones who can do the extraordinary things; they work hour after hour without tiring. You must find something to get hold of so that you are wanted and know that you are giving something, have accomplished something. Find a job you are mentally fitted for, because a person who is in step is happy and a person who is out of step is miserable. If you are not happy, you cannot be well. There are many people who are satisfied with being out of step. They are like a worm in horse-radish. They think they are' in the sweetest place in the world because they have never been anywhere else. They don't know what it is to be happy.

The greatest crime is not being able to touch the thing we could be a success in. You must do the thing you love to do, the thing that will make you happiest. You must find where your success faculty is and how your mental temperament can decide the kind of job you should be in. This has been proven to the point where you can actually chart a person from the physical characteristics, telling the type of work they are capable of doing, their inherent abilities and their capacity for thinking.

There are very few who know that when we are successful mentally, we are happy. We must get into the work we feel we want to do. You cannot be well unless you are happy, and you cannot be happy unless you are well-they work together. When movie star Gene Tierney had a nervous breakdown, she went to the Menninger Clinic in Kansas City and was advised to try a different type of occupation for awhile. She took a clerking job in a store. She realized that the job she wanted to do was to sell clothes to people, that that was what she needed to become peaceful, content, and happy.

A lady in England inherited a huge fortune, but rather than live the life that goes with it, she took a job as a scrub woman, and she was happier doing this than using the fortune that she had inherited.

Your Right Place Is A Happy Place. To be in your right place is to be happy. To serve in what you are able and capable of doing is always the best. If you want anything in life very badly, apply yourself, persevere in that direction and you are bound to be a success, whether it is playing the saxophone or being a doctor. There are a lot of misfit doctors. I think it is better to be a happy musician than a miserable doctor. To be a round peg in a round hole is necessary in order to be happy.

As we go through life, we all have to work. Eight hours a day is a long time if you are working at something that makes you miserable, but it is wonderful if you are happy in your work. To the person who is happy there is no time, but when a person dreads the time spent at work he is unhappy, he is a misfit. He is doing something he doesn't want to do, something he hasn't the mental faculty to enjoy.

Eight hours are for work, eight hours for rest and sleep; the other eight hours should be be for recreation. How many people put eight hours aside to re-create and develop some of their ideas? How many people know that recreation is something that belongs to them; a time to recuperate from the work they do. When people are miserable, their bodies break down fast, and it takes more than eight hours of rest to rebuild them. On the other hand, if you are happy in your work, nine times out of ten, when you start your recreation, your hobby, you will carry your happiness with you.

Balance Your Day with a Hobby. Find out who you are, what you are capable of doing and the kind of hobby you should have in your spare time, your recreation time. I don't believe you can be happy without a hobby. To balance your day well, you cannot live in monotony. There are a few people who can do monotonous jobs and enjoy them, but that is not for the average. The right person in his right place is something for us to think about. And if you have never had a hobby, have never done the things you would really love to do in life, you have never lived. You have missed the very things that make living a bubble of joy.

Develop "Words and Axioms". One of the things we should all start to do is to learn how to handle words. I think everyone should take a word and start working on it. For example, restaurant means "to restore." Emotion means "I move." Worry means "to choke." (That should give us something to think about. Is it worth worrying about? Am I choking myself?)

I think the best advice I can give you is to start developing axioms. One of the greatest axioms I know is "Whatever you assume in life, you live." If you think you are poor and no good, if you assume, "I'm no good, I'll never get there," then that is what you will become.

I remember once when my little girl was about five years old, she came into the house and I asked, "Well, who is pretty in here?" And she answered, "Me." She assumed something. You must assume things. You must assume and feel loved; you must fell wanted. Find the axioms that work for you.

Another great axiom is, "People are more

important than things." That is the reason we are making a study of people, because people are more important than things.

Look for the Good. What about the spiritual things? *Spirit* means, "the intangible which is real." That may be hard to realize. People think because they see the physical thing, it is real, but it is only the end result of the real thing. The real thing we cannot see. The greatest thing that expresses "spirit," the tangible thing which is the real thing, is *prayer*. Pray for those things hoped for. That is the only thing that is real. If only we knew that when we look for the best things in life- that is the godly things, the only things worth seeking- the godly things will come to us. Be sure that that is what you are looking for, because if you look for trouble, that also will come to you.

Develop Love-Consciousness. If you are looking for the good, you can find it, but you have to have "spirit consciousness" to find spiritual things. It is possible that there are higher things in life, as St. Paul expressed so beautifully in his message to the Corinthians. You can recognize them only when you get there. There is never an end to spiritual growth.

This is another wonderful quotation from Paul. "Greet it with pure joy, brethren, any sort of trial." (See 2 Corinthians 7:4; also, James 1:2.) Don't you think there are mental things that are mental trials? Do you think it is only physical endurance? Make sure your endurance is free from all defects. Is a defect only a physical thing? No. We are talking about a spiritual thing, a mental thing. So you see, this spiritual thing is sometimes more important than all the physical things in the world. Again, Paul puts it nicely: "Whatsoever is lovely, whatsoever is good, whatsoever is excellent, think ye on these things." (See Phillipians 4:8.) That isn't always physical.

"You may speak with the tongue of an angel, but if you don't speak with love, it is like the clanging brass." (See 1 Corinthians 13:1.) And, you can give all your money to charity, but if it isn't given for love, it counts for nothing. You can be burned at the stake, but if you aren't burned for love, it counts for nothing.

I feel, that of all the faculties we should learn to develop in our bodies and our minds, love-consciousness is the greatest. Love-consciousness is a universal consciousness and you will find that with it you are accepted by everyone. Anyone with this nature would certainly have the consciousness of the Great One who said, "I am all things to all men." You have to have a Universal Love to be all things to all men. You have to understand all men at all levels. Now that is something to think about.

Mentally Healthy Persons.
Are able to think for themselves and make their own decisions.
Plan ahead, but do not fear the future.
Do not push people around, nor do they allow themselves to be pushed around.
Do something about their problems as they arise.
Shape their environment whenever possible, but adjust to it when necessary.
Neither underestimate nor overestimate their abilities.
Take life's disappointments in stride.
Feel a sense of responsibility to their neighbors and fellow beings.
Are not bowled over by their own emotions — by their fears, anger, love, jealousy, guilt, or worries. [Dr. Rudolph Novick]

Be Humble. There comes a time when we must become absolutely humble. There is a time when we may have to recede and go back into "nothingness." It is necessary to learn how to let go and to give up a little. There is also a time when you have to hang on; and there is a time, too, when you have to tie a knot in the rope and don't let yourself slip; and, finally, there is a time when you just have to let go. It takes a wise person to know the time and season for all things.

The thing we should learn in our quiet time is how to be selective, be positive, be wise. This is what we have to learn in our spare, quiet time. We must learn how to elevate our minds so that when we go into this quiet time, we take the best of us into that world. It is there where we recreate; there, where we cooperate with Divinity; and we come out anew. Without a transformed mind, we will stay in the same place we were before. If we are satisfied with what we were, then this is very serious.

Look To Change. The Moral Rearmament Group has devised a formula for mental compatability. If things are not right, it is time for a change. People are more important than things. To make the proper change, the first thing to consider is getting rid of selfishness; the second thing to consider is purity. Cut out the old and start anew! Third, consider the importance of honesty. And, fourth, consider absolute love. These are the four rules to follow.

One of the greatest rules I know for attracting the very best in this world is to set ourselves straight first. Don't expect to be happy only when everything else in this world is all right. Nothing in this world is "all right." There is nothing in this world that does not need some changing. We should remember that the last decision we made is what we live on.

We need to get away from mean, spiteful people and pick out good companions. Select people who love you. You will have to love them also, so that they will wish to have you around. You cannot expect people to want you around if the association is not mutually uplifting.

I think you should consider what kind of health vacation you should go on as a remedy. Most people use a vacation to compensate for a whole year's work. Most of them will drive four thousand miles during the summer to see some cave in Virginia; and then drive another four hundred miles around the country to see something else, and then turn around and go home to rest.

Vacation means to "vacate" where you have been. Get out of there, seek a new scene, a new place in life, a better time, so that when you return home you will be completely rejuvenated. You will see it with a new mind and can once again handle your life. This is what a vacation should be.

One's emotional life can best be controlled by realizing that you live in a world of action and reaction. It is what you react to that causes your problems, not what you act on. You must be strong mentally. Some people cannot have a bad word said to them without fighting. People will complain at you; people will throw "tomatoes" at you. You have to go through with it and recognize that nothing of an inferior nature should disturb you. This is the emotional side of your health program.

There may be times when you have to go it alone. The more truth you have, the more alone you go, and you will find that you may have to go along a very lonely road. I do know that it is never right mentally to look to someone else for your happiness. There are exceptions to this, however, such as when you take another person to share a soul growth, but that is still acting as one. When you cannot act as one, then you cannot grow together mentally. Unless you walk together agreed, you will walk apart. Love is as strong as its weakest link.

You Were Created for Joy. We must all take the road of joy, because the path of misery is not worth it. Don't worry about things that have happened or things that are coming. If you have been planning for a year at a time and cannot make your plans materialize, plan for a week or perhaps less. There may be a time when you can plan only a day ahead. Sometimes that is all your mind can handle, and in the case of a sick mind, one should not plan even a day ahead. Just take care of the moment, and let everything slip into place. It is important to recognize that "now" is the only thing you will every have to worry about. The past is gone; bury it. The future has not even been born yet; don't start raising it; leave it alone.

Inheritance. Some of us are still suffering from our mother's and father's weaknesses. I don't like to say that , but I know it happened in my case. My mother died of tuberculosis when I was only ten years old. At the age of 20 I too had problems with my lungs. Since then, I have lived 45 years on borrowed time! You have to live a certain kind of life to overcome your weaknesses. As soon as you discover the weaknesses in your body and treat them as weak links in the chain and don't strain them to the place where you break down, then you have the secret of your life. We all have weaknesses. Some have weak stomachs, weak lungs, weak kidneys or bowels; some have weaknesses in the head. Sometimes this weakness in the head is just stubbornness. Many times we have everything we need in the head but we don't use it. I think this is a major problem as far as our heads are concerned.

Setting a Good Foundation. If you put together the value of good diet (six vegetables, two fruits, one good starch, and one protein every day), sunshine, exercise, and good thinking, you find that you start out on a foundation that is bound to keep you well.

Self-Exaltation

One of the most important keys to health self-exaltation, which means to —

Search for our own greatness until we find it.

Convince ourselves that a God actually dwells in our Great Within.

Give ourselves the self-recognition that is due to us to recognize our own high qualities.

Raise ourselves high in our own eyes

Thrill with joy and confidence in ourselves.

Elevate ourselves in self-estimation.

Say as King David of Israel, "Study me, I am fearfully and wonderfully made." Fill our souls with sublime sentiments. Honor ourselves.

Feel noble.

Tell ourselves that we came here from the high heavens, that we have a sacred mission to perform, and that we shall and will perform it nobly.

Convince ourselves that we have a perfect command of our every act, thought, and emotion, and that we have perfect control over our every nerve.

It means to —

Expand in soul and soar like the eagle in space.

Give scope to mind, distinctness to voice, dignity to walk, altitudes to aspiration, control to tongue, peace to soul, nobility to purposes, direction to action, expansion to chest, range to breathing, stillness to personality.

Trust the future.

Hope and watch for success.

Trust ourselves, if only in imagination. Promise ourselves much and joyfully expect it to come in the near future.

Live in a higher soul-altitude.

Forget the past and live in the future.

Forget our own folly, faults, errors.

Find our higher qualities and those of others.

Live in our higher selves and thank God for making us as perfect as we are.

Help others to find their Great Within. Feel and think that we are God-like and made in His image.

Feel lofty.

Convince ourselves that we are masters of every situation.

Sit like a statue of repose and let the world spin as we dwell on exalted sentiments. Long for the communion with our higher selves, with God, angels, saints, and noble-living people.

Reason out our own greatness and find our noble qualities, convinced of the fact that a god lives within us, that our possibilities are so great that we have not the faintest idea of what is NOT possible for us.

These mind-exercises have a tendency to exalt us. This is self-exaltation. They will bring sure results in every case.

What You Should and Should Not Do

And these things further ensure health and well-being:

Never talk in a loud voice, but always gently.

Never tell ugly, unbelievable stories.

Never go to excess in anything.

Avoid questionable associates.

Establish a reputation for honesty and punctuality.

Give your blood freedom to flow unimpeded by corsets, belts, etc.

Keep your own knowledge to yourself until you can use it.

Cultivate courage, but be like an oiled bullet — silent.

Never be noisy.

Guard your character; it is your highest attainment.

Use tact in public by dwelling upon exalted sentiments.

Cultivate cheerfulness of mind.

Keep your own trouble and pains to yourself.

Always be civil, courteous, polite.

Look for the good points in people.

Let no one force you, but do not fight or argue.

Let no one rule you; act and be silent.

Do not read newspapers, or anything of a low nature.

Live much in seclusion and select noble friends.

Avoid promiscuous sex commerce; it is degrading.

Listen to how people speak. Notice how they look, act, what they talk about. Watch their faces when you talk to them and you know *how* it affects them.

ENGLAND—Home of Dr. Bach who created a healing method he called "Flower Remedies."

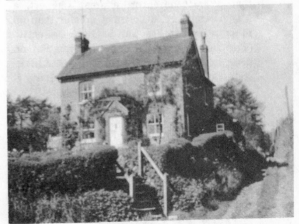

TWENTY SIX

Personology key to self

D ID you ever stop to think why people are not like you? No two people are alike. Everyone is molded differently. Everyone has a different pattern in body, shape, emotions, thinking, and soul growth. Each has a different past and future yet to come.

In *personology*, we study the physical characteristics of the body and their differences. We first determine this difference, and them discover the personality that goes with it.

Differences exist in the mind just as they exist in the body. Is it possible that from the various physical charactersistics in people we can tell just how they are going to react mentally? Is there a relationship between a person's nose and his thinking, a person's ears or eyebrows and his thinking? Is it possible that your physical body expresses what you are capable of doing mentally? Yes, it is possible– through personology.

Personology is a study that will never end. There is always more to know; more than I could possibly tell you; more than I could ever learn in my lifetime. I don't know whether to call personology a science or not, but I do feel man is a scientific phenomenon, that a great Inventor, a great Chemist, a Master Architect, a Scientist greater than all other scientists has put us here on earth. (For those who desire more information on personology than is provided here, write Interstate College of Personology, 1209 Burlingame Avenue, Burlingame, California, 94010.)

Influence Of Parents

Is it possible that our parents influence the thinking we have today? Is it possible our bodies are, more or less, dependent upon the body structure of our mothers and fathers? Is it possible to suffer the sins of our fathers, even unto the fourth generation? How far back does this go? Is it possible to wipe out some of these inherited traits from a health standpoint, from a personality standpoint? Is it possible to change them? Is it possible to out grow them? Are we always going to carry our weaknesses; or will our weaknesses become our strength? Are we going to replace our weaknesses with a philosophy which, in time, will become flesh? Are we going to change our physical weaknesses with foods, which in time will become flesh? I think these questions are worthy of investigation. And I think the answers are there.

While traveling in New Zealand, I had an introduction to a pattern carried down through the parents. A Japanese girl was riding a bicycle while standing on her head and making 30 to 50 turns without stopping. She was considered the world's greatest.

Why should she be so great? Why should it be a girl? Why should she be Japanese? I start ed questioning and the answer came in the fact that both her parents were perhaps the greatest bicyclists the world has ever known.

I sat in the bleachers at a fair in Salt Lake City, Utah, and watched the beautiful work of a cutting horse (if you want to see a beautiful performance, watch a well-trained cutting horse). The cutting horse can do what no other type of horse can do. He can charge the on– coming herd of cattle and cut out any one of a group of cows as the herd comes forward. Cutting horses are very valuable and are often sold before they are born. They are the result of many years of careful breeding.

The mental faculties used by the parents most are usually the ones carried over into the children.   Napoleon was born to a mother married to a general. During the period preceding his birth, his mother was intensely interested in the war and the struggle for freedom of her native island. She followed her husband wherever he went, even living in hay stacks behind the firing line, always close to "war thoughts." She planned and schemed constantly, thought and talked of war. The result, NAPOLEON! — warmaker, conqueror, emperor, exile, and prisoner. What a tremendous train of historical events that mother's thinking was responsible for!

In the year 1577, another mother, throughout her pregnancy, was deeply interested in, and studied, the fine arts. She admired the ability to paint wonderful scenes and faces, portraits, objects, landscapes, all that is beautiful in nature; and the ability to portray sentiment, passion, joy, grief, love, hate, all the human feelings, qualities, and achievements. The result — the great Flemish master, Peter Paul Rubens.

It is not just our parents' thoughts that affect us. We also become what our bodies cause us to be — and, paradoxically, our bodies become what we are. Let's look at some physical characteristics and see what they tell us about personalities.

The Eyes

When we look at a stranger and comment on his nature, we usually use our past experience with outward appearances. To the person with deep-set eyes we are often tempted to say, "Don't be so serious." They are usually serious-minded.

Big eyes are feeling eyes; that person is leading with the heart. They do not rely too much on reason or logic, but go through life on their feelings more than anything else. If the situation feels good, then everything is all right. Of course that isn't always the best way to judge. You should have some good reason for doing things.

If you have a child with large eyes (the child who works with feelings) you cannot whip him or spank him to make him do things; but if someone shows they believe in him, he will go right to the end doing the right thing.

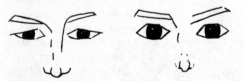

If the outer corners of the eyelids are pulled way down, it indicates a person who is very critical. If such a person spends his days as an inspector, he is very thorough. If the pipes don't fit, you have to take them out. "This is no good; get rid of that!" Then, in the evening if when he walks in the door of

his home his wife greets him with a kiss, he says, "Why didn't you do this? This should be that way; that should be this way." You know what kind of a reception he gets! The

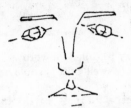

fact is he is using only one of his faculties; his criticalness.

If he has a narrow forehead, he would be more tactful. Tact goes along with a person who has a narrow forehead. These people are the diplomats.

It is the combinations that make these people what they are. Some people are very cruel. Imagine a cruel person giving criticism. They don't care whom they offend. There are people who are very affectionate — this also is indicated in the eyes. A person with a level,

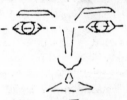

steady look is blessed with great energy in his actions and thoughts. Eyes that are shaped like almonds pledge gentleness and sensitivity.

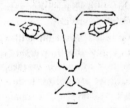

When the upper eyelid doubles over itself it indicates a person who is very analytical.

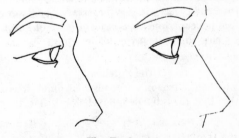

The Eyebrow

People who are very affable have eyebrows that hang down close to the level of the eye it-

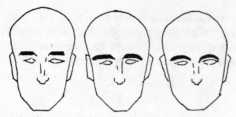

self. They may be called "lowbrows" but they get along very well with people and make friends easily.

The opposite of this is aloofness. The "highbrow" is very difficult to get acquainted with; he doesn't have many friends; but those friends he does have are usually good ones. To get along with these people, you have to live in their kind of world, and they don't take many people in. There is nothing wrong with this type of person or with his thinking. All kinds of people are needed in this world to do the jobs that have to be done.

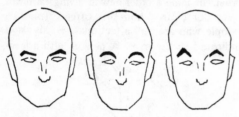

When the eyebrow is high and round, it is a sign of a person with dramatic ability. Usually these people are movie actors or actresses. Look at the magazines and notice the pictures of the actors and actresses. They have this kind of eyebrow.

The person who has an eyebrow that comes to a point is very construction-minded, engineer-minded. He has to have everything in its place or he is disturbed. We find that eyebrows can mean a lot when we are choosing the kind of work we are going to do.

If you have a friend who is an exacting type, watch him work out a problem. What does he do? He furrows his brow and puts in those vertical lines between his eyebrows. This is a sign that he is exacting and it shows in his forehead. This is a very necessary quality for some occupations. If a carpenter is not exact, I'd hate to live in any of his buildings.

The Forehead

When a person's forehead is round, it is a sign that they like people; when it is flat, they

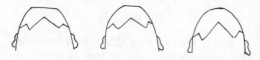

like things. You cannot be interested in both people and things at the same time.

The forehead that goes straight up belongs to people who keep things on their minds, who think their problems out. They will not let the problems out of their minds until they have worked them out. These people are worriers.

The person whose forehead goes backward is the person who gets things off his mind quickly. He is what we would call the objective thinker. He gets things off his mind quickly. He can't hold them; he can't keep them. Many times he doesn't like this. He starts to get hold of an idea and think it out. The more he thinks about it, the longer he will keep it on his mind. In this way, the forehead will be brought out, and in time you will become more of a subjective thinker.

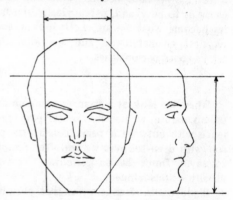

The higher the forehead, the greater the capacity for thinking. Some people are thinkers; others are not. An extremely high forehead indicates a person who has a great interest in the future, in what is to come.

The ego center, the forceful center, is strong in the person whose head is wider across the forehead than the distance from the chin to the eyebrow. Docile birds, for instance, are the ones that have the narrow forehead. The animals with wide heads are the forceful ones who have ego.

There are some people who are so egotistical that they are not wanted. Their attitude is, "I can do this; I am better than you; I am bigger than you; I am more accomplished than you." There are some people who just don't allow you to live or feel good around them because of this ego; yet it is the ego that really gets the job done, that accomplishes things. They have the mental power to get things done.

If a person is narrow across the forehead just above the eyes, then his ego has to be developed. If a person with a small ego was asked

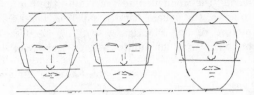

to address a group of people, it would be difficult for him. But public speaking is always an effective way to develop ego.

You cannot be effective and accepted as a leader unless you have ego. Another way of developing ego is to overcome a mental weakness. For instance, if a person is afraid of the water and finally learns how to swim, he has overcome that mental weakness and this helps develop the ego.

You can develop your ego by becoming learned in some direction. Learn one thing very, very well. Albert Hubbard says, "If you will study fifteen minutes a day for five years, on the heart, you will be one of the greatest heart authorities in the world." Now, pick some subject and study it for fifteen minutes a day.

The person with a small ego, who is narrow across the forehead just above the eyes, also has a very poor digestive system. His nervous system does not handle foods well. As we get a bit older, our nerve force goes down.

When people are full in the area between the end of the eyebrow and the temple,

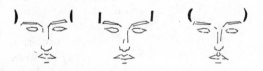

which is the digestive center, it means that they can digest foods well. Fat people are always full there; those who do not digest foods well are thin in that area; they have a slight indentation. They form gas and don't get the good they need from their food. This type of person is finicky and cranky and should eat only when he is feeling good, when there is not tension.

The Jaw

People with a big, square jaw and a square chin are very physical individuals in everything they do. Those who have a narrow jaw are the mental type and haven't much interest in the physical things.

The Lips

Those who have tight lips are curt. They cut off their sentences. When they speak they don't say one extra word. Calvin Coolige was an example. Once when he returned from church, someone asked him what the sermon was about, and he answered, "God." His answers were always yes or no. We have the opposite, the people with thick, big lips. This is a sign of verbosity. They love to talk and they can express themselves well. Examples are: Senator William E. Borah, William Jennings Bryan, and Mrs. Eleanor Roosevelt. We have to have people who talk as well as people who listen.

The Nose

There are people who have a nose with a big knob on the end. This is called a newsy

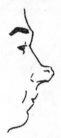

nose. They know everything about their neighbors. They get the news before anyone else. They have their nose in other people's business. They have a nose for news. If you want to know anything, just ask them.

People whose nostrils flare out can be depended upon to get a job done. They are very self-reliant. They will exert themselves to such an extent that they use up their physical and mental energy. They become depleted and need to rejuvenate to restore it again.

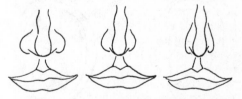

When a person has a big hump on the nose, he loves to acquire things. Ferraro, the richest man that ever lived, had a parrot's beak. This hump on the nose represents the ability to acquire knowledge from books; some like to acquire musical ability. Some people just like to gather salt shakers wherever they go. And some like to acquire money.

Other people have a nose that goes in the opposite direction and we call that the administrative nose. With this type of nose, a person loves to do things for other people.

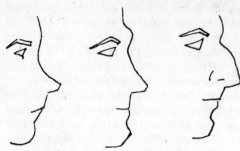

They make good ministers and good nurses. They are never really happy unless they are being a "Helpful Henry." We need to have these people.

Then we have a person with a nose that turns down. This is a very skeptical nose. He

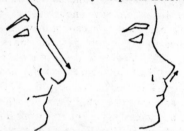

doesn't believe anything he hears; he takes it home and runs it through a sieve. He is a born skeptic. It takes a long time for the good things to come to him, because he keeps them away.

The Ear

An ear round on top, with a long lobe, more or less sharp below, indicates a person with little appreciation for music. If you want to see ears of a person well-developed musically, find a picture of Leopold Stokowski's

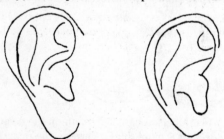

ears or Frank Sinatra's ears, or look at the ears of people who play music "by ear." Perhaps there is something real behind the expression "playing by ear."

The Hands

A pointed hand looks graceful and beautiful, but from the standpoint of coordination,

of doing the greatest amount of work, and of having the mind behind everything the hand touches, the square hand is superior. I saw a picture of Joe DiMaggio waving his hand as he went into an auditorium, and his hand

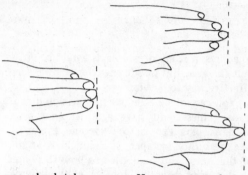

was absolutely square. He was one of the greatest ball players, one who could really pick up the ball, because all of his fingers, not just one, touched the ground.

The Posture

Our posture tells much about us. Are we happy to be alive or bowed down with care? Do we carry ourselves as though we were comfortable with our height — and weight?

Posture can also affect our health. With the most healthy posture one can draw a straight line down the body through the ear, shoulder,

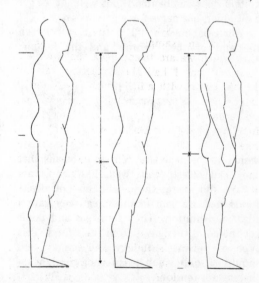

hip, and ankle. When that line is not straight the whole body is misaligned, and pressure symptoms appear in various organs. Abnormal stress is developed on muscles, tendons, and ligaments. This leads to a variety of symptoms, such as neuritis, neck tension, prolapsus, improper chest position and breathing, etc.

One Side More Dominant

One side of the body is more capable of doing things than the other. About 45 percent of all people are left-handed. The reason they are left-handed is that they are left-eyed, meaning that the left eye can see and do things more quickly than the right. We may inherit left-handedness or right-handedness, and it is to our advantage to use the side of the body that has more ability and strength. We usually have a talent that is stronger on one side of the body than the other. A "south paw" can be just as successful as a right-handed pitcher. Imagine taking a left-handed pitcher and trying to make him into a right-handed pitcher.

Very often a child's speech and thinking problems stem from the fact that he is made to use the brain factor that is not the most dominant — it is not the successful or talented one. I have seen many children overcome stuttering just by changing the activity of their hands. There are teachers who teach students to shoot with the right eye and right shoulder, yet some of the greatest marksmen are left-handed. They use their left eye, which is the dominant eye, the successful eye, the strong eye, and they become great marksmen. They use the successful part of their body. This is something to think about.

Natural Talent

Just as an example of how we respond to that which we are talented in, that we are a "natural" in, I had this experience at my health center with a little five-year-old girl. I talked to her about many things and could get no response. Then I looked at her ears. She had large, bell-like round ears, so I said, "You like music, don't you?" She came alive and responded with, "Yes, I'm going to be in a muscial recital; I want to tell you all about it." She loved to express herself in music. It was the thing she loved doing most in her life.

Mother and Father Nature

There are many things we can show to prove that one side of the body is like our mother's and the other side is like our father's.

We inherit characteristics from both mother and father, but there is a dominant side to our body, and this dominant side is the strongest. Many people have a father's day and a mother's day. This gives them "mood swings." If we have a body that has "mood swings" we will make decisions like father one day and like mother the next day. The following day, we may be sorry for having made the previous decisions. The reason that so many people are mixed up and confused within is that they do not understand these swings, these ups and downs.

> *His mother's eyes, his father's chin,*
> *His auntie's nose, his uncle's grin,*
> *His great-aunt's hair, his grandma's ears,*
> *His grandpa's mouth, so it appears.*
> *Poor little tot, well may he moan,*
> *He hasn't much to call his own.*
> *(Author Unknown)*

Leave Problems and Have Better Health

Let's put some of these facts together. First, we must find a way to handle our problems so that our nervous systems are not at a ragged edge all the time; so that when we sit down to eat we have enough nerve force to digest our food. We cannot have anger and revenge in our hearts and feel mean at the world. I tell people to get into a place where they will be happy, because happy people get well quickly. Get on the road to joy. Discover who you are, what your characteristics are — then act accordingly. You will work differently and eat differently, and everything will change. This is so with everyone. I can't promise you money, jewels, or worldly things; but who is the richest man in the world? Isn't he the one who knows how to handle a problem, who has his health in tow, who knows who he is, who knows where he is going and who will finally get there? He is the man who has wealth, who has dominion.

Here is the secret of life: Take some of your weaknesses and make them stronger; but also, don't miss developing the strong points as well, so that you will achieve something more than anyone else. It is only a lack of balance which makes one unacceptable to others.

TWENTY SEVEN

Magic of mind power

THE MAGIC of mind power? Yes! The mind can lead your body into a lot of disturbances, a lot of problems, a lot of troubles. But the mind also has the power to lead us into a lot of joy and a lot of happiness.

The mind can take us into a make-believe world. It can actually help us to tune out some of the things that are disturbing us constantly. We can make a mountain out of a molehill or a molehill out of a mountain.

It is well to recognize that man possesses the ability to view life in two ways — positively or negatively. We have the privilege of going in any direction we wish.

The mind, racing from moment to moment, encompasses thoughts of both a positive and a negative nature; it is influenced by feelings, colors, and emotions; and its action is reflected in the activity of the body.

A man saddled with depression, blue and doomed in his own mind, may walk along singing "Happy Days Are Here Again," but the song won't help him. One's mind can take on only one thought at a time. You can't hate and love at the same time. For this reason, it is necessary that we have some training of the mind so that we don't just do what other people want us to do, or take the frightful and fearful path at every turn of our mind's highway.

We have to set up a program we can follow. We have to roll out our own red carpet. It is difficult to walk the uplifted way in a world set up by negative, sick people. Many times we find that these people are well-meaning. and many times they have a leadership of mind. But we have to develop a program from within that is going to help us out of the doldrums and onto the higher road that leads to a holy land, a spiritual land, a wonderful, new psychological state that is good for our body. Every thought will find every cell in your body.

Are there people around you who just make you feel as if you are all "choked up"? Do some people give you a "pain in the neck"? Do people ever make you "sick to your stomach"? How does this feeling get there? How does it get to this physical body?

The magic of the mind is that it can actually bring on activities in our bodies that are detrimental — or it can bring on activities that are uplifting. Nothing of an inferior nature will come upon you unless you give it your consent. Many a family has gone through life feeling that they have to live in duty. They forget that there should be joy with that duty. We have been created for joy. The mind can lift us and carry us over a hurdle- or it can stop us in our tracks in fear and fright.

We must realize that the mind has the greatest power in the world to make us a success or to make us a failure; to make us healthy or diseased. The magic of mind is something that we should get acquainted with. You know that there are people who can disturb you — but you must develop a positive outlook on life — and use it! No one can disturb you unless you give your consent.

As my mother used to say, "If your outlook isn't right, get a new inlook." We should recognize that there is a relation as far as levels of thinking is concerned. There are some things we can dwell on that may not do us any good, and we have to consider even the spiritual thoughts that come to us. Is it possible that the mind magically could go on to higher things and seek better things in this life? Two men sat in jail behind bars — one saw mud, the other, stars.

I am convinced that whatever happens in life requires an attitude to meet it. I am convinced that in our own mind we can smile, we can laugh, we can seek mirth, cheer, joy, and happiness. Or we can sink into the doldrums; we can see doom; we can exist in a

214

living hell. We can be constantly in mourning and in sorrow. These latter thoughts have a detrimental effect on our physical body, on our breathing, on our heartbeat — on every activity of our physical self.

This experiment in the medical field bears out my statements: A cat was tested in the laboratory to find out how much hydrochloric acid was being secreted from its stomach wall. Something like three drops every three minutes was coming from the cat's stomach. But a dog outside the laboratory barked, and for a solid hour there was no more hydrochloric acid coming from that stomach wall. Think about that.

I am convinced that many times we are not fit to sit down to the dining table to eat. Unless we have a lot of joy, unless we view this meal as a happy experience to our bodies, it will harm us, and can often cause painful indigestion. It is not only the kind of food that goes into the man that is important, but also what kind of a man the food goes into!

The phychologists tells us that we use only ten percent of our brain structure. Well, it is a wonderful thing that we use only ten percent if we are looking for the ugly things in life — the harsh, dirty, mean ideas. Suppose we were to use 90 percent of our mind on all these detrimental effects. I am sure that most of us would not be able to control it, and we would very shortly lose our life physically.

On the other hand, the person who has changed his mind to see beauty, to see culture, to see the higher things in life, to see the God in the people that he meets is constantly uplifting every person he encounters. He knows that only good things are to follow, and he is thankful for what is yet to come. I am convinced that such a person is going to have something fine and magically healthful happen to his body, especially if he can develop himself to use the other 90 percent of his brain. Just imagine using 100 percent of your brain for the adventure of life.

Some years ago, I realized that the most important thing in helping a person attain that magical mind was to recognize that there is no such thing as defeat; that there is no such thing as a stumbling block without a way to overcome it.

In working out this magical mind, I discovered the following axioms that we can live by. Study them and see how true they are. Get them into your consciousness. Live them every day. Practice them. Use them on other people. Repeat them often until they are part of you.

Whatever you are seeking in life; that is also seeking you.

God made food for the birds, but he did not put it in their nests.

We do not have to love what people do, but we do have to love people.

War and hate are made in the hearts of man, but by the same token, peace and love are found in the hearts of men, also.

It is not what we have in life that is important, it is what we enjoy. We have not been given things to enjoy, but we have been given life to enjoy all things.

Get off Poor Street — poor me, poor dog, poor in spirit, there goes a poor soul.

Get on the rich side of the street. See that you are doing something in life that is really worthwhile, that you are accomplishing something fine.

Have a smile that is uplifting to others.

Have a happiness to share with others.

The only stimulation of the body should come from exercise. If we don't use our bodies, we lose them.

We must have a hobby. We must do something we love to do. Get away from mean, spiteful people. Pick your friends from people you like to be with.

Never eat with people who are depressing to you or your guests. Make your meals joy meals.

Do not merely let life happen, but find what the good life is and just let it flow through you.

Time is here to stay; it is we that go. Let us make the most of time.

I feel that as we go over these many axioms and they become part of our everyday living, we will realize that we can face our tomorrow, we can face our problems. And if we don't take care of these problems now, when we wake up tomorrow we will have to face them again. So as we look at these things we realize we become stronger and we become a magic person through changing not only our own life, but the lives of others as well. Truly, this mind is a magical thing. Realize that no man who faces the sun sees his shadow.

You Can Change Your Mind

As man goes through life, he looks outside himself and sees everyone else as mortal; but he considers himself immortal. This is a good thought, but when I stop to think about it, I find that I am mortal also. "If you can do it, so I can do it." If there was anything that could be done, I did it. If there was an impossibility, I did that too. I have never known an impossibility; that is part of my nature. When you have that idea in your mind, you never consider yourself as one who has an age limit.

It is true that wherever there is a disease, there is a remedy right next to it, but it is up to us to use that remedy before we miss the opportunity. That is why I believe that faith without works is dead. Your spiritual concept in life is not worth two cents if you have hate for your fellowman. Don't talk to me about foods unless you exercise; if you don't exercise, food is nothing — it will never circulate in your body.

Don't try to run away from your problems. There are times when you can run away for relaxation, but if you run three thousand miles to get well and don't do anything, you will go home feeling the same. You will find out that if you go to the moon because you are frustrated here, you will be frustrated there. It is not a matter of running off into space, getting away from these things. The space you have to conquer is between your ears.

If you have the mind to work with, you can overcome and do wonderful things. Life is just one exciting challenge after another. The first thing you have to do is meet life head on. Life is going to plow you under if you don't fight it. If you don't want to get up in the mornings, you really don't have to. If you stay in bed long enough, one of these days they will bury you.

I tell you this because we sometimes think that all we have to do is hang around and let the doctor get us well. I sat at the feet of Dr. Henry Lindlahr of Chicago, Illinois, back in 1924. He talked about cures and how a chronic condition could be reversed. Produce a crisis, produce a fever, and you can burn up any infection in the body, regardless of where it is.

Learn what a crisis is. Learn to reverse the disease process, or stay where you are. I once said to a young fellow: "You are going to have to quit smoking or I can't help you."

He said, "I can't quit smoking."

I replied, "Well, I can't help you."

We went down to a medical doctor in Escondido, California, and I said; "Doctor, I can't do anything with this young man. See what you can do."

The doctor said, "Well, with this bronchial problem here, do you smoke?"

The fellow said, "Yes, and I can't quit."

The doctor said, "Then die."

The young man walked out. And he quit!

What kind of shock do you need before you get out of your problems? What can a doctor do but to lead you nicely: "Yes, dear, let's do it this way"? But the thing is this: Sometimes you can be so soft mentally that you don't do anything. I have had people come to me and say: "Doctor, I am sick." And, I can tell right away, and I have to say, "Yes, you look it too." Then I walk off for a minute and let them think about it. I let them stew, and I let my words begin to work. Usually when I come back they say, "Maybe I ought to change."

I can't do anything with anyone who doesn't desire to do the right thing.

What I Learned from the Essenes

I think the greatest lesson I ever learned in my life was from the Essenes. They lived a very natural life. When I say "a natural life," I mean they lived close to the soil, close to the garden, close to the sun and to the earth. These people knew the earth, the odors, and the animals. They knew that water treatments would take away inflammations caused by high fevers. They knew enemas could take a fever down. They never treated with vaccinations to get rid of germ life; they built up the host.

They found that if they built up the body in what we call the image of God, it would be acceptable before God. You cannot be acceptable before God with a cigarette in your mouth. It is an impossibility. You cannot be acceptable to God while you are drinking liquor. You have to come to the Divine, straight and clean. These people knew that. When a child was born in this particular group and community, they revered that child and everything that went with him. They were thankful for the privilege of bringing the child into life; they were thankful for the mother's milk. When the mother gave milk to the child, she had to have food from Mother Earth, so she revered the earth. When she looked down at Mother Earth, she looked up and thanked God. She knew the earth nurtured her, took care of her, and belonged to her and her child.

When a child was born, they planted a tree for that child, because Mother Earth had been so good. At the age of one year, they planted another tree; at the age of two, another. When the child became 18, they said: "We have given you all the knowledge we can — we have taught you how to use water packs; we have taught you how to eat; we have taught you how to take care of the earth and to replenish the earth; how to grow trees; how to eat; how to think; how to meditate; and how to recognize the things that had the approval of God."

Their inheritance for a child of 18 was 18 trees, a piece of land: "We have given you everything we have everything we know. We have given you honesty; we have given you lovely endeavors; we have given you all the health we possibly can. Now your life is your own, to be lived as it ought to be lived." What inheritance could be better than that?

A young girl came to Dr. V.G. Rocine (who was ninety years of age when I studied with him) and said: "I am five months pregnant and I want to start living right to have a good baby," and I remember him saying, "Well, darling, you should have started twenty years ago."

Mind Power

Many people today feel that they have to hoard money and food because they are afraid of starving. They are living until the time they get Social Security. Is this social security? No. Security comes from the mind. It is mind over matter; mind over platter; mind over money; mind over dissension and resentment. If you put your mind in good order, you can control almost anything, regardless of what it is. When you get a strong mind and know in what direction you should be going, you can make the body as perfect as possible. Mind is going to make it or break it.

Let's Get Moving

Then you need to start exercising to get in shape. You need to get fit through physical exercise and get a nice, hard muscle and a strong will working this muscle structure, so that when you want to jump, you can jump, move when you want to. You can do this through muscle structures you build through exercising.

Exercise can come to you in many ways — don't tell me that you are in a wheelchair and that you can't exercise. Through tension relaxation, you can move every muscle in your body, and you can do it with your mind. If you have a mind, you can move anything you want to in your body.

I am not going to ask you to go any place to start a new spiritual or physical life. You can just sit where you are and start a new life right in your mind.

Unless you have this good health, your finances will go down the drain. Everything

you earned while you were well will be lost when you are sick. Just ask a sick person. The only thing you have is what you have to give in life. Your deepest self is the thing that will get you well.

Look Ahead

Let's get away from people who do us no good. Be selective enough to have people around who will uplift you. We need strong people. One reason you are reading this is because you are a seeker; you want to elevate yourself toward better things in life. Let us recognize that, as seekers, we have to have this knowledge to get to the finer things in life.

Read about Father Kneipp — he treated 4,000 people a week. He treated princes and kings from all over the world. At one time the Pope sent for Father Kneipp, and Father Kneipp wrote: "I am too busy healing people to come to see you." So the Pope sent a Commission, which brought Father Kneipp to the Pope. Father Kneipp says in his diary that he sat down next to the Pope, who asked about the weather, asked about this and that, and finally asked Father Kneipp about the Pope's health. "Then," wrote Father Kneipp in his diary, "I was the Pope."

I am trying to bring out that when you are in control, you have the knowledge, you are the Pope, you are the King. Health can never be gained from pills from out of a bottle. It is you who will get it to work.

Know Yourself

Before you try to improve yourself you should come to know yourself. You should study your personality, your mind, how you work, how you give out.

You have to recognize that there are certain kinds of protein that feed every faculty of the mind. Every faculty you have takes a different level of protein. There are amino acid proteins that fit avarice and destructive ability. Some of us have to have more emotional stability to get ahead in this life. You can be so humble and recede so far back in your life that you bcome a meditator. The only thing good for you then is to be a hermit on top of a hill with a fence around you, with your dog inside a fence that has the sign "Don't come in here; the dog will bite you!"

If you want that kind of life, you can have it. However, until you get to the place where you are beyond that fence, until you recognize that you are no good in life until you start doing something for somebody else, you will stagnate. Somebody always needs you. You will never attain real happiness until somebody really needs you and wants you and blesses you. Only then will you realize what real living is all about. The idea of having a good body so that you can jump, have a good heartbeat, and have two bowel movements a day is not total living. There is more to life than that.

We Are More Than Physical

I was once a physical boy and I know what it is to be physical. I know what it is to have only health with nothing else. "Don't talk to me about God. When you show him to me, I will believe in him. I want a demonstration." However, one evening I found the answer. I was sleeping in the desert and as the sun went down, the poppies closed their petals. I wondered what was controlling them. What made them close up?

The next morning as I awakened the sun was coming up over the mountains. I noticed that the poppies were also coming to life. For the first time in my life I realized that there was a divine principle, a divine architect, a divine chemist. The One who controlled this universe had good things to say as far as my life was concerned.

I was thankful for what I saw in myself and those flowers. There is something that keeps you alive and keeps you going. There is something that will keep you from worry, because this something is taking care of you. You must get into the swing of life. You must get close to nature.

We Are Co-Creators

Your life is in the lap of the Gods, and you and your God will work it out. God and you make good health and beauty. You are co-creators. Nothing has to be changed as far as God is concerned because all things in heaven are all right. If you want to have that heaven right here on earth, you must do something about it. For starters you have to have good digestion. Second, you have to have a good nerve system. Third, you have to have a good elimination system. Fourth, you have to have a good glandular system. Fifth, you have to have a good breathing apparatus.

How do you get theses things? It starts with the magic of the mind. Sometime you are going to awaken and say, "What a crazy fool I am." At this time you will quit smok-

ing and start changing your life. This is the time you will drop the bad habits and start replacing them with a new set of good habits. You need the transformation to be in the direction of health. Don't you think you have been on the wrong path long enough?

One of the oldest men, Li Chung Yun, who died in 1930 at the age of 256, said, "We should sit like a rabbit and run like a tortoise." At 190, he claimed he shortened his life by playing tennis. Before he died, he was asked what he attributed his long life to. He gave a sermon in two words: "Inward calm." Without that you are not going anywhere.

How to Get Along with People

Sooner or later the wise man discovers that life is a mixture of good days and bad, victories and defeats, give and take.

Getting along with people is an art, but there are rules to every art. Try these:

1. Keep skid chains on your tongue; always say less than you think. Cultivate a low, persuasive voice. How you say it often counts more than what you say.

2. Make promises sparingly and keep them faithfully, no matter what it costs you.

3. Never let an opportunity pass to say a kind or encouraging thing to or about somone. Praise good work done, regardless of who did it. If criticism is needed, criticize helpfully.

4. Be interested in others: Interested in their pursuits, their welfare, their homes and families. Make merry with those who rejoice and with those who weep, mourn. Let everyone you meet, however humble, feel that you regard him as one of importance.

5. Reserve an open mind on all debatable questions. Discuss, but do not argue. It is a mark of superior minds to disagree and yet be friendly.

6. Let your virtues speak for themselves, and refuse to talk of another's vices. Discourage gossip. Make it a rule to say nothing of another unless it is something good.

7. Be careful of another's feelings; avoid wit and humor at the other's expense. Sometimes it hurts where least expected.

8. Pay no attention to ill-natured remarks about yourself. Simply live so that no one will believe them. Disordered nerves and bad digestion are a common cause of backbiting.

There is a staff of life within you. Find and nourish yourself with it. Regardless of what happens, you will have something to turn to. If someone turns to you, show him the higher way, using the silver key of understanding. It will make him happy to return the favor. getting along with people is conducive to good health. Getting along with others is an important prerequisite to getting along with yourself. Only then can we have the control over our minds that we need to exercise their magic.

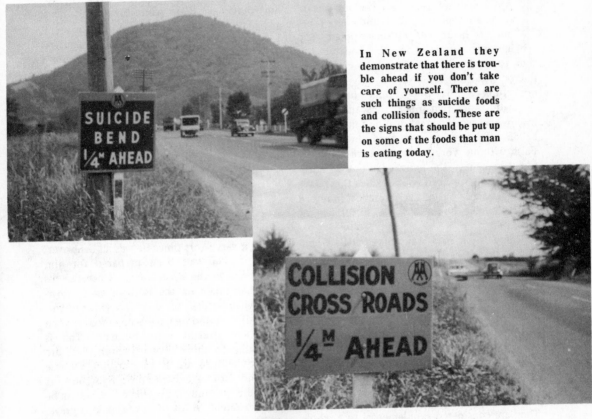

In New Zealand they demonstrate that there is trouble ahead if you don't take care of yourself. There are such things as suicide foods and collision foods. These are the signs that should be put up on some of the foods that man is eating today.

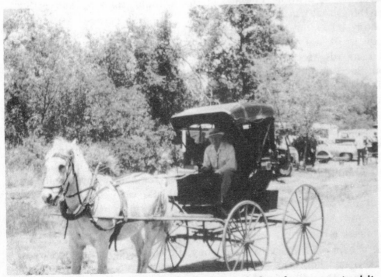

Dr. Jensen in his buggy that many of the doctors had used years ago to visit their patients.

Think good thoughts

I AM convinced that man was not meant to be a cripple or a fool, and many times doctors make a living on crippled, sick, ignorant people. I say this because it is time to awaken. Nature does the curing; the doctor gets the fee. Nature only needs an opportunity. The opportunity lies within yourself. And remember that nature and healing can work a great deal on faith and our beliefs. We have to put them into action. Faith without works is dead. There are many today who have the knowledge but do nothing about it. We need good leaders these days to help lead us out of the ignorance, in regard to the human body, and into fulfillment of good health.

There is no easy way to get well. Whenever I take care of any patient, no matter what the ailment or disease may be, we first start to improve the digestion and elimination. Every organ in the body is dependent upon what you digest, how well you digest, and the elimination of toxic waste. Cleansing is healing. As we improve one organ, we help every other organ in the body to function better. We treat the whole man.

This is a book of remedies, not "cures." None of the remedies in this book will cure. They are considered supplemental to a whole program and all the other things that can be used to build the whole body into a natural state of healthy functioning.

If you asked me what standards we could live by, I couldn't tell you. But I do know if we could find the truth, it would be the best standard I could give you. It reminds me of the time when John D. Rockefeller offered a million dollars to anyone who would help him to digest a ham sandwich. You know, I felt sure that with all my knowledge of food I was going to make a million dollars. In fact, in my mind I was all packed; but then I began to think about it realized what a fool I was. How can you, for any amount of money, get anyone to digest a ham sandwich? No one can digest a ham sandwich. What do they use to make ham? Pork! We cannot digest pork well. More than likely,

he would have it on white bread, and this is a bad combination of starch and protein. I began to think of all the things that he was doing wrong. For a million dollars could I make it right? I knew I couldn't, so there was no reason for me to go. One thing I did learn, though, is that you are never going to make a good thing from a bad start. You have to start right. this is the reason we connot continue to fix up human beings who are breaking down their bodies faster than you can repair them.

Think Straight

A few years ago when I was in London there was a man who was expected to die within a very short time. He was all bent over, and a casket had been prepared for him which was in the shape of an S because his body had taken on the form of an S. However, when he died his body straightened out. Now, why should he have been crooked when living and straight when he died? This is something to think about. I think there are a lot of us who are all tied up like Chinese feet and look like corkscrews right now. If we could just unwind a little we would be quite different. A lot of us are making graveyard material without thinking and eating properly.

I had another experience in London when I visited a graveyard. On one tombstone was this epitaph: "There was one thing I believed in life: that there was no God. I would only believe it should seven trees grow through my tombstone." It was a little late to believe. If you doubt for one minute the power of God and the power of God to heal and give a good life, you are very wrong. There is more perfection, more prosperity, health, and harmony, more tranquility than all the tranquilizing tablets can give, and more good feeling in following a right mental and spiritual program than any other way. A person who does not feel good cannot have a good body. He is tearing himself to shreds; he is breaking himself up bit by bit. I am convinced that a person who doesn't walk in absolute harmony with God cannot be successful in his financial health. The health of his marriage will suffer also. There is such a thing as being financially healthy. Many of us talk about being poor; just where are the riches?

To live well, it is necessary to get to the place where we realize the nature of God; realize we don't have to beg; we don't have to wait. Right now, we have the privilege of changing our lives. Whatever we do today is going to bring us a better tomorrow. Many people would like to change their lives, but they don't march out on this good program.

Dr. Alexis Carrel kept the heart of a chicken living for over 30 years. He gave it constant, meticulous care. Each day, sometimes more often, he had to clip and remove structure as it broke down from age. New structure had to be removed to keep it from growing and expanding — but he stayed with it and proved beyond a doubt that heart structure repairs, rebuilds, and remolds. When Dr. Carrel retired he left the heart tissue and its tending to his students. The heart went right on beating until, through a mixup in duty hours of the attendants, it was not fed for 12 hours. This ended the experiment. The heart died.

This is the history of mankind and his structure. Care for the structure and you will live. Neglect it and you die. When we consider the heart as an organ we must recognize that its function is influenced by many things (worry, fear, joy, and gloom) as well as food. We should know that drugs, drink, heavy meals, acids in the body, gasses in the blood, stomach gasses pressing against the heart, breathing, heavy work, late hours, loss of sleep, heat, cold, athletics, constant oratory, age, body position, air in the lungs, blood pressure, altitude, air pressure, electrical tension, atropine, nicotine — ALL have an effect on the heart.

If we are to have a proper heart-building program, we must provide a sustenance program, not only in our diet, but through peace of mind, self-control, and self-content. It is imperative that we put all these together, and do not expect to build our body only through diet. One religion ends each of its services with these words:"As you leave today, seek a God of contentment." Such an attitude is good for the heart and lightens our heavy burdens. Let us not become too one-sided in chasing after a cure; it's not to be found in one special drink or preparing a potato in a special way. There is much more.

An English physician, Alexander Bryce, wrote in 1912: "Nothing offends patients more than to be asked to change their habits of life. Their desire is to be able to break every known law of health, then when they are called upon to pay the penalty, they accept absolution in a bottle or two of medicine. They do not want to be cured, but are content to be patched up sufficiently to continue their practice of self-indulgence in various forms."

Mental Therapy

It was Professor Brauchle who fasted many people in Dresden, Germany. While they were taken care of with natural methods: Baths, fasting, therapeutic massage, diets, vitamins, and herbs, he assigned a person to talk with these people about their inner problems. They found that the willpower of the patient was strengthened and they overcame many diffculties, hates, destructive thoughts, doubts, resentments, and fears. They replaced those feelings with peace, harmony, and hope. It gave them a motivation and something to live for and put their natural therapeutic activities to work.

Success

Success is not made up of only one section of your body, one organ, or one mental faculty. It is the total use of all your faculties through a maximum use that no one can copy, no one can duplicate or substitute. You are your own when you do this. No one can take your place. It was Longfellow who said, "It is doing what you do well, and doing well whatever you do."

Laughter

Laughter is one of the best things we can do to fight stress. A little nonsense, now and then is relished by the wisest man. He who laughs lasts!

"Seven Tips on How to Control Stress"

Learn to control stress, and you'll work and play better, advises a leading clinical psychologist who offers seven tips on what to do when tension threatens:

1. Learn to recognize in advance situations likely to cause stress. Then when you realize you're going into one of these situations, try to take stock of your tension level. Sometimes, just realizing what you are getting into can help.

2. Try to relax your muscles for 10 minutes,

twice a day. Take a break and concentrate on relaxing leg muscles, then arm muscles, and so on.

3. Direct your attention to non-threatening things. Take a look around you — at the walls, out the window or at the phone — for a moment to distract your mind from the stress.

4. Talk to friends about your tension and anxiety.

5. Rehearse an upcoming stressful situation. Go over the things you know you can do well, and then gradually build up until you can rehearse the whole task or situation.

6. Learn to control your attention by concentrating on a task step by step.

7. Don't try for perfection. Sit back at times and say to yourself that you're not going to be perfect. *(From the National Enquirer)*

"Ten Million Americans Are Scaring Themselves Sick"

The anxiety neurotic has a doomsday attitude that controls his every thought. He goes through life expecting disaster to overcome him at any minute. He is seldom in any real danger, yet all day long, it's fear, fear, fear. He has a racing heart, a churning stomach, a lump in the throat, difficulty in breathing and feelings of mounting panic. Almost everyone has some of these feelings at one time or another, but for the victim of anxiety neurosis these problems are frequent and chronic. The problem generally stems from a troubled childhood, Dr. Pasternack explained. Once the patient realizes that his fears are the result of internal stimulus, and not anything that is happening on the outside, he is better able to cope with the situation. *(From the National Enquirer)*

" 'Dieting Fads Can Drive You Crazy,' Claims Nutritionist"

Dieting fads are responsible for a great amount of the mental distress in the country today. Ten million Americans, who are shedding weight by consuming fewer calories, put themselves in great emotional risk. Dr. Cheraskin said the most popular reducing diets recommend the consumption of about 1200 calories a day. But any adult diet allowing an intake of fewer than 2100 to 2400 calories a day is bound to be deficient in vitamins, minerals and elements vitally needed to maintain good mental health. The truth is the brain cells aren't getting the substances they need and these cells require nutrients more than other cells. The nervous system is the first to react badly to nutrient deficiency. For example, dieters who eliminate all carbohydrates from their diet are also eliminating some high mineral content foods. One result could be a magnesium deficiency, which tends to make people extremely nervous. High protein diets can also cause emotional problems. The more protein you eat, the more you need elements such as calcium and magnesium to help break down the protein in the body. I've heard a lot of dieters say, "I'd rather be dead than fat" but they could be choosing between obesity and sanity. The dieting craze can indeed drive you crazy. *(From the National Enquirer)*

The Art of Getting Along In The Business World

The businessman (and any man) learns that it doesn't pay to be a sensitive soul— that he should let some things go over his head like water off a duck's back.

He learns that he who loses his temper usually loses.

He learns that all men have burnt toast for breakfast now and then, and that he shouldn't take the other fellow's grouch too seriously.

He learns that the quickest way to become unpopular is to carry tales and gossip about others.

He learns that it doesn't matter who gets the credit so long as the business shows a profit.

He comes to realize that the business could run along perfectly well without him.

He learns that it doesn't do any harm to smile and say, "Good Morning!" even if it is raining.

He learns that most of the other fellows are as ambitious as he is, that they have brains that are as good or better, and that hard work and not cleverness is the secret of success.

He learns to sympathize with the youngster coming into the business, because he remembers how bewildered he was when he first started out.

He learns that bosses are not monsters trying to get the last ounce of work out of him for the least amount of pay, but that they are usually fine men who have succeeded through hard work and who want to do the right thing.

He learns that the gang is not any harder to get along with in one place than another and that "getting along" depends about 98 percent on his own behavior.

The king's domain

WHEN I speak of spiritual things, I do so from a health standpoint. However, whatever I do from a mental and spiritual standpoint should be so logical that it would be good in any church. I would like to live so that any church would like to have me.

Don't you think we should be able to find a common denominator so that we can all have good health; so that we can all have good minds; so that we can all be spiritually understood? I have long been a student of comparative religions, and I am convinced that each person can find himself some place along the line.

You can't go very far in the spiritual realm without physical and mental health. We have learned from religious groups the value of vegetarian foods as opposed to a lot of meat in the diet. A religious group in Montreal has taken the acidophilous culture from Romania (which has more people over a hundred years of age than any other place in the world) and is carrying on the culture of this friendly bacteria, which is so good for the bowel.

We had a boy here who had decided he would go all spiritual. He told me he was finished with the physical business. He said, "It is not what goes into the mouth that defiles the body; it is what comes out of it. I am going to live on a spiritual basis." He went all spiritual, going back to coffee and doughnuts. He is all spiritual now, because he isn't with us anymore! You can actually go that far. There are some people so spiritual that they do not fit here on earth.

In delving into all the religious fields, I wanted to know what I had to do first. I found that the scriptures said to "seek first the Kingdom of God, and all things would be added unto you." (Holy Bible, Matthew 6:33) Seek the kingdom first, if you want to live in the king's domain.

Everybody wants to live like a king, but everybody has a different idea of a king. Some have the idea of a king from the health standpoint; some want to enter the king's domain through a mental attitude; some think a king should have a lot of money so that he can have gold and do and be everything he wants. One man had the idea that he wanted the riches of a king, and he was transformed into a king, and he had all the riches. For one month, all he could do was count the king's money; but he got so tired of handling money that he had to get out with the people once again.

Your money should be your talent. I don't think you should have any more than what your talent earns every day. Some of us are making interest on our money, and we are living on other people. This interest that we are getting today will bring on a holocaust.

A king's domain is not health — but it is health. It is not mind. What is the use of having a mind without a body? Wouldn't it be nice to have a deep, loving mind with a sweet breath. I can't conceive of Christ with a cigar in his mouth. This domain is exacting. Almost every night I have to do things because I am looking for this balance that I speak about.

I feel that the king's domain is made up of seven doctors— a good mind, a good spiritual attitude, sunshine, water, good air, good food, and good exercise. Without these things, you don't have the king's domain. If you don't have these, you can have all the money in the world, and it will never do you any good. In this king's domain, you have to get peace of mind. This peace of mind is a wonderful thing. There is no tension in the king's domain, and there are no tranquilizers, either.

The king's domain is what we all seek. It is very practical, because, after all, I could straighten out most of my patients if I could go the king's route. Since you are a king and a queen, don't ever accept anything less. You must walk in beauty.

It is possible to kill ourselves with the pictures that we create in our minds. I will give you a true example in medical history. Seven men were placed before a firing squad with blank bullets in the guns. When the signal was given — one, two, three, FIRE — the blanks went off and one man fell over dead. There were no bullets in those guns. The man knew he was dying then, and he appointed that time for his death. The kingdom that is in your own mind is the king's domain.

If you are the king in this domain, if you have a million dollars, you will know how to use it wisely.

Anyone who knows the spiritual realm and has a million dollars is going to do something wonderful with it. I believe it would be a sin to put a million dollars in a burglar's hands. I feel that if you are going to have money, you should learn the spiritual values from a health standpoint. There are very few rich vegetarians, very few people with money who are vegetarians, because they live in a different domain; they live in a different world. Usually money is not a big object in life for people who go the health way. You don't need a lot of money when you have this king's domain. When your mind gets right, you know how to be happy with ten cents.

I know it is not money that gets you happiness, because I know some people who have money, and they are very unhappy. Others think all they have to do is get married and they will be happy. And they are unhappy. There are those people who must have a fine car — yet look at all the unhappy people driving fine cars. Happiness is something that comes from within.

Most of us live in this king's domain by looking at it as though it were on the outside of the body. The king's domain is on the inside. Many people are going to church and feel nothing. They go to church as if they were an empty bag and when they come out, they find they do not have anything in the bag either. I feel if you are going to get anything out of church, you must have a church within yourself.

Health comes when we are in absolute ease. Health comes when we go through life with a feeling of security. There are few people today who have a feeling of healthy security. Some people are afraid of what is yet to come. In our Father's kingdom, we have to be thankful for what is yet to come, for this is the only way we can have security for tomorrow.

There are some people who fear whether or not they are going to survive, and they believe that in the last days they are going to have pestilence and famine. They don't know that they are living in pestilence and famine at this moment. If they can take care of the conditions they are in right now, they will not have any problems in the future. You must prepare for the future today. What you do right now is going to make tomorrow better. The better your life is today, the better tomorrow is going to be. The more you learn about survival and good health today, the better you are going to be able to handle it tomorrow.

Now, as we look toward seeking the king's domain, we have to do this first. We must be able to walk in peace and harmony. Then we must accept our instruments to receive wonderful things in this world. The first thing we will recognize in this tuning business is that we are not going to say, "Now, give me health; give me a million dollars; give me a good mind." No, we are going to say, "Thy will." We are going to tune in to "Thy will." This is the greatest thing I know from a religious standpoint.

We must realize that we must accept whatever God wills upon us. I would hate to think that I am here on this earth just for my own purpose. I think there must be some divine will in this thing. We accept that we weigh 132 pounds, that we are tall or short, that we are thin or fat, freckled or not, redhead or blond. You will find that you have to agree with your adversary and quickly. You find that you have to agree with things that are not right; and agree with people who are around you.

You will find that there are some people who want to lie, cheat, and steal; and you will let them, until they get finished with it. Haven't we all lied and stolen? Of course we have. There is a freedom that comes, a free feeling that you are honest and you are straight and you are clean and you are completely free and everything is all right. This comes with good health. You can't have a good thyroid gland without that. You can't have a good adrenal gland.

We have so much hypoglycemia today. I would say 50 percent of the people in this country nave hypoglycemia. And do you know what it comes from? People do not build health! People don't know this truth. You have to come out of your troubles the same way you got into them. If you have mental problems, you put in a new thought and come back. If you have used coffee and doughnuts, then you will have to suffer the sins of the flesh. If you have been using degerminated grains, you will have to use whole grains. You will have to use whole foods to compensate for the fragmented foods you have been using. If lack of exercise got you into your trouble, you will have to come back by the way of exercise. *You* will have to come back, no doctor can do it for you. You will have to earn your way back to health. You cannot lift the law of compensation.

In the king's domain there is a God of good consequences. What kind of a God do you want? When you do the right thing, the right thing happens for you. If you have a God of poor consequences, then change your God, because that isn't the way it works. I know that there are foods that are approved by God, and there are foods that are not approved by God. You can't live today on what young people call junk foods and have beautiful, rosy cheeks with beautiful action in your spine. You don't have that kind of body — you may think you have, but I know you haven't.

I am offering you something for the future, and you will have a good future, with better things than you ever had before. You are going to have a better digestion and a better elimination than you have now. Not too long ago a man came in here, and all he talked about was that he had had a natural bowel movement for the first time in 27 years.

Negative, Positive

Those in the king's domain know how to care for their bodies. Years ago I found that the right and left side of the body are never the same. The right side is positive and the left side is negative. If you have trouble on the negative side, negative things will help you. The positive things are necessary if you have trouble on the positive side.

When you get into the study of polarity, you will find that you breathe twenty minutes out of the right nostril and twenty minutes out of the left nostril. You do this to get the positive and the negative electric energy out of the air you breathe. You will find that if you are in a positive attitude, you will breathe out of the right nostril; if you are

negative you will breathe from the left nostril.

I had a man here who hadn't breathed out of the right nostril for three years and had been advised to have surgery. I put him on a right side diet of positive things: sliced tomatoes, and a few leafy vegetables. Three days later he came in to see me and said he was breathing out of the right nostril for the first time in three years. He didn't have to be operated on.

We had a minister here with heart trouble. He had been in bed for three months with heart trouble. We put him on starches and sweet fruits and a few vegetables. In three months he was out of bed and back to work, with no more signs of heart trouble.

We should learn about the positive and negative aspects of health because everything in nature is either positive or negative. The crane and the canary will stand on one leg all night. This is because they have an electrical circuit throughout their systems. When they wish to rest, they stand on one leg, which stops the electricity, and it is then possible for them to rest.

We should learn to recognize the negative and the positive aspects of Nature. We have hot and cold, sunshine and darkness, male and female. We should know that sunshine produces acids in the body, and when we produce all these acids in the body, we find that we can alkalinize the condition — alkaline our bodies. By going to bed early, we can neutralize a lot of the acids from hard work. Those people who work night shifts make an acid condition when the sun is shining in the daytime. Working nights is often referred to as "the graveyard shift." These people walk into these troubles, and this is because they lack knowledge.

Citrus fruit as a daily habit is another example of a lack of knowledge; most people have oranges every day. The fruit is picked two weeks, perhaps two months too early. Your body cannot use a fruit that is picked two months too early. Fruit has a mature date; it has to be picked when it is ripe. You cannot eat a green apricot; you can only eat it when it is ripe. The same is true of citrus fruits; but today no one is able to get a ripe grapefruit unless he lives where it is grown. This is the reason I do not believe in a complete fruit diet; the average person is unable to get fresh fruits. You are going to have a health problem if you allow this green citrus acid to flood your body. It is an irritant to the bladder, stomach, and kidneys.

Seek knowledge through nature; it is your

best teacher. I am interested in knowing what carrots, onions, garlic, parsley can do for you.

Some people are vegetarians to the extent that they won't touch anything unless it is raw, but we find that there is some activity in all food, even if it is cooked. Sixty percent of your daily intake should be raw foods in order to take care of the collodial activity. If wheat is cooked in stainless steel, I can take that wheat and put it in the ground, and it will grow after it has been cooked. You cannot grow it, however, after it has been cooked in the usual way, ground into a cereal, and so forth. It is dead. If you eat it, you won't have too much life either! If you expect to get a good, lively body from dead food, you have another thought coming. You should live on live foods; you shouldn't have anything but good, organic live food! I want you to have as much life as possible.

I am thankful for this knowledge, because there is so much that I can bring to you to show that there is a better way to live.

It comes back to this "King's Domain."

Without this knowledge, we are not going any place!

Use Knowledge for Betterment

A medical doctor here in Escondido, when filling out a death certificate for a youth, wrote that the patient had died from a certain kind of anemia — aplastic anemia, I think it was called. The doctor said, "From drinking too much of the cola drinks." The boy had consumed four bottles of cola drinks a day for a year. I said to the doctor, "Would you dare to put that on a death certificate?"

The doctor replied, "This is only the beginning. One of these days, they are going to put on the death certificate, "Died from a lack of knowledge."

So, what are you going to ask for when you pray; what do you want more than anything else? Knowledge! Then you want to know when to use that knowledge; how to use it; what time of day, whether you are going to use it in the middle of the day. As they say, "Eat like a prince for breakfast, like a king for lunch, and like a pauper for supper." It is wise not to eat a large meal before retiring in the evening. If you have your starch meal in the evening instead of your protein, you will sleep better. For those people who have trouble sleeping, this is just a little idea — just change your meals around a bit. If you don't have wisdom to begin with, it is because you don't have enough experience. Few people learn from other

people's mistakes. My mother used to say, "Learn as much as you can from other people, especially from their bad habits, their bad faults, because you will never live long enough to make all the mistakes yourself." I think you have to learn from others. But do you *want* to learn from others? It's liking saying that you are going to find out if the fire is hot, or eat DDT to prove that it will not kill you. It proves nothing.

If you pray, pray for knowledge. Just ask for wisdom and ask for guidance. Then your troubles will be light. After all, if you asked for a million dollars and got it, you would at this moment be at home guarding it.

If you had asked for freedom instead of health, you would have just health. It is because you are bound, you are mentally bound with certain ideas that you do not have health. We are all bound by customs, some which are inherited from our parents. Sometimes I think that freedom is more important than anything else in the world.

God — Health

The king's domain is God's kingdom. It is the secret place of the Most High. This is where all good health begins. In God's kingdom, we have joy, peace, harmony, happiness, health; we have everything but money. There would be a place for us all, for "I have not given you the spirit of fear." It is the spirit that goes forward. If we were to go forward in the king's domain, this body would really be taken care of. It would go in love, in peace instead of pieces.

We have to accept what is around us and go through life in ease and in peace and in happiness. It gives the Father great pleasure to give us His kingdom; it is up to us to take it. We must first seek the Father's kingdom, and everything else will be added. We don't have to worry about anything if we live in the king's domain; if we have God's kingdom, then what else is there?

Whatever we do should have the approval of God.

A woman came here and said, "I need my eyes taken care of. I didn't come to change my diet; I can transmute food when it comes into my body." I said, "If you can go ten days on coffee and doughnuts and be the same way or better, I will give up my work here."

In ten days, she called up and told me she was sick and would come to the office. After her visit here, she learned that no one can work against nature. It takes a divine architect to make a garden; and it takes a divine architect to make a person. There is no one who can make you change your habits — except yourself.

You will find the real secret of health when you start helping others; I am convinced that I live on what I preach. I believe if you hate, every cell in your body becomes poisoned. Your body feels every note you play and every color you see, and certainly it is to your advantage to reach out for the highest.

Code for Daily Living

Just for today, I will live through the next 12 hours and not tackle my whole life problems at once.

Just for today, I will improve my mind, I will learn something useful. I will read something that requires effort, thought, and concentration.

Just for today, I will be agreeable, I will look my best, speak in a well-modulated voice, be courteous and considerate.

Just for today, I will not find fault with friend, relative, colleague. I will not try to change or improve anyone but myself.

Just for today, I will have a program. I might not follow it exactly, but I will have it. I will save myself from two enemies— hurry and indecision.

Just for today, I will exercise my character in three ways. I will do a good turn and keep it a secret. If anyone finds out, it won't count.

Just for today, I will do two things I don't want to do, just for exercise.

Just for today, I will be unafraid. Especially will I be unafraid to enjoy what is beautiful and believe that as I give to the world, the world will give to me.

Find a Philosophy

Essential to health is a strong philosophy. Most people come to it the hard way. Why does it have to be so? We believe in everything else, try any other path, until at the last minute we are forced to believe in this, the best and only way through the natural way.

In these days of civilization you have to have knowledge. You cannot buy the survival principle. It is priceless! "Yellow gold has a price, but knowledge is priceless," said a Chinese teacher. There is no adversity that cannot be turned into an advantage. We never go backwards. Every experience I have had has been a stepping-stone — never a stumbling block. We have to grow. I believe that man is *going* to grow, regardless. Everyone must find this faith in mankind. Everyone must find this faith in himself. It is possible to change all weaknesses into strengths. So many people are trying to make things happen. It is wiser to let life flow through you. I think we would all be in better health if we would evolve into a philosophy of just letting things take their course.

How would you like to go through life without having a staff — no power from any source but yourself? You can meet any obstacle if you have faith in a greater strength. In your Father's house you have everything. If you take anything less, you are sick mentally and spiritually. We have been given everything for our good and have been told, "I have not given you fear, but I have given you power and strength and love." The Godly things — the Kingdom in which we should live — these treasures are in our hearts. The man who is really rich is the man who has these things. A person can live in misery before he finds them.

We get lost in negative things of life. If we could only realize what the positive things can do for us, we would have something. A man is really poor who says, "I am sick." You are rich no matter how little you have in the bank if you live in the king's domain. it is your faith, your courage; it is what you do that makes you rich or poor. It is entirely up to you; no one gives it to you, you take it yourself. Is this hard to realize? You are walking in the heavenly kingdom all the time. If you don't recognize that it is here for your use, you are truly poor. This is the richest thing I can tell you.

Health Axioms to Live By

I believe that there are health axioms that we can live by that can actually change our lives. Here are some axioms for your collection, to make you a healthier and happier person:

"Man will walk alone until he learns how to walk in agreement with his fellow man."
*

An Indian Axiom: "When brother stands with brother, a war is already half won."
*

"To be strong, speak with one voice. Many voices make confusion."
*

"There is one Father; that makes us all brothers and sisters."
*

"We never miss the water until the well goes dry."

"Love knows not its depth til the hour of separation." — Kahlil Gibran

*

"There is no security in this life, only opportunity."

*

"It is not who is right, but what is right that counts."

*

"Yellow gold has a price, but knowledge is priceless." — A Chinese teacher

*

"You can have anything you want in life, but you must take everything that goes with it."

*

"Waste not, want not: waste it today, go hungry tomorrow."

*

"As you think, so is it."

*

"Judge not, lest ye also be judged."

*

"The measure of a man is not how he fell, but that he got up."

*

"You don't have to *seek* a miracle; you are a miracle." — A Chinese saying

*

"Man merely discovers; he never can and never will invent." — Kahlil Gibran

*

"No one can hurt a spiritual person."

*

"There are no stumbling blocks in life if we use them as stepping stones."

*

"All experiences are experiments, and some mistakes it would be a mistake not to make."

*

"Worry is concentrating on something you don't want."

*

"No one who faces the Sun ever sees the shadow."

*

"What we assume, we become, therefore, let us assume perfection."

*

"To the happy one there is no time" — You have been created for JOY. When you realize this, you have come a long way.

*

"If you have never burnt anything, you have never baked anything." — An Old European saying

In Arabia they say, "Have no regrets. What has happened in the past will be for the good of the future."

*

"As our philosophy enriches us, we learn to recognize "Nothing ever just happens — everything happens just."

*

"Bad thoughts are nervous cares."

*

"We should seek the higher values in life, for what we are seeking is also seeking us."

*

"We come to know that harmony creates and chaos destroys."

*

"We learn there is a time to think, a time to meditate, and a time to let go."

*

Personal Note

Some years ago I was a very sick person, and it was a Seventh-Day Adventist doctor, Ellen G. White, who helped me get well. I studied much of her work through the *Ministry of Healing*, a very fine volume and I recommend it to young people going into the health field. There is another wonderful book, called *Healthful Living*. One of the first things I learned is that whatever we do, whatever we use, it should have the approval of God. I also learned that if we lived close to nature and close to God, there would be no use for doctors, sanitariums, medicine, or drugs. This appealed to me because I was trying to find a way of life, a way to live that would make me as well as possible.

Nature Is an Open Book That Reveals God

He who has given you life knows your need for food to sustain it. In the varied schemes of nature are lessons of divine wisdom for all who have learned to commune with God.

Our happiness will be proportionate to our unselfish works, prompted by divine love.

The work of the Christian physician does not end with healing the maladies of the body. His efforts should extend to the diseases of the mind; to the saving of the souls. Physicians who wish to be successful in the treatment of diseases should know how to minister a diseased mind. The physician in our institutions must be imbued with the living principles of health reborn.

The physician needs more than human wisdom and power that he may minister to

228

the many perplexing causes of disease that he is called on to deal with. If you are suffering with poor health, there is a remedy for you. The condition of the mind has much to do with the health of the physical system. Nothing is so fruitful a cause of disease as depression, gloominess, and sadness. Let the mind become intelligent and you will be placed on the Lord's side. There will be a wonderful improvement in the physical health.

Any abuse put on the Lord's mechanism by disregarding his specified laws for human habitation is a violation of God's law. Eating merely to please the appetite is a transgression of nature's law. Sickness is the result of violating nature's laws.

God will keep human machinery healthful if we will but obey his laws and cooperate with him. When we obey the laws of God we should also include the laws of health.

Health should be as secretly guarded as our character.

We are God's workmanship and His work declares that we are fearfully and wonderfully made.

The living organism is God's property. God is the owner of the whole man.

The physical organism should have special care that the powers of the body may not be dwarfed, but developed to their full extent.

In the Silence of One's Own Being

Inquire of the stranger the earthly road you seek, but ask your higher self for the torch that will light you on your way. In the silence of one's own being, is lighted the candle of will and aspiration. No wind can put it out, no heat can melt it. The flame is of the spirit's quality — pure and of even temperature.

Wait in the morning for inspiration, at noon for guidance, and in the evening for a full understanding of the road thou hast travelled.

— Teachings of the Master

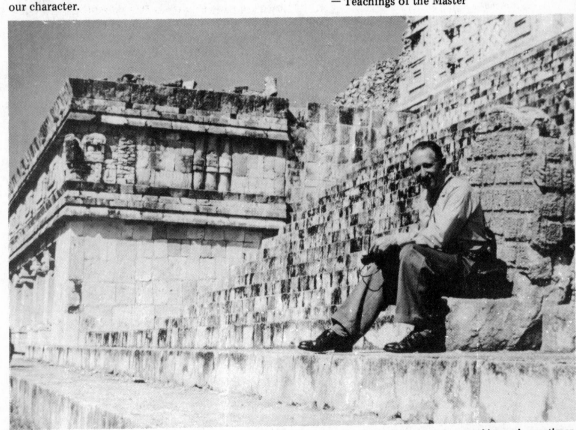

We sit at the temple wondering about the philosophy of the past civilizations, how they existed, why did they fail, why aren't they here today, what can we learn from them. It is through these thoughts that we have put our philosophy together and have developed a way of healing and a pathway of life that man should get acquainted with and try to follow more. As the years pass and we find stumbling blocks on our path, reversals, tragedies not of our making and sometimes of our making, we forget to look up at the stars . . . to higher ideals. A wonderful thought is expressed in the works of Carl Schurz . . . "Ideals are like stars: You will not succeed in touching them with your hands, but, like the seafaring man in the desert of waters, you choose them as your guides, and, following them, you each your destiny."

Index

PRICE LIST AND ORDER BLANK

BERNARD JENSEN, D.C.

Route 1, Box 52, Escondido, CA. 92025, Tel. (714) 749-2727

SHIP TO: Name _____

Street _____

City _____ State _____ Zip _____

BOOKS

BLENDING MAGIC — Blend your way to health and happiness. 650 prize winning recipes. A must for those interested in preparing meals, drinks, and special food combinations by way of blending. **3.95**_____

CREATING A MAGIC HEALTH KITCHEN — A doctor's manual for his patient. Clear directions and lists for the *best* proteins, starches, vegetables, etc. Start your life and health the right way in a revised kitchen prepared by a nutritionist. **1.95**_____

DOCTOR-PATIENT HANDBOOK — Dealing with the REVERSAL PROCESS and THE HEALING CRISIS through Elimination Diets and Detoxification. **3.50**_____

MAGIC SURVIVAL KIT TO YOU!

HEALTH MAGIC THROUGH CHLOROPHYLL — In more than 150 pages clearly outlines the Survival food benefits of Nature's greatest healer. Easy and clearly stated, this book is more than a book about greens, herbs, or wheatgrass, as it presents the beginning of Dr. Jensen's compilation of the Survival Laws that affect all our lives. **3.95**_____

SURVIVE THIS DAY — More than three years in preparation, completes the basic survival foods program Dr. Jensen began in *Health Magic Through Chlorophyll*, and adds 21 more Survival Laws for your study. A classic in the natural healing arts, this book has an extensive bibliography and list of sources for survival day equipment. A must for anyone facing these personal critical times. **5.95**_____

WORLD KEY'S TO HEALTH AND LONG LIFE — Dr. Jensen explores the secrets that have contributed to the well being of the world's healthiest men, and places these keys before you. More than 40 years in research. **5.95**_____

NATURE HAS A REMEDY — Completes the Survival Kit of his 4 best books on acquiring and maintaining the best of health. The remedies have been used in the health practice and teaching patients to live correctly, for the last 50 years. **9.95**_____

TWO NEW BOOKS COMING: Arise and Shine; The Greatest Story on Earth - The Dust Thou Art.

DR. JENSEN'S LECTURES ON CASSETTE TAPES-60 to 90 minutes. Inspirational! Informative!

1. CHEMICAL STORY	**6.95**_____
2. BUILDING A WAY TO EAT	**6.95**_____
3. REPLACEMENT THERAPY	**6.95**_____
4. REGULARITY MANAGEMENT	**6.95**_____
5. DIVINE ORDER	**6.95**_____
6. SEEDS	**6.95**_____
7. NATURAL HEALING	**6.95**_____
8. KEY TO INNER CALM	**6.95**_____
9. BREATHING EXERCISES	**6.95**_____
10. PATHWAYS TO HEALTH	**6.95**_____
11. ARISE AND SHINE	**6.95**_____

IRIDOLOGY

THE SCIENCE AND PRACTICE OF IRIDOLOGY — A 360 page practical course of instruction in analyzing body ailments through the eyes. Full color photographs. (FREE brochure available) **22.50**_____

WALL CHART, 27"x22". Suitable for framing. **7.50**_____

PLASTIC DESK CHART, 4"x8", pocket size. Plastic cover. **3.50**_____
Send for additional information on Iridology and Seminars given.

Subtotal_____

6% Ca. sales tax_____

Total_____

Prices subject to change without notice.